Encyclopedia of
U.S. Biomedical Policy

ENCYCLOPEDIA OF
U.S. BIOMEDICAL POLICY

Robert H. Blank
and
Janna C. Merrick
Editors-in-Chief

Greenwood Press
Westport, Connecticut • London

Library of Congress Cataloging-in-Publication Data

Encyclopedia of U.S. biomedical policy / Robert H. Blank and Janna C.
    Merrick, editors-in-chief.
        p.   cm.
    Includes bibliographical references and index.
    ISBN 0-313-28641-8 (alk. paper)
    1. Medical policy—United States—Encyclopedias.   I. Blank,
    Robert H.   II. Merrick, Janna C.
    RA395.A3E545   1996
    362.1'0973—dc20   95-33969

British Library Cataloguing in Publication Data is available.

Library of Congress Catalog Card Number: 95-33969
ISBN: 0-313-28641-8

First published in 1996

Greenwood Press, 88 Post Road West, Westport, CT 06881
An imprint of Greenwood Publishing Group, Inc.

Printed in the United States of America

The paper used in this book complies with the
Permanent Paper Standard issued by the National
Information Standards Organization (Z39.48-1984).

10 9 8 7 6 5 4 3 2 1

For Chris

Contents

Acknowledgments

There are a number of people who have worked diligently on this encyclopedia. Most notably, we would like to thank the section editors Deborah Mathieu, Jim Bopp, Barry Bostrom, and Pauline Vaillancourt Rosenau, as well as the individual authors. Without the efforts of the section editors and individual authors, this encyclopedia would not exist. Research support was provided by Marcella Mika and secretarial support by Lynn Gilmore, both at the University of South Florida at Sarasota. We also had strong support at Greenwood. Mim Vasan initiated the project, and after her retirement, Jean Lynch ably handled the production duties. We would also like to thank our families and friends, Mallory, Jeremy, Mai-Ling, and Maigin Blank, Christopher Merrick, and Roger Frazee, for their patience and support.

Introduction

SCOPE OF ENCYCLOPEDIA

This volume is a compendium of U.S. biomedical policy primarily since the early 1970s when political activity began to intensify. Although biomedical policy issues are intimately related to bioethics and health policy, the goal of the encyclopedia is to focus on subjects that relate directly to the array of issues on the public agenda raised by biomedical technologies. Although the substantive topics included here overlap with what is termed *bioethics,* the focus is on public policy.

Similarly, although entries concerned with broader questions of health care delivery and funding are included where considered essential to the coverage, the focus of this volume is on the policy issues that accompany the proliferation of technological innovations in biomedicine, not health policy per se. To a large extent the growing health care funding crisis is tied to the diffusion of biomedical interventions. Although there is disagreement as to the extent to which technologies have contributed to the health care crisis, few persons discount their role in escalating costs. Furthermore, as public expectations for access to these highly promising technologies have intensified and interest groups demanding such access have multiplied, biomedical technologies have moved to the center of the health policy agenda.

In their broadest sense, biomedical technologies encompass much of what today is termed *medicine.* From new biologics and drugs, to sophisticated diagnostic machines such as magnetic resonance imaging (MRI) and computerized axial tomography (CAT), to life-support systems used to extend life, biomedical technologies have a tremendous influence over the way we define health care in the 1990s. This encyclopedia focuses on policy developments and issues raised by a broad array of applications of biomedical technology including human genetics, reproduction, neonatal intensive care, organ transplantation, intervention in the brain, and medical interventions at the end of life.

RATIONALE FOR THIS VOLUME

We have entered a dynamic and volatile era of advances in medical technologies that promises to transform the human condition significantly. At least 3 million people worldwide live with artificial implants such as cardiac pacemakers, arterial grafts, hip joint prostheses, middle ear implants, and intraocular lenses. Another 300,000 patients are kept alive by kidney dialysis machines. Vast improvements in surgical procedures, tissue matching, and immunosuppressant drugs such as cyclosporine are making repair and replacement of organs increasingly routine. Whereas in the recent past we were dependent on cadaver organs and low patient survival rates, now transplants from brain-dead individuals, other species such as baboons and pigs, and artificial organs are revolutionizing organ substitution.

Likewise, human genetic technology offers an expanding array of diagnostic and therapeutic applications that are giving us considerably more control over determining the health and the characteristics of future generations. Similarly, biotechnology now offers among many other products unlimited supplies of pure human insulin, interferon, and human growth hormone, as well as monoclonal antibodies that promise widespread benefits to society. Finally, the development of more effective chemicals to enhance physical and mental capacity suggests that there will be few limits to manipulation of the human body in the future.

Until recently, decisions about medicine lay almost entirely in the private realm between physician and patient. Yet the speed of new technologies, their scope, and the dilemmas they raise have all contributed to the idea that public officials ought to be involved in making decisions about who should have access to technologies and whether the techniques should be developed in the first place. The emergence of biomedical decision making on the public agenda in part can be traced to institutional review boards set up in the 1970s, which gave "outsider" oversight to medical protocols involving human subjects. Then in the "right to die" case of Karen Ann Quinlan, a contested decision about whether to withdraw life-support systems gave no clear answer, and the parents and hospital turned to the courts for guidance. This and following decisions motivated the growth of biomedical ethics as a distinct field. Today, bioethicists, who are routinely consulted in hospital decision making, seek a philosophical framework for balancing biomedicine's promise with the broader social welfare.

Biomedical policy, like bioethics, is rooted in rapidly accelerating biomedical innovations and the social issues they raise. It builds on the principles of biomedical ethics and moves into still further uncharted domains. The task of biomedical policy is to create principles for framing public decisions when the form of these decisions, or even the need for making them, is elusive. Biomedicine has brought with it a range of public decisions, some hasty, some ill-thought, some creative, and some quietly effective. Concurrently, medical decision making has become considerably more complex, in part because of questions as to when to use these often life-and-death capacities, who should make such a decision, who should have access to health care, and who should pay.

Although there is a historical tie between the emergence of interest in biomedical ethics and in biomedical policy and the two approaches overlap, the emphasis in policy analysis is critically different from that of bioethics. There are three policy dimensions that have become crucial in biomedical issues. First, decisions must be made concerning the research and development of the technologies. Because a substantial proportion of medical research is funded either directly or indirectly with public funds, it is important that public input be included at this stage. The growing emphasis on forecasting and assessing the social as well as technical consequences of biomedical technologies early in research and development represents one means of incorporating broader public interests.

The second policy dimension relates to the individual use of technologies once they are available. Although direct government intrusion into individual decision making in health care has, until recently, been limited, the government does have at its disposal an array of more or less implicit devices to encourage or discourage individual use. These include tax incentives, provision of free services, and education programs. Biomedical policy has a special importance in contemporary politics because it challenges keenly held societal values relating to privacy, discovery, justice, health, and rights. Biomedical techniques involve the human body and, with it, a deep-seated expectation of privacy.

The third dimension of biomedical policy centers on the aggregate societal consequences of widespread application of a technology. For instance, what impact would the diffusion of artificial heart transplants have on the provision of health care? How would widespread use of reproductive techniques alter our view of children, of families, and of women? Adequate policymaking here requires a clear conception of national goals, extensive data to predict the consequences of each possible course of action, an accurate means of monitoring these consequences, and mechanisms to cope with the consequences if they are deemed undesirable. Moreover, the government has a responsibility in ensuring quality control standards and fair marketing of medical applications. As technologies become widely available that allow for sex preselection, collaborative conception, neural grafting, and extended life spans, social patterns will be affected. Observers question the impact of such capabilities on the family, on demographic patterns, and on the structure and size of the population. Policy planners must account for these potential pressures on the basic structures and patterns of society and decide whether provision of such choices is desirable.

The need for integrated and clearly articulated policy objectives to deal with the expanding array of high-cost technologies is clear. However, it must be acknowledged that their attainment is difficult, given the inextricably complex economic, cultural, social, and political context of biomedical decision making. In a pluralist society, especially on issues as fundamental as those that relate to human life and death, there are many conceivably legitimate but contradictory goals. Moreover, because these issues are not amenable to traditional political techniques of bargaining, compromise, or negotiation, it is a formidable task to attain a rational balance among the competing goals.

Because of their threat to traditional values, decisions concerning the priorities of biomedical research and technology and their clinical applications are being made within a highly politicized context. The politically sensitive nature of the issues raised by these technologies, as well as recent trends in the political arena and increased public awareness, demonstrates that technical decisions are no longer made independently of politics. One major trend in the 1970s was the growing governmental role in biomedical research. This emergence onto the public agenda is a result of a combination of general inflation, uncontrolled health care costs, and the general freedom-of-information climate. As the costs of research and applications have increased, public debate over priorities has expanded. Because a large proportion of the funding comes from public monies, decision makers are likely to scrutinize biomedical expenditures closely, producing an even greater presence of the public sector.

Public decisions by judges, legislators, civil servants, and other officials have special significance for our daily lives and influence the way we see things and define issues. What distinguishes public policy is that public decisions imply the use of public funds, and they thereby broaden the interested constituency. Even when only small amounts of public money are at stake, public decisions are significant because they subsume the backing of the state. Policy decisions represent societal commitments. They are statements that respond to emerging concerns and demands among citizens. When the government allocates hundreds of millions of dollars to map and sequence all the genes in a human cell, it gives genetic inquiry a new legitimacy. Similarly, when a public hospital develops criteria for deciding who should receive scarce organs, it legitimates the priorities underlying those criteria.

In summary, the rapid diffusion of biomedical technologies, in conjunction with social and demographic trends, has led to the need for increasingly arduous decisions as to how to best use them. As we come to realize that we cannot afford to do everything for everybody, we are thrust into policy dilemmas that deal directly with human life and death. Ironically, these dilemmas are all the more difficult because we are now at the brink of developing remarkable capacities to intervene directly in the human condition, from preconception to life extension. Just when we have the technical capacity to do things we only recently dreamed about, rising expectations and scarce resources combine to limit their availability. The resulting need to allocate biomedical technologies, in turn, raises critical concerns over whose needs take precedence, what individual rights and responsibilities entail, and when societal good justifies restricting individual benefit. These policy issues, although by no means new, take on a new importance within the context of these emerging conflicts accentuated by technological successes in biomedicine.

SUBSTANTIVE AREAS OF BIOMEDICAL POLICY

Biomedical innovations are proliferating faster than our capacity to make rational public policy to deal with them. The issue areas below are representative of the potential foci of attention in biomedical policy. While the following list is not exhaustive, it does illustrate the breadth and relevance of biomedical issues in the 1990s.

Issues in Human Genetics and Reproduction

Abortion (RU-486)

Characteristic selection

Contraception (subdermal implants)

Cryopreservation (sperm, egg, embryos)

Eugenics

Gene therapy

Genetic counseling

Genetic screening

Reproduction-aiding technologies (donor insemination, egg fusion, embryo lavage, gamete intrafallopian transfer [GIFT], in vitro fertilization, zygote intrafallopian transfer [ZIFT], etc.)

Sex preselection

Sterilization (reversible procedures)

Surrogate motherhood

Prenatal and Neonatal Issues

Coerced cesarean section

Fetal monitoring

Fetal research

Fetal surgery

Maternal behavior and fetal health (cocaine babies, fetal alcohol syndrome, etc.)

Nontreatment of severely ill newborns

Prenatal diagnosis (amniocentesis, chorionic villus sampling, fetoscopy, ultrasound)

Selective reduction of fetuses

Biomedical Issues Within the Life Cycle

Acquired immunodeficiency syndrome (AIDS) testing, vaccines, and care

Drug therapy

Human experimentation

Neural grafting

Organ transplantation

Problems of allocating scarce life-saving resources

Psychosurgery and electrical brain stimulation

Death-Related Issues

Advance directives

Definitions of death

Futile treatment

Permanent vegetative state

Research on aging/terminal patients

Rights of dying persons

The state of biomedical policy has now matured to the point that a reference work of this type is warranted and timely. Each of the substantive areas above has many dimensions that are reflected in the entries in this encyclopedia. Moreover, the emergence of novel court cases in response to these new capabilities, such as torts for wrongful birth, wrongful life, and prenatal injury, combined with extensive legislation and regulations at the national and 50 state levels provide the basis for this encyclopedia. Although the encyclopedia of bioethics and other reference works in that field are well established and valuable, no other volume published today offers a specific focus on U.S. public policy surrounding biomedicine.

ORGANIZATION OF ENCYCLOPEDIA

This encyclopedia is organized to provide a ready reference to U.S. biomedical policy. Entries are listed alphabetically and are cross-referenced with an asterisk (*) to related entries. The extensive index offers another means of cross-checking entries by subject. The entries vary considerably in length, depending on the extensiveness of existing governmental activity and the complexity of the topic. They include a mixture of legislation and court cases, as well as descriptions of key government agencies, private organizations, technologies, and issue areas. Each entry has a short, selected bibliography of key sources for further reading. Appendix A is a chronology of key events, court cases, and legislation and can be read as a summary of the cumulative development of policy activity in biomedicine. Appendix B provides a directory of key sources of information.

Each entry has been authored by an expert on the particular topic. Authors represent a wide range of disciplines including the social and biological sciences, law, medicine, and bioethics. The contributors of the entries were selected by section editors who were responsible for commissioning entries that they believed covered the most important aspects of the general topical areas. The section editors suggested appropriate lengths of each entry and assured that their respective areas were adequately represented in the volume. Although it is not possible in an area as vast and dynamic as biomedical policy to ensure comprehensive coverage of all topics, the volume editors made every effort to minimize any remaining gaps.

—Robert H. Blank

Encyclopedia of
U.S. Biomedical Policy

A

AGENCY FOR HEALTH CARE POLICY AND RESEARCH

The AHCPR, which was established in December 1989 as part of the Public Health Service within the U.S. Department of Health and Human Services, replaced the national Center for Health Services Research and Health Care Technology Assessment. The agency's mission is to improve the quality, appropriateness, and effectiveness of health care; improve access to health care services; and reduce health care costs. AHCPR accomplishes its mission by supporting and conducting health services research in the areas of cost, quality, access, and medical effectiveness; by the development of clinical practice guidelines; and by the dissemination of research results. AHCPR also provides resources for training in health services research.

AHCPR facilitates the development, publication, and dissemination of clinical practice guidelines, providing clinicians with a tool to improve their medical care decisions and to increase the effectiveness of their services. A multidisciplinary panel—composed of private sector health care providers, consumers, and contracted nonprofit organizations—conducts an extensive literature review to develop clinical guidelines that reflect the best of the current scientific evidence. Guidelines are then peer reviewed and tested onsite by potential users to assess their validity, efficacy, and applicability. Guidelines have addressed, for example, pain management, breast cancer screening with mammography, and pressure ulcer prevention.

AHCPR also supports the largest number of medical treatment effectiveness studies in the United States, including the Patient Outcomes Research Team (PORT) projects. PORTs are five-year, multisite research projects that examine alternative diagnostic, preventive, and therapeutic methods with which to address a certain condition with the aim of determining the best approach for each patient. Studies on stroke prevention, diabetes, and ischemic health disease, among others, have been supported. Other AHCPR outcome projects include the development of outcomes research methods and an analysis of pharmaceutical therapy outcomes.

In addition, AHCPR sponsors programs that address access to health care services, cost and financing of care, and quality of services. Topics in this area have included a national survey on the cost of health care and the out-of-pocket expenditures for health care by individuals and an analysis of where the population obtains health care services and who pays for those services.

AHCPR projects have critically assessed new or unestablished medical devices, procedures, and other health care technologies by evaluating their risks, benefits, and effectiveness. Areas that have been studied include autologous bone marrow transplantation and home uterine monitoring.

AHCPR recognizes the need to improve the quantity and quality of data for use in health services research and health care delivery. To this end, the agency supports establishing uniform methods to develop and collect data as well as interlinking governmental and private sector databases. The agency also supports research aimed at defining the most effective means to detect, treat, and prevent conditions more prevalent in minorities and women.

The agency supports a multitude of investigator-initiated research requests on topics targeted to health policy and health care reform. These topics include primary care, quality assessment and assurance, medical disability, home health care, and rural health care. The agency also supports research on the best ways to disseminate information gained from research and provides training in health services research through the support of doctoral dissertation research and National Research Service Awards in the form of training grants and fellowships to individuals.

REFERENCES: Clinton, J. J. 1994. "Agency for Health Care Policy and Research." *Food and Drug Law Journal* 49:449; Clinton, J. J. 1993. "Financing Medical Effectiveness Research." *Annals of the New York Academy of Sciences* 703:295; Mass, W. B., and Garcia, Isabel. 1994. "Health Services Research and the Agency for Health Care Policy and Research and Dental Practice." *Journal of the American College of Dentists* 61:18; Salive, M. E. 1990. "Patient Outcomes Research Teams and the Agency for Health Care Policy and Research." *Health Services Research* 25:697.

ANA MARIA LOPEZ

AIDS VACCINE AND TREATMENT RESEARCH

Despite the vast research funding and expanding knowledge about the acquired immunodeficiency syndrome (AIDS) virus, finding a cure or vaccine has proven elusive. The first widely prescribed drug was zidovudine (AZT), originally developed in 1964 as an anticancer agent. AZT treatment has had mixed success, with some patients benefiting in the short run and some not at all. Also, the side effects, including organ damage and other toxic effects, can be severe in some patients.

The development of new drugs to treat AIDS has become itself a major issue in the policy debate. Traditionally, it takes approximately 12 years to move a drug from inception to approval by the Food and Drug Administration (FDA). As a result of strong pressures from AIDS activists for immediate access to promising experimental drugs, the traditional research protocol that ensures safety and efficacy has been short-circuited. Clinical trials have been streamlined by combining phase I, II, and III testing. Didanosine, for instance, was approved by the FDA in record time without definitive evidence of any clinical benefit. Moreover, expanded access programs have made promising agents widely available even as the compressed clinical trials proceed. This has created a pattern where new agents are introduced with much publicity and false hope, only to be shown lacking after several years of use.

Some experts believe that the most effective therapy potential rests with combinational or sequential therapies that minimize virus replication. Others, however, remain skeptical. "The chronic nature of HIV-1 infection, coupled with the emergence of drug-resistant mutant viruses, suggests that the road to successful control of this virus will be rocky" (Hirsch and D'Aguila, 1993, 1692).

If the mood on therapy is less than optimistic, the hope over the prospects of developing a vaccine for AIDS in the near future is bleak. Moreover, even if an effective vaccine is developed this decade, it will probably not be 100 percent protective and will certainly not be available to all the world for many years after that. The virus's ability to mutate quickly and to elude immune responses poses serious obstacles to vaccine development. Moreover, success in laboratories is a far cry from demonstrating useful protection against natural infection (Greene, 1993, 73). Although there is preliminary evidence that development of effective human immunodeficiency virus (HIV) vaccines is feasible, many challenges make this unlikely in the near future. Two major problems that must be resolved are the "development of vaccine formulations that induce anti-HIV responses against a broad spectrum of worldwide HIV strains, and maintenance of anti-HIV protective immunity for significant periods [years] after immunization" (Porter, Glass, and Koff, 1993, 190). Therapy that introduces into the infected person's T cells a gene that would make the cells resistant to HIV infection might be possible in the remote future, but we presently lack the gene delivery and expression systems that could make this genetic therapy widely available.

At least 16 HIV vaccine applications have been entered into preliminary safety and immunogenicity testing in several countries. These potential vaccines are being considered in three research areas that include (1) prophylactic vaccines to prevent establishment of the infection; (2) vaccine therapy to prevent progression from infection to disease; and (3) perinatal intervention to prevent transmission of HIV to fetus or newborn. Initial vaccine trials are of the second type, designed to slow or halt the progression of AIDS. The trials involve from 6,000 to 12,000 HIV-infected people. Despite the consensus that a vaccine of any of these types is well in the future, the worldwide scope of AIDS has created a broad international commitment to the development of safe and effective technological responses.

As vaccine trials reach the clinical stage, however, difficult ethical, legal, and policy issues emerge. Although in the end all of society will benefit significantly from development of an AIDS vaccine, the risks to individuals participating in the early phases of vaccine testing are bound to outweigh the benefits, particularly for the prophylactic vaccine. Even if the long-term health risk is minimal, those persons vaccinated will show up positive for HIV. This raises critical social risk, including discrimination, possible breaches of confidentiality, and in some persons, the attitude that the vaccination process of the clinical trial has conferred protective immunity against HIV, thus leading to risk behaviors with tragic consequences (Porter, Glass, and Koff, 1993, 193).

REFERENCES: Goldsmith, Marsha F. 1993. "HIV/AIDS Early Treatment Controversy Cues New Advice but Questions Remain." *Journal of the American Medical Association* 270(3): 295–96; Greene, Warner C. 1993. "AIDS and the Immune System." *Scientific American* (September): 67–73; Hirsch, Martin S., and Richard T. D'Aguila. 1993. "Therapy for Human Immunodeficiency Virus Infection." *New England Journal of Medicine* 328(23): 1686–94; Porter, Joan, Marta Glass, and Wayne Koff. 1993. "International AIDS Vaccine Trials." In Robert H. Blank and Andrea L. Bonnicksen, eds., *Emerging Issues in Biomedical Policy,* Vol. 2. New York: Columbia University Press.

See also **HIV TESTING.**

ROBERT H. BLANK

ALCOHOL, DRUG ABUSE, AND MENTAL HEALTH ADMINISTRATION

From its establishment in 1974 (Public Law [P.L.] 93–282) until its demise in 1992 (P.L. 102–321), ADAMHA was the federal agency principally responsible for supporting research into and treatment of mental and addictive disorders. As an agency within the Department of Health and Human Services (DHHS), ADAMHA conducted biomedical and behavioral research in its own laboratories, supported extramural research, awarded block grants to states to support treatment and prevention activities (P.L. 97–35, P.L. 98–509, P.L. 99–570), provided technical assistance to states and communities, and disseminated information. Among its many notable contributions were research on the mental and addictive disorders associated with acquired immunodeficiency syndrome (AIDS), development of new drug abuse treatment medications, advances in alcohol genetics, studies demonstrating that most alcohol and drug abusers are initially afflicted with a mental illness, and improvement of services for homeless individuals with mental and/or addictive disorders.

In 1992, Congress eliminated ADAMHA and reconstituted its components. The research institutes (the National Institute of Mental Health,* the National Institute on Alcohol Abuse and Alcoholism,* and the National Institute on Drug Abuse*) were transferred to the National Institutes of Health (NIH).* A new entity, the Substance Abuse and Mental Health Services Administration, was created within DHHS to oversee the service components (such as substance abuse prevention and treatment improvement).

REFERENCES: Institute of Medicine. 1991. *Research and Service Programs in the PHS: Challenges in Organization.* Washington, D.C.: National Academy Press; Rice, D. P., et al. 1990. *The Economic Costs of Alcohol and Drug Abuse and Mental Illness.* San Francisco: DHHS Pub. No. (ADM) 90–1694; Rochefort, D. A. 1989. *Handbook on Mental Health Policy in the United States.* Westport, CT: Greenwood Press.

DEBORAH R. MATHIEU

AMERICAN HEALTH SECURITY ACT OF 1993

Health care reform was identified early in the Clinton administration as a primary goal of the president, who announced the outline of his legislative proposal in this regard on September 22, 1993. The essential provisions of the American Health Security Act (AMSA) of 1993 mandate (1) universal coverage, regardless of health, employment, or financial status; (2) employers paying 80 percent of the average cost of insurance for their employees, with employee payment of the remaining 20 percent; (3) a comprehensive benefit package; (4) consumer choice as to providers, plans, and treatments; and (5) implementation by means of so-called regional health alliances, offering health plans approved according to national standards of coverage and cost, overseen by a "National Health Board" composed of seven presidential appointees.

The impression of many is that AMSA would stimulate managed health care arrangements such as health maintenance organizations (HMOs). But the proposed legislation also requires that the secretary of Health and Human Services (HHS) appoint a 13-member Advisory Council on Breakthrough Drugs that would make determinations, to be published in the *Federal Register,* regarding the reasonableness of introductory prices of new drugs based on numerous variables, including the costs of other drugs in the same therapeutic class, cost information supplied by the manufacturer, and the price of the same drug in other countries. In addition, for each Medicare-covered biopharmaceutical dispensed, manufacturers will be required on a quarterly basis to pay HHS rebates of at least 17 percent of the average manufacturer retail price for such biopharmaceuticals. A series of formulas will determine actual rebates to be paid, effectively resulting in government control of the price of Medicare-covered biopharmaceuticals. Thus, any new drugs will be ineligible for Medicare reimbursement until manufacturers negotiate specific price rebates with HHS, which rebates may be more or less than the minimum 17 percent rebate for already-approved drugs. If a manufacturer of a new drug cannot reach a rebate agreement with HHS, HHS may at its discretion exclude the new drug from Medicare coverage.

Some believe that these provisions of AMSA would codify present practice, to the extent that the government already negotiates for cheaper drug prices in the context of Medicare reimbursement. There have been complaints, however, that uncertainty over the impact of health care reform on commercial prospects in the biopharmaceutical sector has driven equity funding away from many companies focused on developing biotechnology-related medicines and treatments.

REFERENCES: "Administration Health Care Reform Bill Still Includes Indirect Price Controls." *Bio Bulletin* (Nov. 9, 1993), at 1 (Biotechnology Industry Organization, Washington, D.C.); National Health Lawyers Association (Washington, D.C.). October 1993. *American Health Security Act of 1993—Summary Outline and Selected Analyses;* Shaw, Donna. "Clinton's Healthcare Plan Is Cramping This Industry's Style." *Philadelphia Inquirer* (Nov. 26, 1993), at A1; Waldhole, Michael, and Udayan Gupta. "Biotech Firms Try to Block Clinton Price-Control Plan." *Wall Street Journal* (Jan. 31, 1994), at B4.

STEPHEN A. BENT

AMERICAN SOCIETY FOR REPRODUCTIVE MEDICINE

The American Society for Reproductive Medicine (ASRM—formerly American Fertility Society) is a nonprofit organization with a membership of over 11,400, including obstetrician-gynecologists, urologists, nurses, and technicians. The society's Practice Committee publishes *Guidelines for Practice,* which addresses problems in areas of reproductive medicine such as vasectomy reversal, tubal disease, endometriosis, and unexplained infertility.

The society publishes a monthly journal (*Fertility and Sterility*) and individual documents such as Guidelines for Human Embryology and Human Andrology Laboratories (1992) and Guidelines for Gamete Donation (1993). Approximately every four years it revisits and updates a supplement to *Fertility and Sterility* on the ethical considerations of assisted reproductive technologies (see, e.g., Ethics Committee, 1994). These supplements address issues and reach conclusions about the ethics of in vitro fertilization (IVF),* donor insemination, sperm and egg donation, embryo freezing, surrogate motherhood, preimplantation genetic diagnosis,* research on preembryos, and other reproductive technologies.

The ASRM's public relations office in Birmingham, Alabama, distributes policy position statements, and its government relations office in Washington, D.C., examines the impact of regulations and seeks to inform debate at state and federal levels. Each year, data collected by ASRM's Society for Assisted Reproductive Technology are published in *Fertility and Sterility.* These reports summarize the number of IVF programs, cycles of assisted reproductive treatment, and pregnancy and birth rates by type of procedure. As such, they contribute to public understanding of assisted conception and its outcomes. The ASRM's Ethics Committee regards public understanding as a prelude to effective policy (Ethics Committee, 1994).

REFERENCES: American Society for Reproductive Medicine. "Professional Education Publications"; American Society for Reproductive Medicine. "Society Profile and Fact Sheet"; Ethics Committee of the American Fertility Society. 1994. "Ethical Considerations of Assisted Reproductive Technologies." *Fertility and Sterility* 62:1–125s.

ANDREA L. BONNICKSEN

AMERICANS WITH DISABILITIES ACT

Congress passed the Americans with Disabilities Act (ADA) on July 26, 1990, and President George Bush signed it into law later that year. The ADA is land-mark legislation that extends legal protections to about one of every six Amer-icans in the areas of employment, public benefits, and physical access to facilities, among others. Since the scope and language of the law are broad, it will take the courts years to resolve many of the ADA's important interpretive issues.

The ADA protects any individual who has or is perceived to have a disability. Drawing heavily on terms and concepts familiar under the Rehabilitation Act of 1973 (which prohibits recipients of federal funds from discriminating against individuals with disabilities), the ADA defines a *disability* as a physical or men-tal impairment that substantially limits one or more of the major life activities of the individual. The definition of *major life activities* is expansive and includes walking, seeing, breathing, and many other activities. The statute excludes cur-rent drug use, most sexual dysfunctions, and gambling disorders from the def-inition. The ADA specifically applies to private employers, state and local governments, labor organizations, places of public accommodation, and a variety of other entities. It contains a relatively small number of exemptions, primarily for religious organizations.

The ADA provides both for federal enforcement and for private rights of action. The courts have wide latitude to provide equitable relief in the form of injunctions, reinstatement, hiring, promotion, and other forms of relief. Courts can also award compensatory and punitive damages, although caps on damages provide some insulation from liability for defendants.

Although the ADA applies to virtually every part of the health care industry, Congress expressed its intentions with very little specificity. Most hospitals and nursing homes were already covered by Section 504 of the Rehabilitation Act of 1973, but it is possible that the ADA will have significant direct impacts on these providers, due to the increased public awareness of the available legal protections. The ADA does apply to health insurance, an industry that had largely escaped federal regulation prior to the ADA. Although health care reform may eliminate many insurance practices that may be vulnerable to ADA chal-lenges, it is likely that certain types of disease-specific caps on coverage—such as limiting coverage for treatment of AIDS (acquired immunodeficiency syn-drome) to a fraction of the coverage for other diseases—will be forbidden by the ADA.

The ADA's greatest impact on health care may result from its application to state and federal health care plans. Both the Bush and Clinton administrations agreed that so-called quality-of-life indicators were inherently biased against persons with disabilities and therefore could not be used as a part of Oregon's controversial health care rationing proposal. Some observers believe that the ADA will be a substantial constraint for all health care rationing schemes, al-though Supreme Court decisions interpreting Section 504 of the Rehabilitation

Act of 1973, such as *Choate v. Alexander*, suggest that the government will have substantial, although not unfettered, discretion in the allocation of health care resources. Other large parts of the health care system, such as the current network for distributing human organs and tissues, also raise ADA issues.

The doctor-patient relationship has always been something of a safe harbor from direct federal government regulation. However, the language of the ADA suggests that it may become a new area for litigation in areas ranging from informed consent to courses of treatment.

REFERENCES: *Alexander v. Choate,* 469 U.S. 287 (1985); Public Law 101–336 (July 26, 1990); U.S. Equal Employment Opportunity Commission. *The Americans with Disabilities Act: Your Employment Rights as an Individual with a Disability* (1991).

MICHAEL J. ASTRUE

AMGEN V. CHUGAI PHARMACEUTICAL

Recombinantly produced erythropoietin (EPO) is one of the very few biopharmaceuticals to have garnered ''blockbuster'' status by the beginning of the 1990s. With a primary focus on the treatment of anemia, for example, in renal disease patients, the worldwide market in EPO, a blood protein that stimulates production of red blood cells, was over $1 billion in 1993. For many years, however, human cadavers were the only source for EPO, and its purification to pharmaceutical-grade homogeneity was a problematic, expensive proposition. During the early 1980s, therefore, several research groups were in competition to isolate the human EPO gene and to express EPO-active protein recombinantly. Scientists at Amgen, Inc. (Thousand Oaks, California) achieved this goal, resulting in the company's filing a U.S. patent application on November 30, 1984, with claims covering, inter alia, isolated DNAs coding for human EPO. In October 1987, the Amgen application matured into U.S. Patent No. 4,703,008, which was assigned to Kirin-Amgen, a joint venture between Amgen and a Japanese company, Kirin Brewery.

On the same day that the patent was issued, Amgen filed suit in Massachusetts Federal District Court, alleging patent infringement by Genetics Institute, Inc. (Cambridge, Massachusetts) and Chugai Pharmaceuticals, Ltd., a Japanese licensee under a U.S. Genetics Institute (GI) patent, No. 4,677,195, directed to homogeneous EPO having a specific activity above a prescribed level. Chugai and GI counterclaimed, asserting that Amgen had infringed the GI '195 patent, and also interposed several affirmative defenses, including invalidity of the Amgen '008 patent by virtue of Amgen's failure to deposit in a public repository certain biological materials allegedly needed to implement the ''best mode'' for carrying out the claimed Amgen invention. This contention was discounted, not only by the trial court and the U.S. Court of Appeals for the Federal Circuit but also by the U.S. Supreme Court, on petition by GI. The trial court also dismissed Amgen's complaint against Chugai, which used EPO-encoding DNA only in Japan to produce recombinant EPO for importation to the United States. But the trial court did find that GI infringed several Amgen patent claims that the court deemed valid. Certain other Amgen claims were held invalid because their coverage, encompassing any polypeptide with an amino acid sequence "sufficiently duplicative" of EPO's to possess red blood cell–proliferative activity, was considered broader than the patent allowed one to practice without undue experimentation ("nonenablement"). The trial court further held that Amgen had infringed the GI '195 patent, but this determination was reversed on appeal when the federal circuit ruled that the GI patent was invalid for nonenablement.

Nevertheless, Amgen's inability to halt importation of recombinant EPO made by Chugai in Japan, even upon resort in 1990 to the U.S. International Trade Commission, highlighted the importance to the biopharmaceutical sector of process-of-production claims, which, under the Process Patent Act of 1988, Public Law 100–418, are infringed by the act of importing into the United States an item made abroad via a process claimed in a U.S. patent. Like many applicants seeking to protect recombinant expression processes per se, Amgen initially was refused claims for EPO production, based on an interpretation by the U.S. Patent and Trademark Office (PTO) of *In re Durden*, 763 F.2d 1406, 226 USPQ 359 (Fed. Cir. 1985) (chemical synthesis process not patentable simply because both insecticide end product and starting reagents are patentable), which prompted Amgen and others to support a proposed amendment to the U.S. patent law. The "Biotechnology Patent Protection Act"—also called the "Boucher Bill" after an original cosponsor, Congressman Rich Boucher (D–Virginia)— would revise Section 103 of the Patent Act to mandate:

Notwithstanding any other provision of this section, a claimed process of making or using a machine, manufacture, or composition of matter is not obvious under this section if . . . the claimed process is a biotechnological process as defined in subsection (d); and . . . [both the product and process] were owned by the same person or subject to an obligation of assignment to the same person; and . . . are entitled to the same effective filing date; and appear in the same patent application, different patent applications or patent which is owned by the same person and which expires or is set to expire on the same date. . . . For purposes of this section, the term "biotechnological process" means any method of making or using living organisms, or parts thereof, for the purpose of making or modifying products. Such term includes recombinant DNA, recombinant RNA, cell fusion including hybridoma techniques, and other processes involving site specific manipulation of genetic material. (*Senate Report No. 82*)

Ironically, calls for the Boucher Bill continued after resolution of the immediate circumstances that spawned the legislative proposal: A PTO interference proceeding, declared to adjudicate who had been the first to invent a process for producing EPO recombinantly, led to a granting of such process claims to Amgen. GI and Amgen thereafter settled their long-running dispute.

REFERENCES: *Amgen Inc. v. Chugai Pharmaceutical Co.,* 9 USPQ2d 1833 (D. Mass. 1989); *Amgen Inc. v. Chugai Pharmaceutical Co.,* 927 F.2d 1200 (Fed. Cir. 1991), 18 USPQ2d 1016 (Fed. Cir. 1991); *Amgen Inc. v. U.S. Int'l Trade Comm.,* 14 USPQ2d 1734 (1990); *Biotechnology Law Report* 12(4): 376–377 (1993); *Fritsch v. Lin Bd. Pat.*

App. and Inter. Nos. 102,096, 102,097, and 102,334, cited in "Patents: PTO's Interference Ruling on EPO Is Bound by CAFC's Validity Ruling." *BNA's Patent, Trademark & Copyright Journal News & Comment* 43:116 (1991); Granados, Patricia, and Stephen Bent. "Senate Subcommittee Considers Biotech Patent Protection Act." *Genetic Engineering News,* September 1991, at 1; Moran, Terence. "On the Political Frontiers of Biotechnology: Court Fight over Genetically Engineered Protein Moves to Congress." *Legal Times,* January 8, 1990, at 1; *Senate Report No. 82,* 103rd Cong., 1st sess. 1993, 1993 WL 244001.

STEPHEN A. BENT

AMNIOCENTESIS

Amniocentesis is a commonly used technique for detection of genetic disorders in utero. In this procedure, usually administered between 16 and 18 weeks after the beginning of the last menstrual period, a long, thin needle attached to a syringe is inserted through the lower wall of the woman's abdomen, and approximately 20 cc of the amniotic fluid that surrounds the fetus are withdrawn. This fluid contains some live body cells shed by the fetus. These cells are placed in the proper laboratory medium and cultured for approximately 3 weeks. At this time, karyotyping of the chromosomes is conducted to identify any abnormalities in the chromosomal complement as well as the sex of the fetus. If indicated, specific biochemical assays can be conducted to identify up to 120 separate metabolism disorders and approximately 90 percent of neural tube defects. Over 90 percent of women undergoing amniocentesis are informed that the fetus is normal. In the event a fetus is diagnosed as having a severe chromosomal or metabolic disorder, therapeutic abortion is typically offered to the mother.

Amniocentesis is regarded as a routine clinical procedure, and successful tests for wrongful births against physicians who failed to advise the procedure for patients over 35 accelerated its use. Approximately 85 percent of amniocenteses are conducted for chromosomal evaluation, about three fourths for women over 35 years of age. The reason for the emphasis on amniocentesis for women over age 35 is that the frequency of chromosomal abnormalities, especially the most common one, Down syndrome, increases dramatically with maternal age. Despite this use pattern, approximately 80 percent of all children with Down syndrome are born to women under 35 years of age. For this reason, some observers argue that prenatal diagnosis should be offered to all pregnant patients.

Other indications for chromosomal evaluation are birth of a previous child afflicted with Down syndrome or other chromosomal anomaly. The remaining 15 percent of prenatal diagnoses are indicated by previous offspring or close relatives with neural tube defects; the possibility of a sex-linked genetic disorder; or carrier status of both parents for an unborn metabolic disorder such as Tay-Sachs disease.

REFERENCES: Eiben, B., R. Goebel, S. Hansen, and W. Hammens. 1994. "Early Amniocentesis: A Cytogenetic Evaluation of Over 1500 Cases." *Prenatal Diagnosis* 14(6): 497–501; Haddow, J. E., G. E. Palomaki, G. J. Knight, et al. 1994. "Reducing the Need for Amniocentesis in Women 35 Years of Age and Over with Serum Makers for Screening.'' *New England Journal of Medicine* 330(16): 1114–1118; Hanson, Frederick W., et al. 1992. ''Early Amniocentesis: Outcome, Risks, and Technical Problems at < 12.8 Weeks.'' *American Journal of Obstetrics and Gynecology* 166(6): 1707–1711; Platt, Lawrence D., and Dru E. Carlson. 1992. ''Prenatal Diagnosis: When and How?'' *New England Journal of Medicine* 327(a): 636–638; Suzumori, K., S. Okada, R. Adachi, et al. 1994. ''Comparison of Chorionic Villus Sampling and Amniocentesis: Current Status.'' *Prenatal Diagnosis* 14(6): 479–486.

See also **CHORIONIC VILLUS SAMPLING (CVS); PRENATAL DIAGNOSIS.**

ROBERT H. BLANK

ANIMAL SUBJECTS IN BIOMEDICAL RESEARCH

Britain was the first country to enact legislation aimed at regulating the use of animals in research with its Cruelty to Animals Act of 1876. Other countries, such as France and the United States, did not pass similarly aimed legislation until almost a century later. And even then, the United States failed to regulate the use of animals in research; the Laboratory Animal Welfare Act, enacted by the U.S. Congress in 1966, licensed dealers, registered research facilities, and prescribed standards for housing and transport, but it explicitly exempted the actual conduct of research from its regulations.

Serious concern about animals used in research arose in the United States in the post–World War II period. In 1952 the Animal Welfare Institute (AWI) was founded, and later in the 1950s other organizations were established, such as the Humane Society of the United States (HSUS), that would later play an important role in affecting policy governing the use of animals in research. Increased concern about the welfare of laboratory animals coincided with vast increases in the number of animals used in research; it is estimated that between 17 and 22 million animals are used annually in research, testing, and education.

In 1960, federal legislation intended to protect research animals was first proposed. This bill, which would have licensed individual investigators, was modeled on the British Act of 1876. It was opposed by the biomedical research establishment and by the chairs of powerful congressional committees. It languished until 1966, when *Life* published a photo-story exposing the inhumane trade in research animals. Because of the high demand for animals to use in research, many dealers were willing to buy dogs from anyone; HSUS estimated that in 1966 half of all missing pets wound up in research labs. The public response to this article was immediate and intense, and Congress began receiving more mail on animal welfare than on Vietnam or civil rights. The powerful forces that had opposed animal welfare legislation now gave up their opposition and tried to weaken the legislation that would inevitably pass. In August 1966, President Lyndon Johnson signed the Laboratory Animal Welfare Act (AWA) into law (P.L. 89–544).

The AWA provided for the licensing of dealers and the registration of research facilities. It vested the secretary of agriculture with power to promulgate and enforce standards for humane care, treatment, and housing of animals. However, *animal* was defined in such a way as to exclude rats and mice, the most common animals used in research. The definition included nonhuman primates, guinea pigs, hamsters, and rabbits, but dealers and other facilities were only required to keep records concerning dogs and cats, thus effectively exempting the other animals from the act's protection. Another limitation of the act was that although it applied to the transportation of animals by suppliers, it did not apply to common carriers.

In 1970 the AWA was amended in order to address these shortcomings (P.L. 91–579). *Animal* was redefined as "any live or dead dog, cat, monkey (nonhuman primate animal), guinea hamster, rabbit, or other such warm-blooded animal, as the Secretary [of Agriculture] may determine is being used, or is intended for use, research, testing, experimentation, or exhibition purposes, or as a pet." Horses not used for research, and other livestock, poultry, and farm animals used for food or fiber production, were specifically excluded from the definition. In addition to this change in definition, the 1970 amendments extended the act's authority to all those engaged in the interstate commerce of nonfarm animals. Enforcement mechanisms were also improved, and provisions were added for exempting research facilities that did not intend to use live dogs or cats, unless other animals covered by the act would be used in "substantial number."

In 1976 the act was further amended to apply to a broader range of research facilities and to animals used in fighting, hunting, breeding, and security. The act's provisions were also simplified. However, as an instrument for constraining experimentation on nonhuman animals, the AWA remained very limited. In addition to applying to only a few species, the act explicitly stated that none of its provisions shall be taken to apply to the actual conduct of research.

Responsibility for enforcing the AWA fell to the Department of Agriculture, which from the beginning worked to shift enforcement responsibilities to other government agencies and subsequently opposed all attempts to further strengthen the AWA. In 1985 the General Accounting Office released a report documenting the department's failure to adequately enforce the AWA.

Since the early 1960s, the U.S. Public Health Service (PHS) had issued its own guidelines governing animal care and use in research funded by one of its agencies, the National Institutes of Health (NIH).* At first voluntary, conformity to these guidelines later became a condition for receiving NIH funding. However, like the Department of Agriculture (DOA), NIH failed to identify and effectively respond to violations of its own rules. During the 1980s several highly visible cases of prestigious, NIH-funded investigators' violating animal welfare regulations were brought to light by animal rights groups. These included well-publicized incidents at the University of Pennsylvania, the City of Hope Medical Center, and Columbia University. In each case, laboratories were raided by animal rights groups, and subsequent NIH investigations resulted in research grants being suspended for animal welfare violations. In 1985, the PHS issued new guidelines.

Also in 1985, Congress significantly strengthened the AWA. Amendments were passed as part of the Food Security Act of 1985 (P.L. 99–198) and the NIH Reauthorization Act (P.L. 99–158). For the first time, these amendments gave the PHS guidelines the force of law and extended their coverage to other agencies, such as the Food and Drug Administration.* These amendments also strengthened standards for animal care, required that animal pain and distress be minimized, increased enforcement mechanisms, made some provision for disseminating information obtained from animal experiments with a view to reducing duplication, and mandated training for personnel who handle animals. Two provisions of the amendments have been especially controversial within the research community: the requirement that dogs be exercised and that primates be kept in a physical environment that promotes their well-being. Some critics have argued that implementing such provisions would be ruinously expensive, while others have argued that concepts such as well-being are meaningless, vague, or unscientific.

DOA delayed issuing draft regulations under these amendments until 1989— and then only under the threat of a lawsuit from the Animal Legal Defense Fund (ALDF). The draft regulations—especially the sections proposing 30 minutes of daily exercise for caged dogs and an hour of "positive physical contact" from humans each day for those animals kept in isolation—were roundly condemned by the research community as expensive and intrusive. The final regulations issued in 1990 gave individual research facilities the responsibility for developing their own plans to exercise dogs and to promote the psychological well-being of primates. These plans would be available to inspectors from the Animal and Plant Health Inspection Service but not submitted to the Department of Agriculture and therefore would not be available to the public under the Freedom of Information Act. The ALDF and AWI went to court, and in February 1993, these regulations were struck down on the ground that by delegating to research facilities plans for exercising dogs and promoting primate well-being, DOA had failed to implement the 1985 amendments that required it to regulate these institutions. The Clinton administration challenged this decision, and in 1994 a U.S. federal court of appeals ruled in favor of the DOA on the grounds that the ALDF and the AWI did not have legal standing.

Potentially the most important provision of the 1985 amendments is the mandate that all research facilities covered by the AWA appoint an Institutional Animal Care Committee that includes one veterinarian and one member not affiliated with the facility. The intent is to "provide representation for general community interests in the proper care and treatment of animals." To fulfill this mandate, the PHS currently requires that all facilities under its jurisdiction have an Institutional Animal Care and Use Committee (IACUC), which is authorized to suspend projects that are not in compliance with PHS rules. This committee must have no fewer than five members, including at least one veterinarian, one nonscientist, and one person not affiliated with the institution. These committees are required to conduct inspections and to review research protocols and can be required to provide reports on their institution's programs and facilities.

IACUCs, however, are constrained in their effectiveness by the attitudes of the institutions they serve. Because institutions vary enormously in the power and authority they vest in such committees, there is a marked lack of uniformity in the protection of animal subjects from one institution to another. Many small institutions complain that establishing IACUCs imposes large costs on them. IACUCs at large institutions often feel overwhelmed by regulations requiring the semiannual inspection of all laboratory animal facilities. Yet despite the fact that current regulations are highly demanding in some respects, a Hastings Center Group concluded that a great deal of research escapes regulation entirely, especially privately funded research, research conducted under the guise of education, and research on rats, mice, and other unprotected animals.

Another difficulty with IACUCs involves tensions between committee members and the scientific community. Scientists often argue that members of IACUCs do not have the expertise to make judgments about research design. Yet if IACUCs take seriously their charge to ensure that alternatives to animals are considered and that no more than the minimum number of animals are used, then they have little choice but to consider research design. There are also tensions between scientific researchers who overwhelmingly dominate the membership of IACUCs and the community members of these committees. Community members report feeling marginalized by the other members of their committees, and dissenting community members are often accused of scientific ignorance or of harboring antiscience, antivivisectionist views. In one study, almost all of the votes against particular research protocols were cast by community members, and in every case, the research went forward despite their objections.

In the near future, there will be attempts to further regulate animal research. The United States has the weakest system for protecting research animals in the industrialized world, and there will be attempts to follow Canada, Britain, and most European countries in regulating research design, practice, and experimental procedures, as well as in requiring explicit weighing of the benefits versus the costs of the proposed research. There will also be attempts to change the composition of IACUCs so that they better reflect community values and attitudes and are not so heavily dominated by researchers, perhaps by adding members whose charge is to explicitly advocate the interests of the animals. Finally, there are ongoing efforts to extend the coverage of the AWA to all animals used in research, including rats and mice.

Ultimately, however, questions about the use of animals in biomedical research will not be settled in the courts and legislatures alone. The policy shifts described here reflect the decreasing power of the traditional Western view that the purpose of animals is to serve human interests, a perspective that has been under serious attack by a generation of philosophers, notably Peter Singer and

Tom Regan. This philosophical work in conjunction with broader shifts in cultural currents explains how the weak animal welfare movement of the 1950s and 1960s was transformed into the muscular animal rights movement of the 1980s and 1990s. Changing attitudes are making animal research increasingly expensive, difficult to carry out, and ethically and scientifically unappealing to many young researchers. Exactly how far we go as a society in minimizing the use of animals in research will depend in part on what sort of cultural and philosophical consensus emerges about our moral relationship to nonhuman animals.

REFERENCES: Orlans, Barbara. 1993. *In the Name of Science.* New York: Oxford University Press; Regan, Tom. 1983. *The Case for Animal Rights.* Berkeley: University of California Press; Rowan, A. N., et al. 1995. *The Animal Research Controversy.* Medford, MA: Center for Animals and Public Policy, Tufts University; Singer, Peter. 1990. *Animal Liberation.* 2nd ed. New York: Avon Books; U.S. Congress, Office of Technology Assessment. 1986. *Alternatives to Animal Use in Research, Testing, and Education.* Washington, D.C. Government Printing Office.

DALE JAMIESON and JACQUELINE L. COLBY

ARTIFICIAL HEART

Most serious efforts to create artificial organs have been aimed toward replacing the heart or parts of it. The first artificial heart replacement was performed on an animal at the Cleveland Clinic in 1957, although serious research on an artificial heart for humans did not begin until the early 1960s. By 1965, the U.S. government had taken an interest in the quest for an artificial heart and allocated $40 million to the project aimed at developing a fully implantable artificial heart.

In 1969 and in 1981, Dr. Denton Cooley of the Texas Heart Institute implanted an artificial heart in two patients. The intention was to maintain life support until a human transplant became available. The first permanent artificial heart, the Jarvik-7, was implanted into Dr. Barney Clark at the University of Utah in December 1982. The patient lived for 112 days. Further attempts to refine the Jarvik-7, however, were unsuccessful, and on January 11, 1990, the Food and Drug Administration (FDA)* withdrew its approval for the device. To date, the totally implantable, artificial heart remains investigational. Current interest is focused on left ventricular assist devices (LVADs), which do not require the replacement of the patient's heart. A preliminary study of totally implantable LVADs was slated to take place in 1993 but was, at the last minute, tabled due to lack of FDA approval.

Currently the artificial heart is used as a bridge until a human heart is available for transplantation. This use is ethically controversial, however, as the artificial devices do not increase the number of hearts available for transplantation; they only change the identity of the individuals who survive long enough to receive a heart transplant.

REFERENCES: Annas, G. 1985. "No Cheers for Temporary Artificial Hearts." *Hastings*

Center Report 15(5): 27–28; Fox, R. C., and Swazey, J. P. 1992. *Spare Parts.* New York: Oxford University Press; Jonsen, Albert R. 1986. "The Artificial Heart's Threat to Others." *Hastings Center Report* 16: 9–11; Phillips, W. M. 1993. "The Artificial Heart: History and Current Status." *Journal of Biomechanical Engineering* 115: 555–57; Strauss, M. 1984. "The Political History of the Artificial Heart." *New England Journal of Medicine* 310(5): 332–36.

LAURA A. SIMINOFF, ROBERT M. ARNOLD, and MOLLY SEAR

ARTIFICIAL INSEMINATION

This technique is the oldest and most widely used form of technology-assisted reproduction. Although artificial insemination (AI) is a relatively simple procedure, its success depends on a number of technical factors such as quality of the semen specimen and the timing of the insemination. Semen obtained by masturbation is deposited by means of a syringe in or near the cervix. Because the exact timing of ovulation is uncertain, insemination is often conducted on several consecutive days. A success rate of 80 percent pregnancy within several months of the start of the treatment is usual in AI.

Although the procedures are identical, there are two basic types of AI, depending on whether the sperm used is the husband's (AIH) or a donor's (AID, now more commonly termed donor insemination, or DI). Although biologically it is irrelevant whether the semen is provided by the husband or a donor, the ethical, psychological, and social problems surrounding DI are more pronounced. It is estimated that over 500,000 children in the United States have been conceived through AI, most with donor sperm. One survey estimated that 172,000 women underwent AI in 1986–1987, resulting in 75,000 births, 30,000 utilizing donor sperm (Office of Technology Assessment, 1988, 3). Although it is the simplest technique, AI still brings into the reproductive process third parties in the form of physicians or other interveners. Also, it introduces the concept of collaborative conception in which sperm or eggs from donors are used.

Although the first reported child who was the product of DI was born a century ago, DI's use has been expanded in the last few decades by the introduction of cryopreservation techniques, which freeze and preserve sperm indefinitely by immersion in liquid nitrogen. In 1988, the American Fertility Society amended its therapeutic donor insemination guidelines, stating that "the use of fresh semen is no longer warranted" in response to reports of transmission of the human immunodeficiency virus (HIV) through donated semen. Although there is a decreased pregnancy rate using frozen as compared to fresh sperm (Subak, Adamson, and Boltz, 1992), most professional fertility services use frozen semen.

Cryopreservation has led to the establishment of commercial sperm banks, some of which now advertise their "products" to the public. These banks also make it possible for a man to store his semen prior to undergoing a vasectomy as a form of "fertility insurance" or prior to chemotherapy or radiation therapy. They also facilitate eugenic programs, such as the Repository for Germinal

Choice, which inseminates women of "high intelligence" with sperm of "superior men."

REFERENCES: Achilles, Rona. 1992. *Donor Insemination: An Overview.* Ottawa: Royal Commission on New Reproductive Technologies; American Fertility Society. 1988. "Revised New Guidelines for the Use of Semen-Donor Insemination." *Fertility and Sterility* 49(2): 211; American Fertility Society. 1990. "Revised Guidelines for the Use of Semen Donor Insemination." *Fertility and Sterility* 53:1s–13s; Daniels, Ken R., and Karyn Taylor. 1993. "Secrecy and Openness in Donor Insemination." *Politics and the Life Sciences* 12(2): 155–170; Depypere, H. T., S. Gordts, R. Campo, and F. Comhaire. 1994. "Methods to Increase the Success Rate of Artificial Insemination with Donor Semen." *Human Reproduction* 9(4): 661–663; Office of Technology Assessment. 1988. *Artificial Insemination: Practice in the United States.* Washington. D.C.: U.S. Government Printing Office; Subak, Leslee L., G. David Adamson, and Nancy L. Boltz. 1992. "Therapeutic Donor Insemination: A Prospective Randomized Trial of Fresh Versus Frozen Sperm." *American Journal of Obstetrics and Gynecology* 166(6): 1597–1606.

See also **AMERICAN SOCIETY FOR REPRODUCTIVE MEDICINE; SEX PRESELECTION.**

ROBERT H. BLANK

B

BABY DOE

Baby Doe was born on April 9, 1982, in Bloomington, Indiana, suffering from Down syndrome and a defective, but surgically correctable, esophagus. Without surgery, Baby Doe could not eat or drink and therefore would die. The parents refused to consent to surgery, and Bloomington Hospital sought a court order to force treatment. The trial court refused to issue the order, and the Indiana Supreme Court refused to hear the case. Baby Doe subsequently died.

This case was much publicized in the news media and became a major factor in the development of a series of rules issued by the Department of Health and Human Services (DHHS) and legislation passed by Congress. On May 18, 1982, DHHS issued a letter to hospitals receiving federal aid advising them that failure to provide disabled newborns with appropriate care was a violation of those infants' civil rights. On March 7, 1983, DHHS published an Interim Final Rule (Nondiscrimination on the Basis of Handicap), based on the 1973 Rehabilitation Act. The Interim Final Rule required that hospitals receiving federal aid post notices describing federal protections against discrimination and advising that DHHS had established a toll-free "hotline" so violations could be reported. The Interim Final Rule was invalidated by the Federal District Court for the District of Columbia in *American Academy of Pediatrics v. Heckler* (1983) because DHHS had not followed appropriate procedural requirements when issuing the rule.

On January 12, 1984, DHHS published a Final Rule (Nondiscrimination on the Basis of Handicap: Procedures and Guidelines Relating to Health Care for Handicapped Infants) that in most respects was similar to the Interim Final Rule in that it (1) advised hospitals that failure to treat disabled newborns was a violation of Section 504 of the 1973 Rehabilitation Act, (2) required the posting of notices with DHHS and state child protective services telephone numbers, (3) allowed for on-site visits so federal and/or state officials could investigate allegations of failure to treat, and (4) encouraged hospitals to create Infant Care Review Committees. This rule was invalidated on June 9, 1986, by the U.S. Supreme Court in *Bowen v. American Hospital Association.*

Congress became involved in establishing Baby Doe policy by enacting Public Law 98–457 (The Child Abuse Amendments of 1984), which was signed into law by President Ronald Reagan on October 9, 1984. The Child Abuse Amendments were not based on the civil rights provisions of the 1973 Rehabilitation Act but instead were premised on the position that failure to treat critically ill newborns was a form of child neglect. The amendments required that states establish programs for reporting medical neglect as a condition of receiving federal funds. This legislation was not challenged in the courts and was reauthorized on October 25, 1992.

REFERENCES: *American Academy of Pediatrics v. Heckler,* 561 F. Supp. 395 (1983); Blank, Robert H., and Janna C. Merrick. 1995. *Human Reproduction, Emerging Technologies, and Conflicting Rights.* Washington, D.C.: Congressional Quarterly Press; *Bowen v. American Hospital Association,* 106 S. Ct. 2101 (1986); DHHS Final Rule. "Nondiscrimination on the Basis of Handicap: Procedures and Guidelines Relating to Health Care for Handicapped Infants." Federal Register, Vol. 49, No. 8. January 12, 1984; DHHS Interim Final Rule. "Nondiscrimination on the Basis of Handicap." Federal Register, Vol. 48, No. 45. May 26, 1982; DHHS Notice to Health Care Providers. "Discriminating Against Handicapped by Withholding Treatment or Nourishment." Federal Register, Vol. 47, No. 116. May 18, 1982; Merrick, Janna C. 1995. "Critically Ill Newborns and the Law: The American Experience." *Journal of Legal Medicine* 16(2):189–210.

JANNA C. MERRICK

BABY K

Baby K was born on October 13, 1992, at Fairfax Hospital, in Falls Church, Virginia. She suffered from anencephaly, a catastrophic birth defect in which most of the brain is missing and which is universally fatal, usually within a short time period after birth. Based on the mother's religious views, Baby K was intubated at birth and placed on a ventilator due to respiratory distress. The hospital recommended "comfort care" only (warmth, nutrition, and hydration) and a "do not resuscitate" order. The mother refused, and when the hospital and mother could not reach agreement on Baby K's care, the hospital ethics committee was consulted and recommended termination of treatment because it (i.e., ventilator support) was futile. The mother continued to refuse this treatment plan, and Fairfax Hospital sought to transfer Baby K to another hospital, but no hospital with an appropriate pediatric intensive care unit would accept the transfer.

In November 1992, the hospital and mother agreed to transfer Baby K to a nursing facility on the condition that Fairfax Hospital readmit her if respiratory failure occurred. As of January 1995, Baby K had been readmitted to Fairfax Hospital for respiratory failure on four occasions. After a readmission in January 1993, Fairfax Hospital initiated action in the U.S. District Court for the Eastern

District of Virginia, seeking an order so that it would not continue to be required to provide what it deemed inappropriate (i.e., futile) treatment. The trial court held that the federal Emergency Treatment and Active Labor Act (EMTALA) required the hospital to stabilize the patient in emergency situations, and therefore ventilator support was required when needed. The trial court also found that Baby K was "handicapped" and "disabled" according to the 1973 Rehabilitation Act and therefore could not be denied mechanical ventilation due to her anencephalic handicap. The court also found that anencephaly qualifies as a disability under the Americans with Disabilities Act.

On appeal to the U.S. Court of Appeals for the Fourth Circuit, only the EMTALA was considered because the appeals court found that the EMTALA required the hospital to provide medical care for Baby K. The appeals court found that the hospital had a duty to provide treatment to prevent the material deterioration of the patient and, in the case of Baby K, that deterioration was due to her respiratory distress, not the anencephaly.

REFERENCES: Blank, Robert H., and Janna C. Merrick. 1995. *Human Reproduction, Emerging Technologies, and Conflicting Rights.* Washington, D.C.: Congressional Quarterly Press; *In re Baby K,* 832 F. Supp. 1022 (E.D. Va. 1993); *In re Baby K,* 16 F.3d 590 (4th Cir. 1994); Merrick, Janna C. 1995. "Critically Ill Newborns and the Law: The American Experience." *Journal of Legal Medicine* 16(2):189–210.

JANNA C. MERRICK

BIOMEDICAL ETHICS BOARD

The 1985 Health Research Extension Act authorized creation of the Biomedical Ethics Board, which was to be composed of six senators and six representatives, with an equal number of members from each party. In August 1987, after considerable delay, the board appointed the Biomedical Ethics Advisory Committee (BEAC). This 14-member committee of experts in law, medicine, and ethics was mandated under the 1985 act to provide counsel to members of Congress on the ethical issues arising in the delivery of medical care and biomedical research. The deadlock in selection of members focused primarily on their views on abortion and other life issues. The BEAC expired in September 1989, having issued no reports.

REFERENCES: Hanna, Kathi E., Robert M. Cook-Deegan, and Robyn Y. Nishimi. 1993. "Finding a Forum for Bioethics in U.S. Public Policy." *Politics and the Life Sciences* 12(2): 205–219; Office of Technology Assessment. 1993. *Biomedical Ethics in U.S. Public Policy.* Washington, D.C.: U.S. Government Printing Office.

ROBERT H. BLANK

BRAIN DEATH

The development of advanced cardiac life support in the 1950s and 1960s resulted in the unprecedented survival of comatose, vegetative, and "brain-dead" individuals. At the same time, otherwise healthy but acutely head-injured individuals with intact organs provided an ideal source for organ donation.

But such individuals did not meet the accepted criterion of death, which was universally and exclusively the irreversible cessation of cardiac function. These two factors led to a need for a new paradigm for the definition of death: cessation of cardiac function *or* irreversible cessation of brain function. Brain death is therefore one of two criteria for death—the other being cardiac—and is defined as irreversible cessation of whole brain function (i.e., brain stem and cerebral cortex).

Historically, wide recognition of the concept of brain death began in the 1950s. In 1958, Pope Pius XII issued a statement in response to a question posed at the International Congress of Anesthesiologists:

[I]t remains for the doctor . . . to give a clear and precise definition of "death" and the moment of death of a patient who passes away into a state of unconsciousness. . . . In general, it will be necessary to presume that life remains, because there is involved here a fundamental right received from the creator, and it is necessary to prove with certainty that it has been lost. . . . Where the verification of fact in particular cases is concerned, the answers cannot be deduced from any religious and moral principle and, under this aspect, does not fall within the competence of the church. . . . But considerations of a general nature allow us to believe that human life continues for as long as the vital functions distinguished from the simple life of organs manifest themselves spontaneously or even with the help of artificial processes. (Pope Pius XII, 1958, 393)

This statement is critical for four reasons. It came from a widely respected orthodox moral authority; it recognized that the technical definition of brain death was a medical one; it asserted that the diagnosis must be made with certainty; and it legitimized the search for an operational definition of brain death. Here Pope Pius XII defines the central theme of brain death—that there is a fundamental difference between a collection of organs and an integrated organism. The brain-dead individual ceases to function as an integrated organism, though some organs may still function independently. It is the brain and brain stem that regulate body temperature, which is severely deranged in brain death. The brain stem regulates respiration in response to changes in carbon dioxide. This regulation and initiation of respiration are absent in brain death. The brain stem modulates cardiac function to augment or reduce cardiac output and blood pressure to meet the metabolic needs of each of the vital organs, especially the brain. In brain death, there is progressive disintegration of cardiac regulation and vascular tone. In brain death, there is complete cessation of sleep-wake cycles, hearing, and visual function, which are frequently preserved even in deep coma and the vegetative state. It is universally accepted that brain death is truly death of an integrated organism, even if that organism has preservation of isolated organ function. Further, the level of integration in deep coma is magnitudes worse than in coma and the vegetative state.

Soon after Pope Pius XII's statement, multiple reports from the French described individuals who were in persistent coma with absent brain stem function (unable to breathe independently) and with absent brain activity on electroencephalography. An increasing number of reports described a variety of neurologic conditions after cardiac arrest, cerebral herniation, or traumatic head injury. Some conditions, such as the persistent vegetative state,* are characterized by eyes open unawareness, usually with brain stem function. Such individuals are severely neurologically disabled but are not truly comatose. Others appear deeply comatose but are actually awake, a term defined as the *locked-in comatose*. Still others remained in persistent or irreversible comas but with persistent brain stem function and preserved (though deranged) electroencephalogram (EEG) activity. The multitude of disparate conditions begged for precise criteria that would define irreversible absence of integrated function of the brain stem and cerebral cortex and carefully exclude other comatose and severely disabled conditions. Such a diagnosis of whole brain death, as opposed to isolated cortical death (higher brain model) or brain stem death, was desirable because it could be verified at the bedside through objective clinical testing of brain stem functions and could be confirmed through objective measures of cortical function, that is, EEG or brain blood flow studies.

Practically speaking, the issue of defining operational criteria for brain death was not satisfactorily addressed until 1968, when the Harvard Criteria were first forwarded. These criteria, which serve in modified fashion as a basis for the President's Commission criteria for brain death, were the first attempt to provide guidelines for the determination of whole brain death. Problematical, the Harvard Criteria were not based on prospective data and were largely empiric; even the manuscript title, "A Definition of Irreversible Coma," reflected the confusion of the day. In reality, the Harvard Criteria represented a definition of brain death, not irreversible coma. True, brain death is a form of irreversible coma, but irreversible coma may exist that has none of the features of brain death. The Harvard Criteria form the basis of the currently practiced whole brain criteria of death. The Harvard Criteria required the following: (1) unresponsiveness; (2) no muscular movements and no respiration; (3) no reflexes; and (4) electrocerebral inactivity (absent brain electrical function). The Harvard Criteria were artificially restrictive and rather arbitrary. For example, the guidelines required a repeat evaluation in 24 hours based solely on the desire to avoid error. They also called for absence of deep tendon reflexes (knee jerk response), which now are universally agreed to persist after brain death and are a function of spinal cord, not brain stem or cortical, function. Nevertheless, the Harvard Criteria were workable and minimized the potential for falsely diagnosing brain death. Problematical, they resulted in continuing life support in those who were definitely brain dead but did not meet the rigid criteria.

The next major advance occurred in 1981, when the President's Commission for the Study of Ethical Problems in Medicine and Biomedical and Behavioral Research* issued guidelines for the determination of death. These guidelines were intended to serve as a statement of accepted medical standards in the diagnosis of cerebral death and are the guidelines in current use. The guidelines provide two independent models of death:

1. An individual with irreversible cessation of circulatory and respiratory function.
2. An individual with irreversible cessation of function of the entire brain, including the brain stem.

The President's Commission guidelines mandate the following in the setting of cerebral death:

1. Deep coma
2. Absent brain stem function (absent pupillary reactivity, absent corneal reflex, absent vestibular response)
3. Absent spontaneous respirations
4. The cause of coma must be established and sufficient
5. Reversible causes (hypothermia, drug overdose, neuromuscular paralysis, metabolic causes) must be treated or excluded
6. The possibility of recovery is excluded
7. Minimum duration of observation is six hours; longer in the absence of confirmation with EEG or anoxia
8. Confirmation with an EEG or cerebral vascular flow study is desirable

What is unique about the President's Commission guidelines is that they provide a practical framework that simplifies and standardizes the approach in a stepwise fashion. Further, they provide (but do not clarify) a method to test respiratory function and eliminate the needless repetition of EEGs to confirm the diagnosis. These guidelines integrate the results of several studies that effectively confirmed the reliability of brain death determination based on unresponsiveness, absence of brain stem function, apnea, and inactive EEGs.

Several other centers have validated the concept of brain death, including Jennet et al. in 1981, who continued 326 patients on life support after a diagnosis of brain death was made. No patients awakened, and all died a cardiac death. The validity of criteria that include cerebral unresponsiveness, absent respiration, and a "flat line" or inactive electroencephalogram was also confirmed by a Collaborative Study of the National Institute of Neurologic Diseases and Stroke.

In diagnosing brain death, the preeminent model is one of whole brain death—that is, death of both brain stem and cerebral cortex. Other models have been proposed but are less satisfactory. One model, the higher brain model or neocortical death model, proposes that one is dead when one loses functions that are uniquely human, such as thought, emotion, or will. This definition would lump together patients in a vegetative state, persistent coma with intact brain stem function, severe dementia, and anencephaly. Problematic, there is no objective way to validate when these functions are absent or irreversibly gone.

In summary, the only valid criterion for brain death in the United States is whole brain death. Such a diagnosis can be made reliably after severe head trauma, herniation, and anoxic injury to the brain. The President's Commission has defined straightforward criteria for the diagnosis, which include absence of *both* brain stem and cortical function. Application of the whole brain death model safely excludes patients with other severe neurologic disabilities, who though disabled still function as an integrated living human being and are not dead.

REFERENCES: Ad Hoc Committee of the Harvard Medical School to Examine the Definition of Brain Death. 1968. "A Definition of Irreversible Coma." *JAMA* 205: 337–340; Bernat, J. L. 1991. "Ethical Issues in Neurology." In *Clinical Neurology.* Vol. 1, sec. 3 (R. J. Joynt, ed.), Pp. 18–42. Philadelphia: J. B. Lippincott; Jennet, B., Gleave, J., and Wilson, P. 1981. "Brain Death in Three Neurosurgical units." *British Medical Journal* 282: 533; "Medical Consultants on the Diagnosis of Death to the President's Commission for the Study of Ethical Problems in Medicine and Biomedical and Behavioral Research. Guidelines for the Determination of Death." 1981. *JAMA* 246: 2184–2186; Multisociety Task Force on PVS. 1994. "Medical Aspects of the Persistent Vegetative State." *New England Journal of Medicine* 330:1499–1508, 1572–1579; "NINDS Collaborative Study: An Appraisal of the Criteria of Cerebral Death." 1977. *JAMA* 237: 982–986; Pope Pius XII. 1958. "The Prolongation of Life." *Pope Speaks* 4: 393; Task Force for the Determination of Brain Death in Children. 1987. "Guidelines for the Determination of Brain Death in Children." *Archives of Neurology* 44: 577–588.

CHRISTOPHER M. DeGIORGIO

BROPHY V. NEW ENGLAND SINAI HOSPITAL, INC.

In *Patricia E. Brophy v. New England Sinai Hospital, Inc.* (1986), the Massachusetts Supreme Judicial Court (SJC) held that a hospital patient who, as a result of irreversible brain damage, had been in a persistent vegetative state* for more than three years and who had expressed his desire not to be maintained in said state could lawfully be removed by his guardian from a hospital that had refused to cease providing him with nutrition and hydration by artificial means, and that the patient could be placed in a different facility or in his home where his expressed wishes could be effectuated. The SJC reached the conclusion by applying the doctrine of substituted judgment set forth in *Superintendent of Belchertown State School et al. v. Joseph Saikewicz,* 373 Mass. 728, 370, NE 2nd, 417 (1977). Three members of the court dissented in whole or in part.

On March 22, 1983, Paul E. Brophy, Sr. (Brophy) suffered a rupture of an aneurysm at the apex of the basilar artery. Prior to that time, he was a healthy, robust firefighter and licensed emergency medical technician (EMT) employed in his hometown of Easton. He enjoyed deer hunting, fishing, gardening, and performing household chores. After the incident, despite surgery, he never regained consciousness. His condition was diagnosed as being a persistent vegetative state. On December 22, 1983, with his wife's consent, a gastrostomy tube (G-tube) was surgically inserted, through which he received nutrition and hydration (food and water). Prior to this time, he had been fed through a nasogastric tube.

In February 1985, the wife in her capacity as legal guardian filed a complaint in the Probate Court for Norfolk County requesting a declaratory judgment, inter alia, granting her the authority to order discontinuance of all life-support treatment for her husband, including nutrition and hydration.

The probate court ordered all life-support treatment continued and appointed a guardian ad litem-investigator and ordered him to report to the court concerning the matter. Mrs. Brophy filed the complaint because the physicians and hospital had refused her request to discontinue life-support treatment.

After extensive hearings, the trial court found that Brophy would, if competent, have agreed with the request of his wife and family to discontinue the life-sustaining treatment; nevertheless, the trial judge denied Mrs. Brophy's request and ordered the life-sustaining treatment continued. Mrs. Brophy appealed, and the SJC on its own initiative transferred the case from the appeals court (id 421–422).

Diagnostic techniques on Brophy revealed subarachnoid bleeding in the posterior fossa surrounding the upper brain stem, as well as an aneurysm located at the apex of the basilar artery. On April 6, 1985, he underwent a right frontotemporal craniotomy. Shortly after surgery, computerized axial tomography (CAT) scans showed extensive damage, namely, complete infarction of his left posterior cerebral artery and infarction of the right temporal lobe of the brain. Although not technically brain dead, he suffered serious and irreversible brain damage. In addition, even though some areas of his brain were undamaged, they were stranded and dysfunctional. The damage made him unable to integrate input from his environment and to commence voluntary activity; he lacked cognitive functioning such as reasoning. His body did respond to certain stimuli, but it was probably from reflexives as opposed to cognitive activity. The trial court found that it would be highly unlikely that he would ever regain cognitive behavior, the ability to communicate, or the capability of interacting purposefully with his environment.

Apart from the extreme injury to his brain, Brophy's other organs functioned relatively well. The trial court found he was not terminally ill, nor in danger of imminent death. He was dependent on his G-tube for his nutrition and hydration but it appeared he could live in his persistent vegetative state for several years.

The trial court also found that the use of the G-tube was not painful, uncomfortable, burdensome, unusual, hazardous, invasive, or intrusive. However, removal of the G-tube would create various effects, resulting from the lack of nutrition and hydration, leading ultimately to death, and said death would be extremely painful and uncomfortable (id 423–427). The trial court found that Brophy would decline the provision of food and water, so as to terminate his life.

The factors the trial court considered were (1) Brophy's expressed preference, (2) his religious conviction, (3) the impact on his family, (4) the probability of adverse side effects, and (5) the prognosis both with and without treatment.

On all the evidence, the trial court, despite what Brophy would do, as stated above, ordered the treatment continued, which was in accord with the recommendation of the guardian ad litem and the treating physician, since to do otherwise would in their opinion constitute a harmful act that would deliberately produce death (id 427–429).

The SJC narrowly drew the issue to whether the substituted judgment of an incompetent patient in a persistent vegetative state to refuse the continuance of artificial means of nutrition and hydration should be honored.

Citing *Saikewicz,* supra, the court stated:

[W]e recognize a general right in all persons to refuse medical treatment in appropriate circumstances. The recognition of that right must extend to the case of an incompetent, as well as a competent patient because the value of human dignity extends to both. . . . We emphasize further, that it does not advance the interest of the State or the ward to treat the ward as a person of lesser status or dignity than others. To protect the incompetent person within its powers, the State must recognize the dignity and worth of such a person and afford to that person the same panoply of rights and choices it recognizes in competent persons.

The SJC then went on to say, however, that "the right to refuse medical treatment was not absolute" (id). It then set forth four countervailing state interests that it had previously recognized: "First the preservation of life; second, the protection of innocent third parties; third, the prevention of suicide; fourth, the maintenance of the ethical integrity of the medical profession" (*Brophy,* supra, 432).

The SJC in *Brophy* then noted that the primary goal of the substituted judgment standard is "to determine with as much accuracy as possible the wants and needs of the individual involved." Since no one contested that the evidence supported the trial court's finding concerning Brophy's subjective viewpoint, and since the SJC accepted that Brophy's substituted judgment would be to discontinue providing nutrients through the G-tube, the only question left for the SJC to determine was whether the commonwealth's interests set forth above require that his judgment be overridden (id 433).

The SJC began with what it called the most significant interest in the case, the interest in the preservation of life. The position of the court was to distinguish, however, between the state's interest when human life can be saved, where the affliction is curable, and when the underlying affliction is incurable and "would soon cause death regardless of any medical treatment" (id 433).

The SJC repeated its stand, set forth in *Saikewicz* (supra), that its decision would not be based on Brophy's quality of life when it stated, "It is antithetical to our scheme of ordered liberty and to our respect for the autonomy of the individual, for the State to make decisions regarding the individual's quality of life. It is for the patient to decide such issues. Our role is limited to ensuring that a refusal of treatment does not violate norms" (id 434).

It then notes that in this case

the State's concern for the preservation of life is implicated, since Brophy is not terminally ill nor in danger of imminent death from any underlying physical illness. . . . While the judge found that continued use of the G-tube is not a highly invasive or intrusive procedure and may not subject him to pain or suffering, Brophy is left helpless and in a condition which he has indicated he would consider to be degrading and without human dignity. In making this finding it is clear that the judge failed to consider that Brophy's judgment would be that being maintained by use of the G-tube is indeed intrusive.

Since this was a case of first impression in the commonwealth, the SJC distinguished it from its other cases and then looked at other jurisdictions for guidance. It finally agreed with the New Jersey Supreme Court's view that "the primary focus should be the patient's desires and experience of pain and enjoyment—not the type of treatment involved" (*Matter of Conroy*, 98 N.J., at 369, 486 A 2nd 1209). Thus, the SJC concluded that the state's interest in the preservation of life does not overcome Brophy's right to discontinue treatment. Nor did it consider his death to be against the state's interest in suicide: "The discontinuance of the G-tube will not be the death producing agent 'set' in motion with the intent of causing his own death. . . . Prevention of suicide is . . . an inapplicable consideration. . . . A death which occurs after the removal of life sustaining systems is from natural causes, neither set in motion nor intended by the patient" (id 439).

Lastly, the SJC held that so long as it declined to force the hospital or its personnel to participate in removing or clamping Brophy's G-tube, there was no violation of the integrity of the medical profession (id 439–440).

The SJC upheld by a vote of 4–3 that portion of the judgment pertaining to the judgment that enjoined the guardian from authorizing a facility to remove or clamp Brophy's G-tube. It then entered a new judgment ordering the hospital to assist the guardian in transferring the ward to a suitable facility, or to his home, where his wishes could be effectuated, and authorizing the guardian to order such measures as she deemed necessary and appropriate in the circumstances. Paul Brophy was transferred to Emerson Hospital in Concord where he died eight days later.

REFERENCES: *Patricia E. Brophy v. New England Sinai Hospital, Inc.*, 398 Mass. 417, 497, NE 2nd 626 (1986); *Cruzan v. Director, Missouri Department of Health*, 497 U.S. 277, 110 S. Ct. 2841 (1990); *Matter of Conroy*, 98 N.J. 321, 486 A 2nd 1209 (1985); *Matter of Jane A.*, 36 Mass. App. Ct., 236, 629, NE 2nd 1338 (1994); *Matter of R. H.*, 35 Mass. App. Ct., 478, 622, NE 2nd 1076 (1993); *Superintendent of Belchertown State School et al. v. Joseph Saikewicz*, 373 Mass. 728, 370, NE 2nd 417 (1977).

PHILIP D. MORAN

BUCK V. BELL

Buck v. Bell was the landmark U.S. Supreme Court decision of 1927 that upheld the sterilization of Carrie Buck for eugenic reasons. In *Buck,* to date the controlling decision in this area, Oliver Wendell Holmes wrote his stinging opinion upholding sterilization for eugenic purposes.

We have seen more than once that the public welfare may call upon the best citizens for their lives. It would be strange if it could not call upon those who already sap the strength of the state for these lesser sacrifices, often not felt to be such by those concerned, in order to prevent our being swamped with incompetence. It is better for all the world, if instead of waiting to execute degenerate offspring for the crime, or to let them starve for their imbecility, society can prevent those who are manifestly unfit from continuing their kind. The principle that sustains compulsory vaccination is broad enough to cover cutting the fallopian tubes. . . . Three generations of imbeciles are enough. (at 207)

Given the powerful forces behind the eugenics movement in 1927, especially within the intellectual community, Holmes's dictum was not surprising. It should be noted that the only dissent in *Buck* came from Justice Butler, who did not write a dissenting opinion. Conversely, the justices joining in support of Holmes's opinion read like a who's who of the Supreme Court: civil libertarian Louis Brandeis, former president William Howard Taft, and former Columbia University Law dean Harlen Stone. The opinion was, however, bitterly attacked by commentators of the day, including a leading authority on sterilization who was "surprised by the lack of a thorough understanding of the field of eugenics" demonstrated by the Court. There is also considerable doubt as to the accuracy of the facts in the case, that is, that Carrie Buck's child was "feeble-minded."

Holmes's dictum that "three generations of imbeciles are enough" is a cogent reminder of the impact of even faulty medical theory on the courts. In light of subsequent events and the deflation of many foundations of the eugenics movement, however, it is difficult to imagine why this decision has had so much staying power. Despite major changes in the way we view the mentally retarded, criminality, and alcoholism, and the many legal attempts to reverse *Buck,* none to date has been successful, except to clarify and narrow the boundaries within which involuntary sterilization may be applied.

REFERENCES: *Buck v. Bell,* 274 U.S. 200 (1927); Macklin, Ruth, and Willard Gaylin. 1981. *Mental Retardation and Sterilization: A Problem of Competency and Paternalism.* New York: Plenum Press.

See also **STERILIZATION—INVOLUNTARY**.

ROBERT H. BLANK

C

CENTERS FOR DISEASE CONTROL AND PREVENTION

An agency of the Public Health Service within the Department of Health and Human Services, the CDC is the nation's primary disease prevention agency. The CDC was established in Atlanta, Georgia, in 1946 as the Communicable Disease Center. Its goals were to control the spread of infectious disease (such as malaria and yellow fever) and to encourage the immunization of children. Over the years its focus expanded to include other diseases, and its name was changed to the Centers for Disease Control; in 1992, its emphasis on disease prevention brought another name change. Its current mission is to promote health and quality of life by preventing and controlling disease, injury, and disability. The CDC accomplishes these goals by working in cooperation with national and international organizations to track disease outbreaks, generate and implement prevention strategies, develop sound health policy, and train health workers.

Recognizing the role of chronic disease in morbidity and mortality, the National Center for Chronic Disease Prevention and Health Promotion works to promote health behaviors and to prevent morbidity and mortality from chronic diseases by (1) conducting research to define, prevent, and control chronic diseases, (2) developing, disseminating, and evaluating health promotion, school health education, and risk reduction programs, (3) conducting a national public education campaign against smoking, and (4) assisting the surgeon general in publishing the annual report on smoking and health.

As environmental factors are increasingly determined to be significant factors in the promotion of disease processes, the National Center for Environmental Health seeks to prevent death and disability due to environmental factors by (1) utilizing surveillance systems, surveys, registries, and other data to evaluate associations between environmental exposures and adverse health outcomes, (2) cooperating with the states in the prevention and control of environmental public health problems, and (3) conducting special programs (such as reviewing Environmental Impact Statements).

Injury has been documented to be a major cause of morbidity and mortality in the United States, particularly in those under the age of 40. The National Center for Injury Prevention and Control aims to prevent unintentional and intentional nonoccupation-related injury and death by (1) conducting research on the causes of common injuries and the ways to treat them and (2) proposing and evaluating objectives for national injury prevention and control programs.

The National Center for Infectious Disease focuses on preventing and controlling the morbidity and mortality of infectious diseases by maintaining surveillance of infectious diseases as well as by developing vaccines, antitoxins, and immune system globulins.

Actively supporting the importance of prevention services, the National Center for Prevention Services is charged with developing and implementing preventive health services. Among its goals are (1) expanding knowledge about preventable health problems, (2) supporting states' efforts to establish and maintain disease prevention and control programs, and (3) training U.S. Immigration and Naturalization Service and Customs officers to screen arriving foreign visitors for communicable diseases.

The National Institute for Occupational Safety and Health examines efforts to prevent work-related injury, disease, and death caused by occupational hazards. It conducts epidemiologic and laboratory research to identify occupational hazards, recommending acceptable exposure limits for toxic substances in the workplace; it evaluates health conditions and worksites at the request of employers and employees; and it develops new methods of approaching occupational safety and health problems.

The Epidemiology Program Office seeks to integrate epidemiology into the general workings of the CDC by (1) training experts in epidemiology and providing epidemiologic assistance through their field assignments; (2) managing the Preventive Medicine Residency Program; and (3) preparing the Morbidity and Mortality Weekly Report, a result of an 1878 act of Congress requiring that states inform the federal government of infectious diseases.

The Public Health Practice Program Office aims to increase the efficacy of the public health delivery system by working with academic institutions to develop and evaluate prevention practices and by ensuring that the quality of laboratory services is consistent with requirements for the implementation of high-priority prevention and control programs.

Recognizing that disease does not respect country boundaries, the CDC's International Health Program seeks to support other nations' efforts to control disease, disability, and death. In cooperation with international agencies such as the World Health Organization, this program provides assistance to those countries facing outbreaks of infectious diseases and coordinates requests for international assistance for natural and man-made disasters and refugee relief. The program also works to prevent diseases in other countries from entering the United States.

REFERENCES: CDC. 1994. "Attitudes Toward Smoking Policies in Eight States." *Journal of the American Medical Association* 273:531; CDC. 1994. "Vaccines for Children Program." *Journal of the American Medical Association* 272:1316; Erickson, J. D. 1993. "CDC: Congenital Malformations Surveillance." *Tetratology* 48:545.

ANA MARIA LOPEZ

CHEMICAL CASTRATION

Depo-Provera* (DMPA) is a pharmacological alternative to surgical castration. An injectable progestogen principally used as a female contraceptive, the drug is also characterized as "chemical castration" because it presumably suppresses testosterone levels in men. Depo-Provera was first used at the Biosexual Psychological Clinic of Johns Hopkins Hospital in 1966 to treat sexual deviation disorders, or paraphilias. John Money and other biosexual researchers have used a dosage varying from 100 to 600 milligrams (mg) per week to treat deviant sexual behavior, with most patients receiving 200 to 300 mg. "[B]y calculating the dosage," he found that "the frequency of ejaculation, erection, and erotic behavior could also be calculated" (Money et al., 1976, 111). Once testosterone levels were decreased to one fourth of initial levels, Pierre Gagne reported that "the patients became sexually impotent" (Gagne, 1981, 645).

Initially, these studies held out the promise that Depo-Provera could play a leading role in the pharmacological control of sexual disorders and sex offenders. At the same time, however, this research also revealed that men who took Depo-Provera experienced short-term adverse side effects including fatigue, weight gain, hot flashes, cold sweats, hypertension, headaches, hypogonadism, and insomnia. Depo-Provera may also have long-term adverse side effects because it must be continuously administered to control the paraphiliac's behavior; but no studies have explored its carcinogenic potential in men even though the drug's approved contraceptive use of a 150-mg dose every three months may cause breast cancer, and the amount of Depo-Provera given to men with each injection may vary from 12 to 50 times the amount given to women for contraception.

Depo-Provera has never been Food and Drug Administration* (FDA) approved for the treatment of sexual disorders, nor have these studies been conducted on the basis of FDA experimental authorization but on the basis of the FDA practice-of-medicine exception that allows a drug approved for one purpose to be prescribed by physicians for other uses they believe are consistent with appropriate patient care. In this questionable experimental setting, Drs. Money and Fred Berlin and other biosexual researchers are not able to make any scientifically valid statements about the drug's safety and effectiveness because their findings are not based on controlled group studies but on case reports and single-case experimental designs that provide only anecdotal evidence. As a consequence, there is no scientific evidence that Depo-Provera acts as a sexual appetite suppressant by lowering testosterone levels and that it is effective for the treatment of male sex offenders, nor are there any data concerning the drug's long-term safety for men including the risk of cancer, cardiovascular disease, or permanent sterility. Depo-Provera has been used to treat rape offenders, but these studies do not directly address the question as to whether Depo-Provera that has been used to treat sexual deviates is applicable to rapists. So far, research focuses almost exclusively on subjects with a variety of paraphilias but not rapists. If rape stems from a sexual impulse, it may be treatable with Depo-Provera, but popular and professional opinion suggests that rape is the sexual manifestation of violence and that Depo-Provera would be a doubtful rape therapy.

Depo-Provera has been used as a probation condition for sex offenders, including rapists, in spite of these questions about its safety and effectiveness. The drug's use as a probation condition gained national attention when Roger Gauntlett, an Upjohn heir, was convicted on a plea of nolo contendere to a charge of first-degree criminal sexual conduct for the rape of his 12-year-old stepdaughter and was sentenced to five years probation on the condition that he submit himself "to castration by chemical means patterned after the research and treatment of the John[s] Hopkin[s] Hospital" (*People v. Gauntlett,* January 30, 1984).

On appeal, Gauntlett argued that his probation condition violated the state's probation statute and, as a form of sterilization, violated a broad range of his federal constitutional rights, including his freedom of thought, right to privacy, freedom from cruel and unusual punishment, and right to equal protection of law. The Supreme Court of Michigan found it unnecessary to examine his constitutional arguments and held that in the absence of statutory authorization for treating sex offenders with Depo-Provera, the trial court did not have the discretion to impose the probation condition because of the drug's experimental status, the limited professional literature on its use, and its failure to gain acceptance in the medical community as a safe and reliable medical procedure. In spite of the court's decision on the drug's mandatory use, Depo-Provera continues to be used as a probation condition if defendants knowingly and voluntarily accept it even though the risks are unknown and the choice is inherently coercive.

REFERENCES: Berlin, Fred S., and Carl F. Meinecke. 1981. "Treatment of Sex Offenders with Antiandrogenic Medication: Conceptualization, Review of Treatment Modalities, and Preliminary Findings." *American Journal of Psychiatry* 138: 601–7; Gagne, Pierre. 1981. "Treatment of Sex Offenders with Medroxyprogesterone Acetate." *American Journal of Psychiatry* 131: 644–46; Green, William. 1986. "Depo-Provera, Castration, and the Probation of Rape Offenders." *University of Dayton Law Review* 12: 1–26; Money, John, Claus Wiedeking, Paul A. Walker, and Dean Gain. 1976. "Combined Antiandrogenic and Counseling Program for the Treatment of 46XY and 47XYY Sex Offenders." In Edward Sachar, ed., *Hormones, Behavior, and Psychotherapy.* New York: Raven Press; *People v. Gauntlett,* January 30, 1984. Order of Probation. No. D 824–00–

076 FY. Circuit Court, Kalamazoo County, Michigan, and 353 N.W.2d 464 (Mich. 1984); Peters, Kimberly A. 1993. ''Chemical Castration: An Alternative to Incarceration.'' *Duquesne Law Review* 31: 307–28.

WILLIAM C. GREEN

CHOICE IN DYING

Choice in Dying (CID) is the nation's oldest and largest champion of patient rights at the end of life. CID is a national, not-for-profit organization dedicated to protecting the rights and serving the needs of dying patients and their families, caregivers, and health providers and has been working for more than 55 years to ensure individual choice and compassionate care at the end of life. More than 25 years ago, CID's parent organizations (Society for the Right to Die and Concern for Dying) developed the living will and since then have distributed 10 million free advance directives. The work of CID led to legislation in all 50 states and the District of Columbia that recognizes some form of advance directive (Choice in Dying, 1994). CID also was involved in the development of the federal law, the Patient Self Determination Act (PSDA) in 1991.

Much of the organization's work is centered around individual patient, family, and health care provider counseling, advocacy for appropriate legal support, professional and public education, and the distribution of advance directives. *Advance directives* is a general term that applies to two kinds of legal documents, living wills and medical powers of attorney. The purpose of these documents is to let individuals give instruction about their future medical care in the event of incapacity due to serious illness or injury, although each does so in a different way. Living wills allow individuals to specify their treatment wishes in writing. Medical powers of attorney allow individuals to appoint a trusted person to make medical decisions in the event of incapacity. Each state regulates the use of advance directives differently. Although the use of these forms is generally associated with the refusal of medical treatment, they can also be used to request specific treatments, including all treatment possible be provided.

The mission of Choice in Dying is to achieve full societal and legal support for the right of all individuals to make decisions regarding the nature and extent of life-sustaining measures, as well as the conditions under which dying occurs, based on their personal preferences and values, and to have those decisions recognized and honored. To carry out its mission, CID advocates and promotes informed advance planning about end-of-life decision making by distributing free advance directives and providing free counseling to individuals who request assistance in completing their documents. CID also provides 24-hour access to its Living Will Registry, the most comprehensive computerized registration service of its type.

CID champions individuals' rights at the end of life relative to determining and receiving the most humane care, including measures that relieve pain and suffering, in the environment of choice and commensurate with their end-of-life treatment decisions. Through CID's free counseling service, lawyers, health care professionals, and educators provide assistance to families who are having difficulty getting their loved ones' wishes honored and to health care providers who have questions about specific individuals' advance directives. This service is provided to more than 2,000 callers each month.

CID also educates and informs the public and provider communities about the importance of informed decision making about end-of-life options, advance planning within a family context, and ensuring that advance health care directives are honored and that death occurs as peacefully and comfortably as possible. Professional staffs, including lawyers, nurses, social workers, health care providers, and educators, create curricula for professional school students, teach special courses, lecture, and train practicing providers. Specially trained volunteers from the public and state legislatures provide education to the public through community-based groups (e.g., churches, schools, libraries).

In addition to its direct service (counseling) and educational programs, CID promotes its mission by providing legislative and public policy recommendations and by representing the public directly in court or through amicus briefs. CID's legal services department tracks all legal initiatives in the country relating to end-of-life decision making (i.e., living wills, durable powers of attorney for health care, nonhospital "do not resuscitate" orders, surrogate decision making, and assisted suicide) and provides up-to-date information about these matters to Choice in Dying members in the jurisdictions affected by changes in legislation.

Finally, through a variety of avenues including publications, public forums, and public and professional conferences, CID supports continued discussion and analysis of the ethical and legal issues involved in emerging issues such as physician-assisted suicide, medical futility, euthanasia, surrogate decision making, and pregnancy exclusions. CID's quarterly newsletter reaches approximately 70,000 people, and hundreds of other individuals order its educational publications and videos. New booklets, such as "You and Your Choices," "Dying at Home," and "Artificial Nutrition and Hydration," are all comprehensive guides that deal with issues related to end-of-life decision making. *Questions and Answers: Advance Directives and End-of-Life Decisions* addresses the most commonly asked questions about advance directives and end-of-life decision making.

CID's headquarters are at 200 Varick Street (10th floor) in New York City (10014). All services are available through CID's toll-free telephone line (1-800-989-WILL).

REFERENCES: Choice in Dying. 1994. *Right-to-Die Law Digest.*

See also **"LIVING WILL" STATUTES.**

KAREN ORLOFF KAPLAN

CHORIONIC VILLUS SAMPLING (CVS)

CVS is a prenatal diagnostic procedure in which a biopsy is taken from the placenta, which has DNA identical to that of the fetus. Transabdominal CVS extracts a small amount of placental tissue from a needle that is put through the pregnant woman's abdomen. Transcervical CVS uses a pump-type sampler to aspirate a specimen of placental tissue under direct view of a laparoscope. The advantage of CVS over amniocentesis is that CVS can be conducted as early as the ninth week of pregnancy, thus providing first trimester diagnosis. Although earlier studies found elevated miscarriage rates, improvements in technique have resulted in optimistic findings in recent studies, making it just as safe as amniocentesis for mother and fetus (Williams et al., 1992); CVS undoubtedly will replace amniocentesis as the preferred approach in the near future. The advantage for the pregnant woman is to give her the same information at a time when a much safer abortion is possible than the midterm abortions associated with amniocentesis.

REFERENCES: Brandenburg, Helen, Coen G. Gho, Milena G. J. Jahoda, et al. 1992. "Effect of Chorionic Villus Sampling on Utilization of Prenatal Diagnosis in Women of Advanced Maternal Age." *Clinical Genetics* 41: 239–244; Elias, Sherman, J. L. Simpson, L. P. Shulman, et al. 1989. "Transorbital Chorionic Villus Sampling for First-Trimester Prenatal Diagnosis." *American Journal of Obstetrics and Gynecology* 160: 879–886; Kickler, T. S., K. Blakemore, R. S. Shirley, et al. 1992. "Chorionic Villus Sampling for Fetal Rh Typing: Clinical Implications." *American Journal of Obstetrics and Gynecology* 166(5): 1407–1411; Williams III, John, Boris B. T. Wang, Cathi H. Rubin, and Dawn Aiken-Hunting. 1992. "Chorionic Villus Sampling: Experience with 3016 Cases Performed by a Single Operator." *Obstetrics and Gynecology* 80(6): 1023–1029.

See also **AMNIOCENTESIS; PRENATAL DIAGNOSIS.**

ROBERT H. BLANK

COCAINE-ADDICTED NEWBORNS

Available information does not give a clear picture of the impact of prenatal cocaine exposure on an infant's future growth and development. A number of problems arise in determining the effect of prenatal cocaine exposure. First, estimates of the incidence of prenatal cocaine exposure are hampered by testing difficulties. Interviews of the mother may miss up to 24 percent of cocaine-exposed infants and correlate poorly with laboratory measures of maternal drug use. Depending on testing conditions, maternal or neonatal urinalysis alone may miss up to 60 percent of exposed infants. Urinalysis provides evidence of only recent exposure (several days) and fails to determine the duration and extent of in utero exposure. Newborn blood testing suffers from these same limitations. Testing an infant's meconium may indicate cocaine exposure during the last 20 weeks of gestation, with metabolites detectable up to the third day after birth. Finally, testing maternal and neonatal hair samples may be able to quantitate an infant's exposure to cocaine in the last 12 weeks of antepartum hair growth.

However, testing of newborn hair still failed to identify 25 percent of exposed infants (Callahan et al., 1992).

Second, it is difficult to establish the timing, quantity, and duration of in utero cocaine exposure. Patterns and route of maternal cocaine use may impact on the nature and extent of fetal injury.

Third, confounding variables such as polydrug exposure and social disruption make it difficult to study the isolated effects of maternal cocaine use. Alcohol is almost always used with other drugs such as cocaine. Cocaine use is often associated with poor maternal nutrition, inadequate prenatal care, and poverty. Also, it is difficult to control for environmental factors after birth that may impact significantly on infant development.

Fourth, standard measures of infant development and cognition do not measure neurologic and behavioral functions that are likely affected by cocaine, such as attention, arousal, motivation, and social interaction.

Fifth, and finally, there has been a selection bias in favor of publishing positive rather than negative studies, leading to a misimpression of extensive and devastating effects of prenatal cocaine exposure.

Nevertheless, it is accepted that cocaine use during pregnancy leads to an increased incidence of premature labor and delivery, an increased risk of placental abruption, and intrauterine growth retardation of the fetus. These general effects are thought secondary to impaired placental blood flow and nutrient transfer, increased uterine contractility, increased fetal metabolism, and the depletion of fetal nutrient stores and increased fetal vascular resistance (Volpe, 1992).

Microcephaly and symmetric intrauterine growth retardation are accepted as teratogenic effects of fetal cocaine exposure. Lesions consistent with fetal vascular disruption, such as limb defects and cardiac, cranial, and genitourinary malformations, also have been attributed to in utero cocaine exposure. Animal models suggest that cocaine disturbs central neuronal differentiation, leading to persistent defects in learning and memory. A clear correlate in human infants remains to be defined, although one study of cocaine-exposed infants found abnormalities in arousal and attention mechanisms and another described a syndrome of "hypertonic tetraparesis" correlated with the degree of microcephaly (Mayes et al., 1993).

Cocaine-exposed infants are thought to be at increased risk for destructive cerebral lesions. Brain infarctions, cavitary lesions, and hemorrhages have been reported (Singer et al., 1994). Both ischemic and hemorrhagic lesions may occur and are thought to be secondary to fetal hypoxemia, impaired cerebral autoregulation, and abrupt alterations in fetal cerebral blood flow. In spite of the belief in the increased risk of these lesions, one large-scale study failed to show any increase in intraventricular or intracerebral hemorrhage in infants less than 1,500 grams (Dusik et al., 1993).

Only a minority of infants exposed to cocaine experience a neonatal abstinence syndrome, which may reflect neurotoxicity rather than addictive withdrawal. The infant may exhibit abnormal sleep patterns, tremor, poor feeding, irritability, seizures, and difficulties with motor behavior, state control, and orientation to the environment. The syndrome is usually not severe, peaks on the second day, and is short-lived, though it can be variable and extend over a longer period. It is unclear if the observed symptoms in cocaine-exposed infants may actually be the sequelae of alcohol, marijuana, or tobacco exposure.

Abnormalities in the regulation of respiration and arousal may lead to an increased risk of sudden infant death syndrome (SIDS). The rate of SIDS among cocaine-exposed infants is between 5.4 and 12.7 per 1,000. Routine home apnea monitoring is not recommended, as the risk is not substantially increased.

Given the increased incidence of prematurity, intrauterine growth retardation, and associated neurological complications as well as the variable impact of maternal depression, sexually transmitted diseases, and potential child abuse and neglect, the lack of a clear understanding of cocaine's unique contribution to an infant's medical conditions makes establishing an identifiable pattern of in utero cocaine exposure difficult at best. There have been no consistent findings related to specific newborn behavioral abnormalities in full-term, healthy, cocaine-exposed infants.

Estimates of the incidence of cocaine use during pregnancy range from 10 to 45 percent of women cared for at urban teaching hospitals (Volpe, 1992). In a suburban setting, over 6 percent of infants with insurance born at a private hospital had a cocaine metabolite in their meconium (Schutzman et al., 1991). In 1989, it was estimated that at least 100,000 infants were affected by the maternal ingestion of cocaine during pregnancy.

Cocaine readily crosses the placenta. With maternal ingestion shortly before delivery, newborn infants excrete cocaine for 12 to 24 hours and cocaine metabolites for up to five to seven days. Cocaine acts on both the central and peripheral nervous systems. Peripherally, cocaine activates adrenergic systems with subsequent hypertension, tachycardia, and vasoconstriction. Decreased uterine artery blood flow may lead to marked fetal hypoxia. The stimulation of smooth muscle, and thus uterine contractions, is conducive to premature delivery of the fetus. Cocaine causes a local anesthetic effect by preventing the expected increase in sodium permeability in peripheral nerves. Centrally, cocaine causes the accumulation of the neurotransmitter dopamine at nerve receptors through the inhibition of normal reuptake. It is thought that the dysphoria that follows the initial euphoria of cocaine use is due to the progressive depletion of dopamine at nerve endings. Cocaine also impairs the homeostasis of the central neurotransmitter serotonin, leading to striking alterations in sleep-wake cycling and a decreased need for sleep. These central neurotransmitters are involved in modulating such functions as attention, activity level, and regulation of anxiety and other emotional states. As a result, one may hypothesize that prenatal cocaine exposure could affect an infant's ability to regulate the response to continued environmental stimulus. Experimental findings, however, have been inconsistent. In addition, cocaine rapidly crosses into breast milk, with measurable levels of cocaine and its metabolites in the breast milk for up to 48 hours after the last maternal ingestion. Accordingly, mothers of cocaine-exposed infants should be counseled against breast feeding.

The neurological and cognitive outcomes of infants exposed to cocaine in utero are unclear. Although abnormalities in habituation in infancy should predict Bayley performance, language production, comprehension, and intelligence test performance at four years of age, Bayley scores usually detect no significant difference between cocaine-exposed and nonexposed infants. Most of the tests used do not effectively quantify arousal, attention, emotional control, and related behaviors—that is, the tests used may not adequately measure those functions that cocaine may affect most profoundly. There are no available studies of the development and behavior of cocaine-exposed infants beyond three years of age; in fact, one study found no difference in the overall performance of cocaine-exposed and drug-free children at two years of age. Thus, some (if not most) cocaine-exposed infants, given prenatal maternal drug treatment and intensive infant intervention, may function within normal developmental limits within the first three years of life (Azuma and Chasnoff, 1993). As compared to the in utero impact of maternal cocaine use, the cocaine-exposed infant may be at more physical and developmental risk from the postnatal environment and the mother's continued use of cocaine, given the increased potential for medical neglect and abuse, failure to thrive, decreased maternal responsivity, and lower social involvement.

If our therapeutic goal is to prevent harm to the fetus and subsequent infant, our focus must be on the prevention of drug abuse in women of childbearing age or on the prevention of pregnancy in drug-addicted women. If our goal is the prevention of harm to the fetus and subsequent infant, we should focus on the problem of prenatal exposure to the effects of maternally ingested alcohol as a major preventable cause of mental retardation, and on the lack of adequate maternal nutrition and health care. Regardless of the difficulty in establishing a specific fetal cocaine syndrome, the finding of cocaine exposure does indicate a significant though potential risk to the developing infant. However, this risk is not inevitable, given the evidence that current intervention available for other high-risk children may prove helpful for cocaine- and drug-exposed children. In the absence of neonatal signs or symptoms, the relationship between cocaine and an effect on the infant is unclear. The majority of cocaine-exposed infants neither are premature nor of low birth weight, especially in the absence of other risk factors such as poor prenatal care and inadequate nutrition.

REFERENCES: Azuma, S. D., and Chasnoff, I. J. 1993. "Outcome of Children Prenatally Exposed to Cocaine and Other Drugs: A Path Analysis of Three-Year Data." *Pediatrics* 92:396–402; Callahan, C. M., Grant, T. M., Phipps, P., et al. 1992. "Measurement of Gestational Cocaine Exposure: Sensitivity of Infants' Hair, Meconium, and Urine." *Journal of Pediatrics* 120:763–768; Dusik, A. M., Covert, R. F., Schreiber, M. D., et al. 1993. "Risk of Intracranial Hemorrhage and Other Adverse Outcomes After Cocaine Exposure in a Cohort of 323 Very Low Birth Weight Infants." *Journal of*

Pediatrics 112:438–445; Gingras, J. L., Muelenaer, A., Dalley, L. B., et al. 1994. "Prenatal Cocaine Exposure Alters Postnatal Hypoxic Arousal Responses and Hypercarbic Ventilatory Responses but Not Pneumocardiograms in Prenatally Cocaine-Exposed Term Infants." *Pediatric Pulmonology* 18:13–20; Kliegman, R. M., Madura, D., Kiwi, R., et al. 1994. "Relation of Maternal Cocaine Use to the Risks of Prematurity and Low Birth Weight." *Journal of Pediatrics* 124:751–756; Mayes, L. C., Granger, R. H., Frank, M. A., et al. 1993. "Neurobehavioral Profiles of Neonates Exposed to Cocaine Prenatally." *Pediatrics* 91:778–783; Schutzman, D. L., Frankenfield-Chernicoff, M., Clatterbaugh, H. E., and Singer, J. 1991. "Incidence of Intrauterine Cocaine Exposure in a Suburban Setting." *Pediatrics* 88:825–827; Singer, L. T., Yamashita, T. S., Hawkins, S., et al. 1994. "Increased Incidence of Intraventricular Hemorrhage and Developmental Delay in Cocaine-Exposed, Very Low Birth Weight Infants." *Journal of Pediatrics* 124:765–771; Volpe, J. 1992. "Effect of Cocaine Use on the Fetus." *New England Journal of Medicine* 327:399–407; Zuckerman, B., and Frank, D. A. 1994. "Prenatal Cocaine Exposure: Nine Years Later." *Journal of Pediatrics* 124:731–733.

ROBERT M. NELSON

COMPULSORY CESAREAN SECTIONS

Prior to 1980, *Williams' Obstetrics* stated that the obstetrician's patient is the pregnant woman. In 1980, the revised edition stated for the first time that the obstetrician has two patients: the pregnant woman and the fetus (Pritchard and MacDonald, 1980, vii). For the most part, the change does not reflect a change in attitude but reflects advances in perinatal medicine. A physician's ethical duty toward the pregnant woman requires the physician to act in the interests of the fetus and the woman. This responsibility, however, does not empower physicians to impose a medical risk on one patient to preserve the health of the other. The physician is also ethically obligated to respect a competent patient's informed autonomous decision, including an informed refusal. To act against her will is tantamount to battery and assault.

Typically, a woman who decides to carry a fetus to term is willing to go to great extremes to promote the health and welfare of the future child. Today, approximately one fourth of all pregnancies will be delivered by cesarean section. The procedure has increased morbidity, the recuperation period is longer, and the expense is much greater. For the delivery of a healthy full-term fetus, there are no significant advantages to either method of delivery. However, there are many conditions in which a cesarean section is recommended to avoid the risk of fetal morbidity. This includes a premature infant in the breech position, a full-term fetus with hydrocephalus (an enlarged head secondary to increased fluid), or a fetus with spina bifida (a neurological condition in which part of the spinal cord protrudes through the baby's back).

Sometimes a vaginal delivery can be life threatening to both the woman and the fetus. For example, in complete placenta previa the placenta covers the cervical as such that a vaginal delivery would result in serious hemorrhage to both the fetus and the woman. The mortality risk of vaginal delivery to the fetus is close to 100 percent; the risk to the woman as high as 50 percent. In these cases, the cesarean section is recommended to protect the pregnant woman and the fetus. Cephalopelvic disproportion, in which the fetus is too large to fit through the woman's pelvis, is a more common medical indication for a cesarean section to protect both the fetus and the pregnant woman.

The competent pregnant woman will usually consent to an obstetrician's recommendation for a cesarean section to promote the well-being of the fetus and/or her own health. The question is what to do if a competent woman persistently refuses a cesarean section that a physician believes is medically indicated.

Between 1981 and 1986, there were at least 21 documented petitions for court orders by physicians to perform cesarean sections on competent women. Of these, 18 (86 percent) were granted (Kolder, Gallagher, and Parsons, 1987, 1193). The justification for the court orders was to protect or promote the well-being of the fetus; in some of the cases, the woman's well-being was threatened as well. In at least 6 of these cases, the prediction of harm to the fetus was overstated if not wrong (1195). In 2 cases of compulsory cesarean section, the pregnant woman had to be restrained with force (see Gallagher, 1987, 10; Elkins et al., 1989, 151).

The major objection to forced cesarean sections is that competent patients have a right to refuse medical treatment, even if it will result in death (*In re Quackenbush,* 1978; *In re Melideo,* 1976). The right to refuse medical treatment is supported in the common law by the right to bodily integrity (*Schloendorff v. Society of New York Hosp.,* 1914) and the right to privacy (*Griswold v. Connecticut,* 1965). Is there anything distinct about pregnancy that can justify overriding a woman's informed refusal?

One suggested difference is that the compelled cesarean satisfies a valid state interest in protecting innocent third parties. The argument can take one of two forms. First, although Anglo-American law imposes no duty to easy rescue, persons who have special obligations due to special relationships have a duty to easy rescue. The relationship of a mother to her born child is such a relationship (Prosser and Keeton, 1984, § 56, 375–77). Nevertheless, the obligation does not require the parent to undergo any bodily risk. No adult has ever been coerced to donate an organ to someone already born, even when the risk is small (see *McFall v. Shimp,* 1978). Since a cesarean section entails a moderate degree of risk, a pregnant woman's moral responsibility to her fetus would exceed her legal duty to her living child, which is unjustified, particularly since the personhood of the fetus has not been legally or morally settled.

The second argument holds that the state has a compelling interest in the well-being of the fetus postviability. This argument is based on a misinterpretation of *Roe v. Wade* (1972). In *Roe,* the Supreme Court argued that the state interest in preserving life becomes compelling at viability. As such, *Roe* allows states to prohibit fetal destruction postviability *unless* it is necessary to protect the woman's life or her health. So the woman never actually waives her right to an abortion. Furthermore, nowhere does *Roe* state that the state can require invasive medical procedure to promote fetal health. Rather, in a later abortion ruling, *Colautti v. Franklin* (1979), the Supreme Court overruled a Pennsylvania statute that would have required physicians to make trade-offs between maternal and fetal well-being: "women's life and health must always prevail over the fetus's life and health when they conflict" (*Colautti v. Franklin,* 1979, 400).

A related argument is that although third parties can be held liable in tort for harming a fetus, third-party liability does not apply to the pregnant woman (*Stallman v. Youngquist,* 1988). To hold a pregnant woman liable for harms to the fetus would severely restrict her freedom to act in even normally innocuous ways. But it still would not empower states to restrict a pregnant woman's conduct to prevent such harms; it would only allow the state to hold the woman liable if fetal compromise occurred and could be shown to have been directly caused by her refusal to undergo a cesarean section. In addition, parental immunity laws prevent the state from holding parents liable for injury to their born children. To hold the pregnant woman liable to the fetus would exceed her legal duty to her living children.

Some theorists have also suggested applying the child abuse and neglect statutes to the fetus if the pregnant woman refuses to undergo an invasive procedure to promote the fetus's well-being. But there is a significant difference between court-imposed medical treatment on a child versus a fetus. In the former, the courts impose treatment on the child for the child's well-being. In the latter, the courts must impose treatment on the pregnant woman in order to treat the fetus. This ignores the right of the woman to refuse treatment, and it ignores that the treatment that will benefit the fetus might endanger her own health. (See *In re A.C.,* 1990.)

None of this is to deny moral responsibility to make reasonable efforts toward preserving fetal health. It is merely a denial that moral responsibility entails a corresponding legal duty. Physicians have a moral responsibility to both the woman and the fetus, but they are under no affirmative legal duty to seek a court order (American Medical Association Board of Trustees, 1990, 2664–66). Rather, seeking court orders may be destructive of the physician-patient relationship and create undesirable societal consequences (ACOG, 1987). It is also unjustified because of the limitations and fallibility of medical judgments (ACOG, 1987; Kolder, Gallagher, and Parsons, 1987, 1195).

Compelling a cesarean section may also be unconstitutional. Court-ordered cesareans have received little judicial review. Despite the numerous court orders, only two cases have reached an appellate court. In *Jefferson v. Griffin Spalding County Hospital Authority* (1981), the appellate court based its arguments on *Roe* (for problems with this approach, see Finamore, 1983). In *In re A.C.,* the court distinguished itself from *Jefferson* and, as such, did not consider its merits (*In re A.C.,* 1990, 1243). The court concluded, however, that the pregnant woman's competent decision should be respected in virtually all cases (1252).

Further judicial review will need to address two other constitutional issues. First, a woman's right to bear a child is constitutionally protected (*Skinner v. Oklahoma,* 1942). To legally enforce a pregnant woman's moral obligation to her fetus is unjustifiable because it creates an undue burden or penalty on pregnancy (Annas, 1989, 213–32). Second is the issue of equal protection. The demographics of the women against whom petitions were sought in Kolder's study are suspicious. Most of the women were from minority groups, half were unmarried, and one fourth did not speak English as their primary language. All of the women were treated in teaching hospital clinics or were receiving public assistance (Kolder, Gallagher, and Parsons, 1987, 1192). In contrast, the courts have been hesitant to impose bodily intrusions on all other citizens, including suspected criminals. For example, the Supreme Court refused to compel a suspect to undergo surgery to remove a bullet (*Winston v. Lee,* 1985) or even to have a nasogastric tube placed in his stomach (*Rochin v. California,* 1952).

Like all competent individuals, the pregnant woman does not make health care decisions in a vacuum. She must weigh her medical needs against the needs of the fetus and the needs of other family members. Her decision must balance her health care needs with other important values, including deeply held religious beliefs. To honor the rare case of a woman's refusal may have tragic results. But to do otherwise tolerates "forcible physical violations of women by coercive obstetricians and judges" and fails to protect the rights of *all* competent adults, of which pregnant women are one subclass (Annas, 1982, 45).

REFERENCES: American College of Obstetricians and Gynecologists (ACOG), Committee Opinion from the Committee on Ethics. 1987. "Patient Choice: Maternal-Fetal Conflict" (ACOG Committee Opinion 55). Washington, D.C.; American Medical Association Board of Trustees. 1990. "Legal Interventions During Pregnancy: Court-Ordered Medical Treatments and Legal Penalties for Potentially Harmful Behavior by Pregnant Women." *Journal of the American Medical Association* 264 (20): 2663–70; Annas, George. 1982. "Forced Caesareans: The Most Unkindest Cut of All." *Hastings Center Report* 12(3): 16–17, 45: Annas, George. 1989. "The Impact of Medical Technology on the Pregnant Woman's Right to Privacy." *American Journal of Law and Medicine* 13 (2–3): 213–32; *Colautti v. Franklin,* 439 U.S. 379, 99, S. Ct. 675, 58 L.Ed.2d 596 (1979); Elkins, Thomas E., et al. 1989. "Court-Ordered Cesarean-Sections: An Analysis of Ethical Concerns in Compelling Cases." *American Journal of Obstetrics and Gynecology* 161(1): 150–54; Finamore, Eric P. 1983. "*Jefferson v. Griffin Spalding County Hospital Authority:* Court-Ordered Surgery to Protect the Life of an Unborn Child." *American Journal of Law and Medicine* 9(1): 83–101; Gallagher, Janet. 1987. "Prenatal Invasions and Interventions: What's Wrong with Fetal Rights." *Harvard Women's Law Journal* 10: 9–58; *Griswold v. Connecticut,* 381 U.S. 479 (1965); *In re A.C.,* 573 A.2d 1235 (D.C. 1990); *In re Melideo,* 88 Misc.2d 974, 390 N.Y.S.2d 523 (Sup. Ct. 1976); *In re Quackenbush,* 156 N.J. Super 282, 383 A.2d 785 (1978); *Jefferson v. Griffin Spalding County Hospital Authority,* 247 Ga. 86, 274 S.E.2d 457 (1981); Kolder, Veronika, Gallagher, Janet, and Parsons, Michael. 1987. "Court-Ordered Obstetrical Interventions." *New England Journal of Medicine* 316 (19): 1192–96; *McFall v. Shimp,* 10 Pa.D. & C.3d 90 (C.P.Ct. 1978); Nelson, Lawrence, and Milliken, Nancy. 1988. "Compelled Medical Treatment of Pregnant Women: Life, Liberty and Law in Conflict." *Journal of the American Medical Association* 259 (7): 1060–66; Pritchard, J., and MacDonald, P. 1980. *Williams' Obstetrics.* 16th ed. Norwalk, CT: Appleton and Lange; Prosser, W., and Keeton, W. 1984. *The Law of Torts.* 5th ed. St. Paul, MN: West Publishing: Rhoden, Nancy. 1986. "The Judge in the Delivery Room: The Emergence of Court-Ordered Caesareans." *California Law Review* 74: 1951–2030; Robertson, John. 1983. "Procreative Liberty and the Control of Conception, Pregnancy and Childbirth." *Virginia Law Review* 69: 405–20; *Rochin v. California,* 342 U.S. 165 (1952); *Roe v. Wade,* 410 U.S. 113 (1972); *Schloendorff v. Society of New York Hosp.* 211 N.Y. 125, 105 N.E. 92 (1914); *Skinner v. Oklahoma,* 316 U.S. 535 (1942); *Stallman v. Youngquist,* 531 N.E.2d 355 (Ill. 1988); *Winston v. Lee,* 470 U.S. 753 (1985).

LAINIE FRIEDMAN ROSS

CONFIDENTIALITY OF GENETIC INFORMATION

The relevant law concerns the confidentiality of medical information generally and the boundaries of the "right to privacy" protected by the U.S. Constitution. At common law, courts in many jurisdictions protected the confidentiality of medical information by allowing patients to recover damages for unauthorized disclosure on a variety of theories, example, breach of contract, invasion of privacy, public disclosure of a private fact, malpractice, breach of fiduciary duty, and/or intentional infliction of emotional distress. Most states now have statutes that provide that physicians and other health care providers may not release medical information or medical records to third parties unless the patient has consented in writing or an exception applies, such as the common exceptions allowing disclosure to governmental agencies as required or authorized by law (e.g., for state birth defect registries) or to any party responsible for payment. A few states have passed legislation that specifically addresses the confidentiality of genetic information.

In 1974, Congress passed the United States Privacy Act, 5 U.S.C. 552a et seq., which places limits on the collection of personal information by federal agencies, but the language of the act is not terribly restrictive. Further, it expressly permits collection of certain classes of information without consent, including the collection of medical information from a health care provider without notice to the patient. Id. at 552a(e)(3) Thus far, all attempts to pass federal legislation to regulate the collection, storage, dissemination, and/or use of genetic information have failed, although further work in this area is expected in connection with the national health care reform effort. The prospect of computerization of all medical records makes the search for comprehensive nationwide standards to control access all the more urgent.

The constitutionally protected "right to privacy" may be invoked wherever governmental intrusion is an issue. As first articulated by the U.S. Supreme Court, the right to privacy shields decisions concerning procreation and other fundamental interests from state interference unless the state can demonstrate that it has a compelling interest that can only be advanced through the challenged regulation or activity. In addition to decisional privacy, the Court has recognized an interest in informational privacy and has suggested that there may be limited constitutional protection against unauthorized governmental disclosure of personal information. See *Whalen v. Roe,* 429 U.S. 589 (1977).

In the context of genetics, ethicists and legal scholars are particularly concerned about the release of genetic information to insurance companies and employers. Because such information is typically released by consent, or disclosed as part of the billing and payment process, it falls outside the scope of existing statutory protections, but consent can scarcely be termed "voluntary" when it is made a condition of employment or insurance. Further, a few commentators have tried to heighten sensitivity concerning the possible misuse of genetic information by law enforcement and educational authorities. They fear a new wave of reductionism and biological determinism, and note a tendency to overlook the limitations of scientific knowledge and medical technology.

In addition, the ethical and legal appropriateness of the disclosure of genetic information to a (potentially) affected spouse, child, or other relative is currently the subject of much debate. The earliest legal precedents for a *duty* to disclose involved infectious diseases and reflected a concern to protect those foreseeably at risk of serious harm, usually a spouse or other close family member. The acquired immunodeficiency syndrome (AIDS) epidemic added concerns about stigmatization and the incentive effects of disclosure (from a global or public health perspective) to the calculus of harms and benefits. AIDS confidentiality legislation varies by state, but most laws permit a physician to notify a spouse at risk without consent and establish procedures for anonymous notification of others at risk with consent. The much discussed case of *Tarasoff v. Regents of the Univ. of Cal.* established that health care professionals may also have a duty to breach confidentiality where a patient has threatened to commit an act of violence against an identifiable individual. Since genetic disease can only be transmitted through procreation, and the patient who declines to inform a relative that he or she is at risk is more properly characterized as refusing to benefit another than threatening to harm, the disclosure dilemma created by genetic testing does not fit neatly into either line of cases (see, e.g., Andrews, 1992). There is also the possibility that the relative may prefer to remain in ignorance. It is nevertheless true that genetic information, unlike most other medical information, will frequently be relevant to medical decisions of related third parties.

Most commentators have concluded that at most the physician or other professional should be regarded as having a conditional *privilege* of disclosure. Oft-cited is the recommendation of the President's Commission:

A professional's ethical duty of confidentiality to an immediate patient or client can be overridden only if several conditions are satisfied: (1) reasonable efforts to elicit voluntary consent to disclosure have failed; (2) there is a high probability both that harm will occur if the information is withheld and that the disclosed information will actually be used to avert harm; (3) the harm that identifiable individuals would suffer would be serious; and (4) appropriate precautions are taken to ensure that only the genetic information needed for diagnosis and/or treatment of the disease in question is disclosed. (President's Commission, 1983, at 44)

Some ethicists argue that informed consent to testing should include disclosure of the conditions for breach of confidentiality. The President's Commission has also recommended that adoption laws be modified to allow for the exchange of information about serious genetic risks between adoptees and their biological families, with appropriate safeguards to preserve confidentiality. Forty-five states and the District of Columbia had sealed record statutes for adoption as of 1988, though in a small but growing number of cases courts have allowed access to records where the adoptee is seeking information concerning hereditary genetic disease (Lamport, 1988). Similar concerns are raised in the context of gamete donation, where genetic screening of donors and permanent recordkeeping of any kind may be the exception rather than the rule.

An unexpected finding as to paternity in the course of genetic testing poses a related question: Who should be informed, if anyone? The consensus among geneticists seems to be that where a couple has requested prenatal testing or testing of a minor child—the hardest case given that the information is medically relevant, but the interests of the parties may conflict—the information should only be given to the mother. On the other hand, the President's Commission favors full disclosure combined with careful counseling. Finally, in addition to concerns raised by genetic information as an especially sensitive category of medical information, the storage of genetic material in DNA banks creates a new range of problems because the content of the stored "information" will change as genetic knowledge increases. Some commentators argue that regulation of DNA banks should be more stringent than existing regulation of tissue banks.

REFERENCES: Andrews, Lori B. 1992. "Torts and the Double Helix: Malpractice Liability for Failure to Warn of Genetic Risks." *Houston Law Review* 29: 149–184; Annas, George, and Sherman Elias, eds. 1992. *Gene Mapping: Using Law and Ethics as Guides.* New York: Oxford University Press; Institute of Medicine. 1994. *Health Data in the Information Age: Use, Disclosure, and Privacy.* Washington, D.C.: National Academy Press; Lamport, Anne T. 1988. "The Genetics of Secrecy in Adoption, Artificial Insemination and In Vitro Fertilization." *American Journal of Law & Medicine* 14(1): 109–124; McEwen, Jean E., and Philip R. Reilly. 1992. "State Legislative Efforts to Regulate Use and Potential Misuse of Genetic Information." *American Journal of Human Genetics* 51: 637–647; Nelkin, Dorothy. 1992. "The Social Power of Genetic Information." In *The Code of Codes: Scientific and Social Issues in the Human Genome Project,* ed. D. Kevles and L. Hood. Cambridge: Harvard University Press; President's Commission for the Study of Ethical Problems in Medicine and Biomedical and Behavioral Research. 1983. *Screening and Counseling for Genetic Conditions: A Report on the Ethical, Social and Legal Implications of Genetic Screening, Counseling and Education Programs.* Washington, D.C.: The Commission; *Tarasoff v. Regents of the Univ. of Cal.,* 551 P.2d 334 (Cal. 1976); United States Privacy Act of 1974, P.L. 93–579, 5 U.S.C. 552a et seq.; *Whalen v. Roe,* 429 U.S. 589 (1977).

MARY R. SCHLACHTENHAUFEN

CONSCIENCE CLAUSES

"Conscience clauses" are laws designed to protect health care providers' rights to refuse to provide or participate in medical procedures to which they have moral or religious objections. Forty-four states have enacted conscience clauses of some kind. Most conscience clauses in the United States (those in 28 states) apply in the case of only one procedure—abortion. Other states extend protection for rights of conscience to abortion and some other procedure, including contraception or sterilization, usually. The Illinois Right of Conscience Act, Ill. Ann. Stat. ch 111–1/2, ¶ 5301 et seq., provides the broadest protection of all the American laws, with California and federal statutes providing relatively broad protection—in relatively limited contexts.

Most conscience clauses protect both individual and institutional health care providers, meaning that hospitals may decline to allow elective abortions to be performed, as well as that nurses, doctors, and medical technicians may personally decline to participate in performing abortions. Some states provide no or very little protection to health care institutions, however. While the most comprehensive protections for rights of conscience of health providers cover all persons who, for moral or religious reasons, object to providing, performing, assisting, counseling, paying for, or otherwise providing or participating in a medical procedure, many conscience clauses restrictively limit the particular individuals that are protected.

Conscience clause laws have been enacted primarily in response to the U.S. Supreme Court's decision in *Roe v. Wade,* 410 U.S. 113 (1973), which provides that women have a fundamental constitutional right to have elective abortions. Concerns that medical personnel and facilities might be forced to facilitate abortions that were morally or religiously repugnant to them stimulated the enactment of conscience clauses. Likewise, the federal conscience clause, 42 U.S.C. § 300a–7, originally called the Church Amendment, was enacted in 1973 in response to *Roe* and to a federal court decision two months before *Roe* to compel a Catholic hospital in Montana that had received federal funds to allow the use of its facilities for performance of elective sterilizations. *See generally* 1973 U.S. Code Cong. & Admin. News 1465, 1473.

There is growing evidence of a wide range and significant number of violations of the rights of conscience of health care providers. Nurses, collateral employees, and medical school students are particularly vulnerable because of their relatively inferior and dependent position in the medical world.

Most courts have shown significant hostility to conscience clauses and have given them narrow, restrictive, begrudging interpretations. For instance, in *Spellacy v. Tri-County Hospital,* 18 Empl. Prac. Dec. (CCH) ¶ 8871 (Pa. C.P. De. Cty.), *aff'd,* 395 A.2d 998 (Pa. 1978), Pennsylvania courts held that Pennsylvania's conscience clause did not protect a part-time admissions clerk who claimed that she was fired because she refused to participate in abortion admissions. In *Brownfield v. Daniel Freeman Marina Hosp.,* 208 Cal. App.3d 405, 226 Cal. Rptr. 240 (1989), a California Court of Appeals ruled that California's facially broad conscience clause did not protect a Catholic hospital from providing information or services about the "morning after" abortifacient pill to a rape victim, even though on its face the statute applied to the provision of abortion. And several cases, including a questionably conclusory opinion of the U.S. Supreme Court, have held that institutional conscience clause protections do not apply to public (or even all private) hospitals. *Doe v. Bolton*, 410 U.S. 179, 197 (1973); *Doe v. Bridgeton Hosp. Ass'n, Inc.*, 71 N.J. 478, 366 A.2d 641 (1976); *see further Doe v. Charleston Area Medical Center*, 529 F.2d 638 (4th Cir. 1975). A series of cases in New York and New Jersey have highlighted the need for protection of conscience rights of health providers who for moral or religious reasons do not wish to participate in withdrawal of artificial life support or nutrition and hydration. *Matter of Jobes*, 529 A.2d 434 (N.J. 1987); *In re Requena*, 517 A.2d 886 (N.J. Super), *aff'd*, 517 A.2d 869 (N.J. App. 1986); *Elbaum by Elbaum v. Grace Plaza of Great Neck, Inc.*, 544 N.Y.S.2d 840 (App. Div. 1989).

Three notable cases have interpreted conscience clauses liberally. In *Watkins v. Mercy Medical Center*, 364 F.Supp. 799 (D. Idaho 1973), *aff'd*, 520 F.2d 894 (9th Cir. 1975), the federal court held that the federal conscience clause protected a Catholic hospital from having to permit a doctor to perform sterilizations at the Catholic facility. In *Swanson v. St. John's Lutheran Hospital*, 597 P.2d 702 (Mont. 1979), the Montana Supreme Court held that a nurse who had been fired after eight years of employment when, after assisting a particularly gruesome abortion, she informed her supervisors that she would participate in no more sterilizations was protected by the Montana conscience clause. And in *Kenny v. Ambulatory Centre of Miami, Florida, Inc.*, 400 So.2d 1262 (Fla. App. 1981), a Florida appellate court ruled that a nurse who was asked to resign, threatened with firing, and finally demoted because she would not participate in abortions was protected by the Florida conscience clause.

REFERENCES: Leslie Cannold, *Consequences for Patients of Health Care Professional's Conscientious Action*, 20 J. Med. Ethics 80 (1994); Judith F. Daar, *A Clash at the Bedside: Patient Autonomy v. a Physician's Professional Conscience*, 44 Hastings L.J. 1241 (1993); Bruce G. Davis, *Defining the Employment Rights of Medical Personnel Within the Parameters of Personal Conscience*, 3 Det. Coll. L. Rev. 847 (1986); Cole Durham, Mary Anne Wood, & Spencer Condie, *Accommodation of Conscientious Objection to Abortion: A Case Study of the Nursing Profession*, 1982 B.Y.U.L. Rev. 253; Harriet F. Pilpel & Dorothy E. Patton, *Abortion, Conscience and the Constitution: An Examination of Federal Institutional Conscience Clauses*, 6 Colum. Human Rts. L. Rev. 279 (1974–75); Marc D. Stern, *Abortion Conscience Clauses*, 11 Columbia J. L. & Soc. Probs. 571 (1975); Lynn D. Wardle, *A Matter of Conscience: Legal Protection for the Rights of Conscience of Healthcare Providers*, 2 Cambridge Q. Healthcare Ethics 529 (1993); Lynn D. Wardle, *Protecting the Rights of Conscience of Health Care Providers*, 14 J. Legal Med. 177 (1993).

LYNN D. WARDLE

CONSUMER PRODUCT SAFETY COMMISSION

An independent federal regulatory agency located in Bethesda, Maryland, the commission was established in 1972 by the Consumer Product Safety

Act (86 Stat. 1207). It has five principal areas of responsibility. First, it works to protect the public against "unreasonable" risks associated with consumer products by, for instance, banning the sale of hazardous products, establishing packaging requirements for poisonous substances, and requiring manufacturers to recall, repair, or replace hazardous products. Second, it develops uniform safety standards for consumer products (e.g., flammability standards for fabrics). Third, it assists consumers in evaluating the comparative safety of consumer products through consumer and industry education programs. Fourth, it promotes research into the causes and prevention of product-related injuries. And fifth, it maintains several computerized databases on product-related deaths and injuries (such as the Death Certificate System, the Medical Examiners and Coroners Alert Program, and Accident Investigations).

The commission's biomedical responsibilities are overseen by its Directorate of Health Sciences, which has two primary functions: (1) directing the chemical hazards program and (2) developing and evaluating the scientific content of product safety standards and product testing methods, especially those involved in the Poison Prevention Packaging Act, which requires special packaging to protect children (84 Stat. 1670).

REFERENCES: Collins, Cardiss. 1993. "The Child Safety Protection and Consumer Product Safety Commission Improvement Act." *Loyola Consumer Law Reporter* 5:36; Kitzer, W. F. 1991. "Safety Management and the Consumer Product Safety Commission." *Professional Safety* 36:25; Rodgers, G. R. 1990. "Evaluating Product-Related Hazards at the Consumer Product Safety Commission." *Education Review* 14:3.

DEBORAH R. MATHIEU

CRUZAN V. DIRECTOR, MISSOURI DEPARTMENT OF HEALTH

In 1988, Lester and Mary Cruzan petitioned the state courts of Missouri for authority to discontinue nasogastric feeding for their adult daughter Nancy, rendered persistently unconscious from injuries sustained in a 1983 car accident. The Cruzans, acting as Nancy's court-appointed guardians, asserted that even though Nancy was incapacitated, they could vicariously exercise her constitutional right to make medical decisions by refusing nasogastric feeding on her behalf. A trial court ruled in their favor, but a divided Missouri Supreme Court reversed because the parents failed to produce "clear and convincing" proof of a prior informed refusal by Nancy.

In a decision issued in June 1990, a five-member majority of the U.S. Supreme Court upheld the Missouri Supreme Court. Writing for the majority, Chief Justice William Rehnquist held that Missouri could presume that patients lacking the capacity to make their own medical decisions would choose life-sustaining treatment. The state could require a surrogate seeking to discontinue a patient's life-sustaining treatment to produce evidence proving that the patient herself no longer would accept treatment before this presumption for life could be rebutted. In addition, the state could disregard "substituted judgments" imputing to a patient the desire to die when such judgments were not based on the patient's prior-expressed directives.

Generally, five aspects of the *Cruzan* ruling contributed significantly to the "right to die" debate. First, the Supreme Court acknowledged that the logic of prior constitutional rulings would implicate a protected interest in refusing life-sustaining treatment. However, the majority characterized this interest as a "liberty" rather than a "generalized right of privacy." Thus, under *Cruzan* the states have broad leeway to regulate medical treatment decisions, especially by surrogates. In addition, the exercise of this liberty could only be "hypothetical" in the case of persons lacking capacity, thus warranting greater state protections against abuse for this class of persons.

Second, the Supreme Court did not distinguish between tube feeding and medical treatment, but the majority found that the states could take into account whether refusals of treatment would result in death and, in such circumstances, could impose heightened state scrutiny. Third, the majority recognized that unconscious individuals are "persons" under the Constitution with the right to live. Thus, the states could defend these individuals from wrongful or erroneous treatment denials. Fourth, the Supreme Court concluded that it was better to err in favor of surrogate decisions prolonging life at the risk of frustrating a patient's not fully expressed desire to reject treatment. This preference for life was not arbitrary or unreasonable since, upon discovering the error, erroneous decisions for treatment could be reversed by removing the treatment, while erroneous decisions to forgo treatment would result in irreversible death. Fifth, the Supreme Court held that surrogates could not rely on their own negative judgments about the patient's quality of life as a basis for forgoing treatment.

The Cruzans returned to the state courts with new evidence purporting to show that Nancy did in fact refuse her present care in advance of her accident. The same trial court that initially ruled in the Cruzans' favor accepted this evidence and authorized the removal of Nancy's feeding tube. Nancy died on December 28, 1990 (Bopp and Avila, 1992).

In the 1994 landmark decision of *Hobbins v. Attorney General*, the Michigan Supreme Court rejected a claim that by recognizing a liberty to refuse life-sustaining treatment the *Cruzan* decision established a constitutional right to "hasten death" broad enough to include a right to assisted suicide.

REFERENCES: Bopp, Jr., James, and Daniel Avila. 1992. "Cruzan II: A Clear and Convincing Travesty." *National University Law Review* 1:1–47; *Cruzan v. Director, Missouri Department of Health*, 497 U.S. 261 (1990) (U.S. Supreme Court decision); *Cruzan v. Harmon*, 760 S.W.2d 408 (Mo. 1989) (Missouri Supreme Court decision); *Hobbins v. Attorney General*, 63 U.S.L.W. 2393 (Mich. Dec. 13, 1994) (Nos. 99752, 99758).

DANIEL AVILA

CRYOBANKS

Cryobank facilities provide a means of freezing and storing semen, ova, and embryos. The most common method of cryopreservation is the immersion of the gametes or embryos in liquid nitrogen. Cans with ampules are suspended over the vapors of liquid nitrogen; the freezing temperature is −80°C. The cans are then submerged in the liquid nitrogen container, lowering the temperature to −196.5°C. Prior to use, the materials are slowly thawed.

Although the initial development of cryobanking was inhibited by warnings from the American Public Health Association and Planned Parenthood–World Population in the early 1970s, research confirming its safety defused some opposition and increased appreciation of the potential beneficial uses. Cryobanks are available in most U.S. cities and may operate as nonprofit, university based, or commercial facilities. Initial commercial interest was based on the largely unrealized expectation that millions of men undergoing vasectomy would elect to store their semen as a form of "fertility insurance." However, cryobanks have diversified and offer many services including timed multiple inseminations for donor insemination (DI) and in vitro fertilization (IVF), storage pooling and concentration of sperm, retention of fertilizing capacity in death or hazard exposure of donor, or on-demand DI, IVF, or embryo transfer with a wide selection of genetic traits.

Despite initial concern over the possibility of long-term genetic damage to the sperm during freezing and decreased fertilization capacity of frozen semen, its use for DI is widespread. By 1988, the number of births from frozen semen totaled over 30,000. Most practitioners (74 percent) who use frozen sperm obtain it from commercial sperm banks (OTA, 1988, 43). The need for a somewhat greater number of inseminations to achieve pregnancy is outweighed by the convenience of frozen sperm because the donor need not be physically present to provide the sample. Also, the freezing aspect tends to depersonalize the process of DI, thus making it more acceptable for some people. Importantly in the era of acquired immunodeficiency syndrome (AIDS), the use of frozen semen allows for more thorough screening of donors and of the semen sample directly.
REFERENCES: Office of Technology Assessment (OTA). 1988. *Artificial Insemination: Practice in the United States.* Washington, D.C.: U.S. Government Printing Office; Subak, Leslee L., G. David Adamson, and Nancy L. Boltz. 1992. "Therapeutic Donor Insemination: A Prospective Randomized Trial of Fresh Versus Frozen Sperm." *American Journal of Obstetrics and Gynecology* 166(b): 1597–1606.

See also **ARTIFICIAL INSEMINATION; EGG DONATION; IN VITRO FERTILIZATION (IVF).**

ROBERT H. BLANK

D

DAVIS V. DAVIS

This is a Tennessee case in which the genetic father fought with the genetic mother after their divorce over the disposition of seven frozen embryos that remained after their unsuccessful attempt at in vitro fertilization. Reversing the lower court decisions, which held that the embryos should not be destroyed, the Tennessee Supreme Court ruled that the father's right not to be a parent took precedence over the mother's right to have the embryos transferred to her uterus and carry the resulting pregnancy to term.

REFERENCE: *Davis v. Davis,* No. 190, slip op., 1990 WL 130807, 842 S.W.2d 588 (Tenn. 1992).

See also **IN VITRO FERTILIZATION (IVF);** *YORK V. JONES.*

ROBERT H. BLANK

DEATH

Prior to 1968, physicians used the irreversible cessation of cardiopulmonary functions to determine death. However, various technological advances encouraged the adoption of a new definition of death. A patient undergoing open heart surgery illustrates how technology can outstrip the cardiopulmonary means of determining death; the patient does not breathe or pump blood on his own, yet he is not considered to be dead. The advent of organ transplantation also encouraged a reexamination of the criteria for determining death, since waiting until cardiopulmonary function ceases in patients with irreversible neurological damage results in damage to the organs, limiting their usefulness for transplantation. The lack of a consensus regarding when a patient could be declared dead limited procurement and led to a public controversy regarding the ethics of organ procurement.

In 1968, a committee convened at Harvard Medical School to develop new criteria for declaring death, at least in part to quell the controversy regarding organ procurement. The neurological criteria that they developed, known generally as the Harvard Criteria for "brain death," quickly became accepted by the religious, legal, and medical communities. In the 1970s, a number of slightly different laws were passed that tried to incorporate these neurological criteria. Unfortunately, these laws never established the relationship between the cardiopulmonary and neurological criteria for death, thus intimating that there was one definition for most people but a more lenient standard when organ procurement was being considered. Thus, in 1980, the President's Commission for the Study of Ethical Problems in Medicine and Biomedical and Behavioral Research,* along with the American Medical Association (AMA) and the American Bar Association (ABA), established a common ground for statutory and judicial law related to determining death using neurological criteria. The President's Commission concluded that "death is a unitary phenomenon which can be demonstrated either on the traditional grounds of irreversible cessation of heart and lung functions or on the basis of irreversible loss of all functions of the entire brain." Both of these criteria were tied to a unitary definition of death as "the permanent cessation of integrated functioning of the organism as a whole." This view was incorporated into the 1978 Uniform Determination of Death Act (UDDA), which said that patients who met either of the above two criteria—the irreversible cessation of cardiopulmonary function or brain function—are dead. While the act specified the general physiological standards for death, it did not specify the actual criteria or tests to be used. Recognizing the rapid changes in medical technology, the law says only that the determination must be made in accordance with accepted medical standards.

All states recognize cardiopulmonary death, and by 1990, 41 states and the District of Columbia recognized neurological criteria for death as well. Despite the widespread legal acceptance of the neurological criteria for death, there is still much conceptual uncertainty regarding the meaning of "brain death." Many people are ambivalent about the status of a patient whose brain has ceased functioning but whose attachment to mechanical support systems keeps his heart beating. This is evidenced by studies describing how people talk about death, distinguishing, for example, between "brain death" and "real death." Confusion regarding when the patient is dead may, despite the legal consensus, lead many families to misunderstand the patient's medical status and thus refuse to donate his organs or to insist that "treatment" be continued. It should be emphasized, however, that both "brain death" and "cardiopulmonary death" are reliable indicators that the individual is indeed dead.

REFERENCES: Ad Hoc Committee of the Harvard Medical School to Examine the Definition of Brain Death. 1968. "A Definition of Irreversible Coma." *Journal of the American Medical Association* 205: 337; Black, P. M. 1991. "Conceptual and Practical Issues in the Declaration of Death by Brain Criteria." *Neurosurgery Clinics of North America* 2: 493–501; Capron, Alexander M. 1986. "Legal and Ethical Problems in Decisions for Death." *Law, Medicine and Health Care* 14: 141–144; Farrell, M. M., and

Levin, D. L. 1993. "Brain Death in the Pediatric Patient." *Critical Care Medicine* 21: 1951–1965; Halevy, Amir, and Brody, Baruch. 1993. "Brain Death." *Annals of Internal Medicine* 119: 519–525; President's Commission for the Study of Ethical Problems in Medicine and Biomedical and Behavioral Research. 1981. *Defining Death: Medical, Legal and Ethical Issues in the Determination of Death.* Washington, D.C.: U.S. Government Printing Office; Younger, S. J., et al. 1989. "Brain Death and Organ Retrieval." *Journal of the American Medical Association* 261: 2205–2210.

LAURA A. SIMINOFF, ROBERT M. ARNOLD, and MOLLY SEAR

DECADE OF THE BRAIN: POLICY ISSUES

In 1989, Congress passed Public Law 101–58 declaring that the decade beginning January 1, 1990, be designated the "Decade of the Brain." According to the joint resolution, an estimated 50 million Americans are affected each year by disorders and disabilities that involve the brain. Treatment, rehabilitation, and related costs of brain disorders and disabilities represent a total economic burden of $305 billion annually, according to the resolution. The decade of the brain is timely in the context of rapid advances in brain research and a technological revolution in the brain sciences, manifested by positron emission tomography and magnetic resonance imaging, which allow noninvasive observation of the living brain. Although our knowledge of the brain is yet rudimentary, within this decade many of the new initiatives are bound to move to fruition and provide answers concerning brain activity and dysfunction. The technological boundaries at this point seem vast.

Experimental and clinical interventions in the brain have always elicited controversy from many directions. One need only look at issues surrounding past innovations such as frontal lobotomies, electroshock therapy, and abuses of psychotropic drugs to see the sensitivity of intervention in the brain. Although these new advances promise considerable benefits in treating a wide array of mental disabilities and behavioral problems, the revolution in brain science challenges social values concerning personal autonomy and rights and, for some observers, raises the specter of mind control and an Orwellian-type society.

Another concern centers on the dilemma of informed consent, a concept at the base of medical decision making. Because consent for treatment of brain disorders must come from the damaged organ itself, brain intervention differs from intervention in other organs. If the damage is severe enough to warrant high-risk experimental treatment, is the person really capable of exercising free, informed consent? Although this problem probably can be dealt with through existing mechanisms to protect human subjects or patients, it is often confused in new areas such as neural grafting, where the line between experimentation and therapy is often nonexistent—that is, where the experimentation is done in a clinical setting.

Brain intervention is also politically sensitive because of the stigmatization that often accompanies persons identified as having disorders or disabilities of the brain. This is especially the case where certain treatments are focused on members of identifiable groups in society that are already the targets of discrimination. Although brain disorders and disabilities affect all parts of the population, past experience with more primitive types of brain intervention such as frontal lobotomies suggests a need for constant vigilance to minimize stigmatization and discrimination so easily associated with disorders of the brain, particularly those with obvious behavioral manifestations.

A more theoretical concern is a hesitancy on the part of some persons to alter that organ, which is viewed as the center of personal identity, autonomy, and determination. If there is an inviolability of the human body, it is likely to be conceptualized either in the human genome or in the brain. How far can we go in altering the brain without inextricably altering the person himself or herself? Again, while the increased knowledge about the brain and the capacity to alter it in themselves are not threatening, the heightened ability of researchers and surgeons to intervene in the brain raises genuine fears over the inability to draw lines between acceptable treatment and potential abuse of these techniques.

REFERENCES: Mahowald, Mary B. 1993. ''Brain Development, Personal Identity, and Neurografts.'' In Robert H. Blank and Andrea L. Bonnicksen, eds., *Emerging Issues in Biomedical Policy.* Vol. 2. New York: Columbia University Press.

See also **NEURAL GRAFTING; PSYCHOSURGERY.**

ROBERT H. BLANK

DELEGATED HEALTH CARE DECISION-MAKING STATUTES

Delegated health care statutes authorize the execution of a document by an adult principal that appoints another person, an agent, to make the health care treatment decisions for the principal, should the principal become unable to do so. Usually described as power of attorney for health care statutes, but sometimes described as health care proxy laws or in some other manner, these statutes were enacted in 49 states and the District of Columbia by 1994. Alabama has no such law at present; Alaska's statute permits the health care proxy to consent to the provision, but not the forgoing, of treatment or care.

General powers of attorney permit a principal to appoint an agent, proxy, or attorney-in-fact to make decisions governing the disposition of real and personal property as where, for example, the principal will be away and appoints an agent to manage affairs in his or her absence. At common law, the agent's authority expired when the principal became incompetent. Thus, ''durable'' power of attorney statutes were enacted to extend the authority of the agent in such circumstances, should the principal believe this desirable.

It is at least doubtful that such financial powers of attorney can properly be used to govern health care decisions that affect the principal. Hence, delegated health care or durable power of attorney for health care statutes were enacted specifically to authorize the appointment of a health care agent to make decisions for the principal. Unlike financial powers of attorney statutes, however, delegated health care statutes authorize the agent to act only when the principal becomes incompetent.

Generally, delegated health care statutes empower the agent with the same decision-making authority that the principal might exercise if he or she were competent, subject only to the requirement that the agent act in accord with the principal's known wishes and otherwise in the best interest of the principal. As such, the agent acts with the same general authority as a court-appointed guardian, although not subject to the same direct court supervision as a guardian. Appointment of an agent under a delegated health care statute also avoids the cumbersome necessity of pursuing the appointment of a guardian, permits the affected person to choose his or her own decision maker (not usually authorized by guardianship statutes), and provides the opportunity to provide specific instructions on health care to the agent. Failure of the agent to act in the best interest or comply with the known wishes of the principal generally might be challenged by another interested person.

The decision-making authority of an appointed agent under a delegated health care statute is broader than the authority that the declarant might exercise directly through a "living will" authorized by statute. Living wills generally govern only the forgoing of life-sustaining treatment when the declarant has a terminal condition or, in some states, is in a persistent vegetative state.* Unless indicated otherwise by the principal in the instrument appointing a health care agent, the agent may make all health care decisions for the incompetent principal, whatever the principal's condition, subject only to the requirement that the agent act in accord with the principal's known wishes or, if the principal's wishes are unknown, in the principal's best interest. Delegated health care statutes thus effectively provide for appointment of a health care advocate (as living will statutes do not) able to act on all health care matters affecting the principal.

In view of the broad scope of authority statutorily provided to the agent by delegated health care statutes, however, it is advisable to provide some instructions in the appointing instrument to the agent on the nature of the treatment or care the principal may wish in certain circumstances. This is so both because it cannot be assumed that the appointed agent will always automatically know the principal's wishes and in order to memorialize the principal's wishes in the event the agent is unwilling or unable to act. The latter prospect also makes it advisable to appoint one or more successor agents.

REFERENCES: Meisel, Alan. 1989, 1994. *The Right to Die.* New York: Wiley Law Publications; *Right to Die Law Digest.*

THOMAS J. MARZEN

DEPO-PROVERA

Depo-Provera is the trade name of an injectable drug whose active ingredient is medroxyprogesterone acetate (DMPA). Developed by Upjohn researchers in 1954, the drug was serendipitously discovered to prevent conception. Depo-Provera's contraceptive effectiveness has never been in question. A single 150-

milligram injection is 99.8 percent effective in suppressing ovulation and in preventing pregnancy for three months. Safety has been the issue. Studies have shown that women suffer adverse reactions from Depo-Provera use. The drug's most common short-term side effect is highly irregular menstrual bleeding. Some women develop amenorrhea, while 25 percent experience heavy and prolonged menstrual bleeding with the first injection. In fact, menstrual disturbances are the most common reason for discontinuing use. Women also experience adverse reactions common to hormonal contraceptives, including depression, decreased libido, dizziness, headaches, nausea, nervousness, and weight gain. All of these side effects are more disturbing because they cannot be easily reversed. Given the contraceptive's long-acting character, a woman cannot terminate its use immediately but must wait, sometimes more than three months, for the effects of the injection to wear off. Even more frightening, the drug is suspected of producing fetal malformations and having long-term side effects including osteoporosis and breast, cervical, and endometrial cancer.

Depo-Provera has been available for the past quarter century and is currently used by nearly 10 million women in 90 countries worldwide, but the U.S. Food and Drug Administration (FDA) did not grant the drug a marketing license until 1992. In the interim, perhaps 10,000 women used it as a contraceptive because the agency has limited control over pharmaceutical company marketing and physician prescription practices, once it has approved a drug for any purpose. The FDA had approved Depo-Provera for other purposes, including palliative treatment and adjunctive therapy for terminal kidney and endometrial cancer. In this setting, Upjohn made the drug available for contraceptive use, and private physicians, family planning clinics, and mental health facilities gave it to women, but women who received the drug did not always make informed contraceptive choices if they were not provided with information about how it might put their personal health at risk.

Women who suffered short-term side effects from Depo-Provera's unapproved use brought product liability and medical malpractice suits against their physicians and Upjohn, but their cases were either dismissed or settled, except for one. In 1986, a Florida trial court found that Upjohn had negligently failed to provide Anne MacMurdo's physician with adequate warnings in the drug's package insert about the heavy and prolonged menstrual bleeding she suffered and awarded her $188,700 in damages. Four years later, however, the Florida Supreme Court reversed the judgment because it concluded that the package insert's warnings were "accurate, clear, and unambiguous" (*Upjohn v. MacMurdo*, 1990, 682–683).

At the FDA, Depo-Provera's lengthy and complex approval process began in 1967 when Upjohn submitted a marketing application. In brief, the agency first approved the drug for limited marketing in 1973, withdrew its approval the following year, reversed itself in 1978 and disapproved the drug for general marketing, convened a Public Board of Inquiry on Depo-Provera, accepted the board's report and denied Depo-Provera general marketing approval in 1986, and then in 1992 approved the drug for general marketing. All during this time, the FDA was at the vortex of a scientific and political struggle over the drug's safety that was driven by medical, health, consumer, and women's organizations, by members of Congress, and by Upjohn, population control organizations, and the Agency for International Development. Their wide-ranging debate focused on the value of Upjohn-sponsored animal experiments and human clinical trials in assessing Depo-Provera's risk to healthy women and on the drug's political, social, and economic acceptability for women in this country and overseas. In general, participants disagreed over their assessment of the drug risk, not for its science alone but because of their fear of its potential abuse and its promise of population control. The FDA's efforts to manage Depo-Provera's risk have reflected these fears and promises. The agency's decisions, on occasion, have also reflected its awareness of the shortcomings of Upjohn experimental procedures and its concern about the drug's unapproved use. Overall, however, the FDA has not been particularly concerned about the short-term side effects women have had to endure in using the long-acting injectable contraceptive but has focused its attention on an assessment of the drug's carcinogenic properties.

Upjohn sponsored human and animal studies to assess the drug's safety and effectiveness. As early as 1971, one clinical study reported that use of the drug might lead to an increased risk of cervical cancer. In 1975, a seven-year beagle dog study reported malignant breast tumors in 2 animals. Two years later, another clinical study suggested that fetal exposure to Depo-Provera might increase the risk of birth defects. Then in 1979, two rhesus monkey studies cast further doubt on the drug's safety. One ten-year study reported endometrial cancer in 2 animals, and another found breast cancer in 24 animals. At the same time, the FDA discovered serious flaws in the conduct of an Upjohn-sponsored clinical study. In 1978, an FDA audit of one of the principal domestic clinical testing sites, the Grady Memorial Hospital's Family Planning Clinic in Atlanta, concluded that there were major deficiencies in the design and conduct of the testing protocol including inaccurate screening, defective informed consent procedures, and no follow-up in a study involving 11,000 to 15,000, principally lower-class black women, between 1967 and 1978 (U.S. FDA, 1979). These failures led to the abandonment of the Grady program and, spurred by the FDA's disapproval of Depo-Provera the same year, moved Upjohn to collect data in a systematic fashion and to request the FDA to create a public board of inquiry to review Depo-Provera's medical, scientific, and technical issues. The FDA appointed three eminent scientists, Judith Weisz as chairperson and Griff T. Ross and Paul Stolley as members, to examine the human and animal studies. In 1983, the Depo-Provera Public Board of Inquiry heard five days of testimony from all the major participants.

In its report, issued the following year, the board of inquiry limited itself to an assessment of the scientific evidence. First, it turned to the animal evidence and rejected Upjohn's argument that the beagle dog was an inappropriate test model because it metabolized progestogens differently from humans and was prone to mammary tumors. Very little research supported the position that the beagle responded differently to progestogens than a woman. The board also rejected Upjohn's argument that the monkey studies should also be discounted because endometrial cancer developed from a cell type that had no human counterpart. No research supported the argument that monkeys possessed a special cell type that made them more prone to endometrial cancer. Furthermore, Upjohn's second dog study provided "evidence that the mammary carcinomas in the dogs were drug-related . . . [and the] malignancies developed both more *frequently* and *earlier* with increasing doses of DMPA" (Weisz, Ross, and Stolley, 1984, 7).

When the board turned to Upjohn's clinical studies, it concluded that Upjohn's human data did not successfully refute the risk of human breast, cervical, or endometrial cancer suggested by the animal data. Moreover, the human data were inadequate because they were not based on studies that addressed the issue of cancer; they were derived from clinical reports, not from epidemiological studies; and if they were, they suffered from major research design and execution limitations. Whether retrospective or prospective studies, they were based on data collected from subjects at various research centers representing different populations and frequently included too few long-term users, too short a period of follow-up, a lack of information about the subject's medical history, inadequate or inappropriate controls, and a lack of documentation (Weisz, Ross, and Stolley, 1984).

In the years after the FDA's decision to deny Depo-Provera general marketing approval on the basis of the public board of inquiry's report, the drug's prospects for approval were altered dramatically by two developments. The first occurred in 1986 when the FDA's Fertility and Maternal Health Drugs Advisory Committee accepted the World Health Organization (WHO) recommendation not to require monkey and beagle toxicological studies for the development of steroidal contraceptives because these studies were not considered relevant to cancer in humans. The FDA agreed and eliminated the monkey studies requirement but reduced the beagle dog requirement from seven to three years and delayed eliminating it pending the WHO studies on Depo-Provera and breast cancer. As a consequence, the FDA's assessment of Depo-Provera's carcinogenic risk would depend on the results of the human studies. Five years later, the second development occurred when the results of the World Health Organization case control studies, initiated in 1979 and conducted in Kenya, Mexico, and Thailand, were reported in leading medical journals in 1991. These WHO studies confirmed some fears about Depo-Provera. They found a slightly higher risk of breast cancer and osteoporosis, but they also dispelled other criticism of the human data because they found no increase in the risk of liver or cervical cancer and a slightly reduced risk of endometrial cancer. The WHO studies also left questions about prenatal exposure unanswered; two studies that suggested that exposure in utero might inhibit fetal growth and lead to a substantial increase in neonatal mortality rates were challenged on methodological grounds.

These World Health Organization studies encouraged Upjohn, once again, to apply for FDA approval in April 1992. When the Fertility and Maternal Health Drugs Advisory Committee held hearings several months later, women's and health organizations argued that the research data did not dispel the concerns about Depo-Provera's link to breast cancer, fetal malformations, and osteoporosis, nor did it address the drug's short-term side effects. They also argued that FDA approval was unacceptable because of the drug's potential for abuse by physicians and health professionals who may fail to provide mentally retarded, poor, and illiterate women with informed consent or who are willing to pressure them to use the drug. But the Advisory Committee paid scant attention to these arguments and agreed with the WHO researchers' assessment of Depo-Provera's cancer risks. The committee also accepted the views of the World Health Organization and International Planned Parenthood Federation that the drug was preferable for women who breast feed because, unlike oral contraceptives, it did not suppress lactation. It was also a desirable contraceptive for Third World women where fertility and maternal mortality rates were extremely high, other methods of contraception were less available and desirable, and the health care system was less advanced and less extensive.

The FDA accepted its advisory committee's unanimous recommendation and approved Depo-Provera for general marketing in October 1992 on the condition that Upjohn conduct postmarketing research on the effect of the drug's use on bone density and the risk of osteoporosis. The FDA and Upjohn later agreed on Depo-Provera's labeling, and in January 1993, the company announced that the drug would sell for $29.50 a shot, roughly equal to the annualized cost of the contraceptive pill. The FDA's decision is, however, unlikely to end the controversy that plagued the drug's administrative odyssey for the past quarter of a century. Depo-Provera's critics and advocates will continue to monitor its use and analyze the results of future research on breast cancer and osteoporosis.

REFERENCES: Gold, Rachel, and Peters D. Willson. 1981. "New Developments in a Decade Old Controversy." *Family Planning Perspectives* 13: 35–39; Green, William. 1987. "The Odyssey of Depo-Provera." *Food Drug Cosmetic Law Journal* 42: 567–587; Green, William. 1991. "Miscarriage of Justice: Depo-Provera Case May Insulate Drug Makers." *Trial* 27: 61–66; Klitsch, Michael. 1993. "Injectable Hormones and Regulatory Controversy: An End to the Long-Running Story?" *Family Planning Perspectives* 25: 37–40; *Upjohn v. MacMurdo,* 562 So.2d 680 (Fla. 1990); U.S., Congress. House Committee on Interior and Insular Affairs. August 6, 1987. *Oversight Hearing: Use of the Drug, Depo-Provera, by the Indian Health Service.* 100th Cong., 2nd Sess. Washington, D.C.: Government Printing Office; U.S., Congress. Senate Committee on Labor and Public Welfare. February 21, 1973. *Quality of Health Care—Human Experimentation: Hearings Before the Subcommittee on Health.* 93rd Cong., 1st Sess. Washington, D.C.: Government Printing Office; U.S. Food and Drug Administration (FDA). January 3, 1979. *Data Audit of IND #9693 (Depo-Provera as an Injectable Contraceptive) at Grady Memorial Hospital.* Rockville, MD: FDA; U.S. Food and Drug Administration (FDA). Fertility and Maternal Health Drugs Advisory Committee. June 19, 1992. *Transcript of Public Hearing on Depo-Provera.* Rockville, MD: FDA; Weisz, Judith,

Griff T. Ross, and Paul D. Stolley. October 17, 1984. *Report of the Public Board of Inquiry on Depo-Provera.* Rockville, MD: FDA.

See also **CHEMICAL CASTRATION**.

WILLIAM C. GREEN

DIAGNOSTIC RELATED GROUPINGS

DRGs are classifications of illness categories identified in the International Classification of Diseases. There were 469 original categories in 1983, the first year of implementation. DRGs are used in a pricing formula for Medicare's Hospital Insurance Program that replaced an earlier formula generally based on the operational costs of a hospital plus profit. The new method of reimbursement using DRGs is a prospective pricing list altered each year and administered by the Health Care Financing Administration (HCFA). The prospective payment is based on a complex formula that considers (1) the principal diagnosis, (2) any surgical procedure, (3) any other complications and comorbidities (earlier this referred to age), and (4) the type of discharge. Cost factors associated with various combinations are drawn from 20 percent of all Medicare cases in 1981. Provisions are made to update cost factors and appropriate categorization for each DRG as well as take into account any recalculation necessitated by new technologies and medical procedures that improve the quality of health.

In 1981 and early 1982, hospital inflation exceeded 12 percent. Both the Democratic congressional leadership and the Republican-controlled White House recognized that comprehensive change in Medicare financing had to be legislated quickly before the health care industry could marshal traditional opposition to pricing regulation for Medicare. Toward the end of the 1970s, some nine states participated in HCFA-sponsored research for prospective reimbursement as a consequence of dissatisfaction with the per diem cost plus profit formula. This research became the basis of a plan submitted by secretary of the former Health, Education, and Welfare (HEW) Department Richard Schweiker. The plan for prospective payment of Medicare was appended to Social Security amendments in December 1982. The amendments had support from the leadership of both parties in Congress and from the president. The legislation was joined to the Tax Equity and Fiscal Responsibility Act of 1982 (TEFRA), and DRGs were implemented in October 1983 in many hospitals.

Overcharging private payers under Blue Cross and Medicare patients in order to subsidize care for the indigent was an open practice in hospitals prior to DRG reimbursement. It was anticipated by federal administrators of the DRG reimbursement system that hospitals would have a strong incentive to make up for their loss of income to cover nonpaying patients (and general profitability) by using a variety of measures that were illegal and carried potential civil and even criminal penalties. Local Professional Review Organizations (PROs) were to oversee the validity of the diagnostic information, admissions, discharges, and the quality of care, but an important external check against illegal and fraudulent practices was the Central Office and the Regional Dispersal Terminal Network, or CORDT. This office monitors each hospital's case-mix history and admission pattern (Shaffer, 1984, 48–51).

Medicare is paid out of Social Security tax and is made up of two parts: (part A) Hospital Insurance Trust Funds and (part B) Supplemental Medical Insurance Trust Fund for doctors' bills and related services. Hospital profits were not seriously reduced right away by DRGs. The reasons are demographic, political, and economic. The population continued to age, and Medicare needs continued to grow. Additionally, prospective payment costs for DRGs were generously calculated initially. Finally, reimbursement formulas contained adjustments for variables such as labor costs, teaching functions performed and indigence of treated patients, and historic per diem costs. Although adjustments were supposed to be eliminated under the original legislation by 1987 with payment based on national rates, Congress assumed responsibility for setting formulas and continued to protect reimbursement for those hospitals with historic high costs. This function was preempted from the start by congressional microman-agement, and congressional authority over the formulas was made official in the Omnibus Budget Reconciliation Act of 1986, taking into consideration hospital service inflation, productivity, technology, quality of care, and cost-effectiveness (Russell, 1989, 14, 19–20).

As a pricing list, DRG payment suffers from the limitations of most pro-spective pricing mechanisms. One way creative hospital administration could augment profitability (illegally) was to increase admissions. Consequently, HCFA carefully monitored any statistically aberrant patterns of admission. Med-icare admissions did decline in 1984, and the average length of stay, which had been dropping for two generations, accelerated its decrease to 8.8 days by 1985, where it has bottomed out (Russell, 1989, 26). But Medicare spending per en-rollee only slowed in the first three years. Real per capita Medicare hospital services dropped from just under 10 percent in 1980 to 7 percent in 1985, still well above inflation for the nation as a whole (CBO, 1993, 19–20, 45). Cost shifting is also a problem. Local hospitals shifted costs from DRGs by devel-oping outpatient services not covered by DRGs and then increasing those prices.

Prospective payment under Medicare may have its most lasting contribution as actuary research encouraging other financing institutions to control prices. Variations of DRGs have been adopted by Medicaid, Veteran's hospitals, and private insurance vendors. Many "all payer" proposals for health care reform are conditioned on our ability to calculate accurate cost factors for treatment (CBO, 1991, 1–4).

REFERENCES: Congressional Budget Office (CBO). 1991. *Universal Health Insurance Coverage Using Medicare's Payment Rates*. Washington, D.C.: U.S. Government Print-ing Office; Congressional Budget Office (CBO). 1993. *Trends in Health Spending: An Update*. Washington, D.C.: U.S. Government Printing Office, Superintendent of Docu-ments, 19–20, appendix A, figure A–22, 45; Russell, Louise B. 1989. *Medicare's New Hospital Payment System: Is It Working?* Washington, D.C.: Brookings, table 3–1, 26;

Shaffer, Franklin A. 1984. "A Nursing Perspective of the DRG World, Part I." *Nursing and Health Care*, 48–51.

ROBERT P. RHODES

DIAMOND V. CHAKRABARTY

A U.S. patent application was filed in 1972 in the name of Dr. Ananda Chakrabarty, whose claimed invention related to a genetically engineered bacterial strain capable of degrading many components of crude oil. Five years later, a closely divided U.S. Supreme Court held that the Chakrabarty claims were not properly rejected on the theory, advanced by the U.S. Patent and Trademark Office, that a composition of "living matter" was not statutory subject matter and, hence, was unpatentable as a matter of law. A fledgling biopharmaceutical sector was the principal beneficiary of the wave of entrepreneurial investment prompted by the *Chakrabarty* ruling.

REFERENCES: *Diamond v. Chakrabarty,* 447 U.S. 303 (1980); Kass, Leon R. 1981. "Patenting Life." *Journal of the Patent and Trademark Office Society* 63:571.

STEPHEN A. BENT

E

EGG DONATION

Egg (oocyte) donation is an option in in vitro fertilization (IVF),* first used successfully in 1984. During egg donation, a woman donates eggs to a couple trying to conceive through IVF. The eggs are fertilized with the sperm of the male partner or a donor, and the resulting embryos are transferred to the recipient's uterus for a possible pregnancy. In 1992, 137 IVF programs used donated eggs. Nearly 2,000 cycles were initiated with the eggs of anonymous or known donors. Over 500 women delivered single babies (63 percent), twins (32 percent), or triplets (4 percent) (American Fertility Society, 1994).

Eggs are donated to women born without ovarian function or who lost that function prematurely and to couples at risk for bearing a child with a genetic disorder who want to circumvent the risk by using donor eggs or sperm. More recently, practitioners have recommended that women over age 40 who are trying IVF should consider using donated eggs from a younger woman to increase their chances of pregnancy (Yaron, et al. 1995), inasmuch as birth rates for women over 40 in IVF programs approximate those of younger recipients when donated eggs are used (Sauer, Paulson, and Lobo, 1992). With hormonal therapy and donated eggs, even postmenopausal women have given birth.

Egg donors include women trying IVF who donate extra oocytes, women having tubal ligations or other medical procedures who donate incidental to the procedure, relatives or friends who donate to named recipients, and strangers who are recruited to donate anonymously (Ethics Committee, 1994). Women who donate incidental to their own IVF attempt assume no extra burden in donating, but the others are stimulated with hormones, give blood repeatedly, undergo ultrasound tests, and receive local anesthesia for the oocyte retrieval itself. Ovarian cysts, which can rupture and require hospitalization, are one infrequent side effect of hormonal stimulation (Quigley, 1992). Recruited donors will spend up to 56 hours from start to finish, which includes pre- and postinterviews and travel to the clinic (Seibel and Kiessling, 1993). Known donors and repeat anonymous donors spend less time if psychological profiles are not conducted.

Women who donate as part of their own IVF attempt may be compensated indirectly through a cut in IVF costs (Braverman, 1993). Some clinics use only volunteer donors, but others solicit donors for pay. Responding to a survey, clinicians reported paying $750 to $3,500, with an average of $1,548 (Braverman, 1993). Seibel and Kiessling (1993) calculate that if men receive $50 for donating sperm, which takes approximately two hours, women should expect to receive around $1,400 for donating eggs, assuming they receive $25 for each of 56 hours.

Egg donation is not regulated in the United States, and the interests of donors and recipients are protected indirectly through market forces, professional association guidelines, and the possibility of lawsuits. Some European nations have responded to ethical issues by enacting restrictive laws. For example, laws in Sweden and Norway forbid egg donation altogether. Sweden's Law No. 711 (1988) forbids the transfer of an embryo to a woman if the egg is not her own or if the sperm is not that of her partner, and Norway's Law No. 68 (1987) states that "[t]he fertilized egg may be placed only in the woman in whom it originated."

Medical groups and ethics commissions in the United States and other nations recommend voluntary restrictions. For example, the Swiss Medical Academy recommends that only ten children be born from the gametes of any one ovum or sperm donor. The Ethics Committee of the American Society for Reproductive Medicine (ASRM—formerly the American Fertility Society) recommends that donors be of legal age and the number of births from any one donor be limited. Expressing "serious reservations about any attempt to produce pregnancy beyond the ordinary childbearing age" (Ethics Committee, 1994:49S), the Ethics Committee nevertheless would not exclude egg donation solely on the basis of age. The ASRM Guidelines for Oocyte Donation recommend, among other things, that women over 40 undergo thorough psychological and physical evaluation and be apprised of pregnancy risks for women over this age (American Fertility Society, 1993).

Egg donation is eased by legislation defining the relations between donor, recipient, and offspring and specifying the responsibilities of the involved parties. Egg donation produces complex relations in assisted conception because it creates a situation in which the baby has both a genetic mother and a gestational mother. If relatives donate eggs, other unusual ties arise, as when a sister donates to a sister and becomes the child's genetic mother but social aunt.

By 1993, North Dakota and Virginia had adopted the Uniform Statutes of Children of Assisted Conception Act (USCACA), a model law drafted to protect the "security and well being" of children born from assisted conception. Among other things, the USCACA declares that "a donor is not a parent of a child conceived through assisted conception." Clarifying, it notes that "an egg donor would not be the child's mother." In general, the law on egg donation is less well developed than that of sperm donation. The Uniform Parentage Act, adopted wholly or in part by one half of the states, shifts the duties and privileges of paternity from the sperm donor to the male partner, who is presumed to be the natural father if he is married to the recipient and consents in writing to the donor insemination and if a physician performs the procedures (Uniform Parentage Act, 1973).

The absence of clarifying policy for egg donation prompted the ASRM to warn donors and recipients about legal uncertainty and to encourage parties to use an attorney to write documents specifying who bears the duties and enjoys the privileges of parenthood (American Fertility Society, 1993). To be included are decisions about when the donor's claim to her eggs ends; the claims, if any, she has over embryos frozen after her donated eggs are fertilized; and clinic arrangements about confidentiality, anonymity, and recordkeeping. Conflicts may also arise in intrafamilial donation if, presuming altruism, parties neglect to sign legal documents ahead of time.

Among the policy questions raised by egg donation are the following: Should donor screening for psychological and genetic profiles and for sexually transmitted diseases be mandated by law? Should compensation be regulated to avoid exploitation of women through underpayment or the appearance of tissue trafficking through overpayment? Should the number of donations, age of donor, age of recipient, and rights of the donor be specified by law? Should administrative regulations be enacted specifically for egg banks?

Although commissions and professional associations have debated the ethics of egg donation, public policy is rare. Future conflicts over screening, parental authority, payment, and safety may generate demands for legislation, either singly or as part of a broader policy on assisted conception. Suggestions that eggs or ovaries from aborted fetuses be used in assisted conception (Shushan and Schenker, 1994) are certain to promote inquiry into the seriousness of the presumed shortage of eggs and into ethically acceptable ways of securing eggs for donation.

REFERENCES: American Fertility Society. 1993. "Guidelines for Oocyte Donation." *Fertility and Sterility* 59:5s–7s; American Fertility Society, Society for Assisted Reproductive Technology. 1994. "Assisted Reproductive Technology in the United States and Canada: 1992 Results Generated from the American Fertility Society/Society for Assisted Reproductive Technology Registry." *Fertility and Sterility* 62:1121–28; Braverman, Andrea Mechanick. 1993. "Survey Results on the Practice of Ovum Donation." *Fertility and Sterility* 59:1216–20; Ethics Committee, American Fertility Society. 1994. "Ethical Considerations of Assisted Reproductive Technologies." Fertility and Sterility 62(5): 1S–125S. Supplement 1; Quigley, Martin M. 1992. "The New Frontier of Reproductive Age (Editorial)." *JAMA* 268:1320–21; Sauer, Mark V., Richard J. Paulson, and Rogerio A. Lobo. 1992. "Reversing the Natural Decline in Human Fertility: An Extended Clinical Trial of Oocyte Donation to Women of Advanced Reproductive Age." *JAMA* 268:1275–79; Seibel, Machelle M., and Ann Kiessling. 1993. "Compensating Egg Donors: Equal Pay for Equal Time? (Letter)." *NEJM* 328:737; Shushan, Asher, and Josef G. Schenker. 1994. "The Use of Oocytes Obtained from Aborted Fetuses in Egg Donation Programs."

Fertility and Sterility 62:449–51; Uniform Parentage Act. 1973. 9B U.L.A. 287; Uniform Status of Children of Assisted Conception Act. 1988. 9B U.L.A. Suppl. 87; Yaron, Yuval, Ami Amit, Steven Brenner, et al. 1995. "In Vitro Fertilization and Oocyte Donation in Women 45 Years of Age and Older." *Fertility and Sterility* 63:71–76.

ANDREA L. BONNICKSEN

ELECTROCONVULSIVE TREATMENT (ECT)

ECT is a procedure in which a patient is administered a series of 70- to 130-volt shocks to the nervous system, resulting in violent convulsions. Although ECT is often criticized as an inhumane and very crude form of therapy, in 1989 the American Psychiatric Association called the treatment "safe and very effective for certain severe mental illnesses," including major depression, mania, and schizophrenia. ECT should be used only after standard treatment alternatives have been considered. Psychiatrists using it have a "serious obligation" to obtain the informed consent of the patient.

Although in the past the patient was awake, now the patient is given a short-acting anesthetic and an injection of a strong muscle relaxant before the current is applied. After ECT the patient awakens, remembering nothing about the treatment. The usual ECT regimen entails about ten treatments given over a period of several weeks. In 1980, approximately 30,000 patients received ECT. Not surprisingly, despite its potential benefit for selected patients, ECT in the past has often been used for control, not therapy, thus leading to strong opposition to its use. Because of its shotgun effect and its violent image, ECT remains a highly controversial therapy.

REFERENCES: Bootzin, Richard R., Joan Ross Acocella, and Lauren B. Alloy. 1993. *Abnormal Psychology: Current Perspectives.* New York: McGraw-Hill, 564; Durst, R., K. Jabotinsky-Rubin, and Y. Ginath. 1994. "Electroconvulsive Treatment: The Right to Accept Versus the Right to Refuse." *Harefuah* 126(2): 80–84; Staver, Sari. 1989. "ECT Stigma Remains, Despite Effectiveness, Panel Says." *American Medical News* (May 26): 12.

See also **ELECTRONIC BRAIN STIMULATION (ESB).**

ROBERT H. BLANK

ELECTRONIC BRAIN STIMULATION (ESB)

ESB therapy (named for "electronic stimulation of the brain") consists of thin insulated wires implanted in the brain, allowing electronic messages to be sent and recordings to be made from areas deep inside the brain; for therapeutic reasons, the most common placement is in the septal region. ESB has been used successfully in the treatment of epilepsy, intractable pain, violent aggressiveness, and chronic insomnia. ESB does not induce a permanent beneficial change but instead an emotional tranquility. It is also effective in relieving psychological pain caused by severe anxiety and depression by evoking a feeling of euphoria.

When used to treat abnormal aggressiveness, periodic ESB treatment is required. Once the electrodes are implanted, brain activity can be monitored and warning signs of an impending crisis identified. This diagnostic capacity might be the only means of revealing abnormal patterns of electrical activity deep inside the brain. The development of miniaturized electronic devices—stimoceivers—permits instantaneous radio transmission to and from the brains of subjects. Computers are used to permit remote monitoring of brain activities. By allowing complete control of general mood of the subject, ESB raises basic concerns of personal autonomy and self-determination.

REFERENCE: Bootzin, Richard R., Joan Ross Acocella, and Lauren B. Alloy. 1993. *Abnormal Psychology: Current Perspectives.* New York: McGraw-Hill.

See also **ELECTROCONVULSIVE TREATMENT (ECT).**

ROBERT H. BLANK

ELI LILLY V. GENENTECH

In 1979 the Indiana-based pharmaceutical giant Eli Lilly and Company agreed to a consent order proposed by the U.S. Federal Trade Commission (FTC) that affected a wide-ranging research and development (R&D) arrangement between Lilly and Genentech Inc., a San Francisco luminary in the nascent biopharmaceutical sector. The FTC had asserted that Lilly was in violation of Section 5 of the Federal Trade Commission Act, 15 U.S.C. § 45, and Section 7 of the Clayton Act, 15 U.S.C. § 18, with respect to a "finished insulin" market that included, inter alia, "insulin produced by . . . microbes genetically manipulated using recombinant DNA techniques." To obviate the FTC allegation, Lilly agreed not to enforce for ten years any patent or know-how so as to restrict commercialization of recombinant insulin and for five years to grant a nonexclusive license to any domestic company seeking to produce or sell recombinant insulin. The FTC consent decree in fact did not derail Lilly's extending its dominance of the U.S. insulin market, previously based on extraction from animal pancreas glands, to the new field of recombinant insulin production. The Lilly/Genentech relationship proved less than harmonious, however, and litigation began in 1987 over Lilly's alleged use of licensed Genentech materials for an unauthorized purpose, namely, the development of a recombinant human growth hormone product to compete with Genentech's own. The ensuing dispute, the longest running and most expensive to date in the area of genetically engineered pharmaceuticals, has expanded to accommodate Lilly's challenge to the validity of several U.S. Genentech patents, as well as efforts by Lilly abroad to revoke foreign counterparts to those patents, and countercharges by Genentech that Lilly not only infringed the challenged patents but also violated both federal antitrust laws and state tort and contract laws, by virtue of certain exclusive-licensing arrangements between Lilly and the University of California. The portion of this litigation relating to human growth hormone has concluded in a settlement.

REFERENCES: *Eli Lilly and Co. v. Genentech Inc.,* 5 USPQ2d 1902 (S.D. Ind. 1987); *Eli Lilly & Co. v. Genentech Inc.,* 17 USPQ2d 1531 (S.D. Ind. 1990); 44 *Fed. Reg.* 54726 (Sept. 21, 1979) ("Eli Lilly and Co.; Consent Agreement with Analysis to Aid

Public Comment''); *Genentech Inc. v. Eli Lilly and Co.*, 27 USPQ2d 1241 (Fed. Cir. 1993); ''Insufficient Pleadings Doom Biotech Firm's Conspiracy Claim.'' *Antitrust & Trade Regulation Reporter (BNA)* 65:163 (1993).

STEPHEN A. BENT

END-STAGE RENAL DISEASE PROGRAM

A unique part of the U.S. government's Medicare program, the End-Stage Renal Disease Program covers most of the health care costs of most persons suffering from chronic renal failure, an incurable condition that is always fatal without treatment; it is the only federal entitlement program designed in response to a particular disease.

In 1972, Congress decided that Medicare, which covers the health care costs of persons 65 years old and older, should pay for the health care of virtually all individuals with end-stage renal disease (ESRD), the permanent failure of the kidneys to collect and dispose of bodily wastes (Section 2992 of P.L. 92–603). Treatment is either by some form of dialysis—filtering and cleansing the blood—or by organ transplantation. The Medicare program had already been paying for some ESRD care—patients who were eligible for Medicare benefits could receive treatment for ESRD—but now Congress widened Medicare's eligibility criteria to include almost all sufferers of this condition, regardless of their age.

Although the congressional vote on the ESRD Program was preceded by only a very brief formal discussion, the debate about appropriate federal policy regarding ESRD had been active for over a decade. Between 1965 and 1972, for instance, more than 100 bills had been submitted to Congress regarding funding for ESRD, and a variety of public programs covering the costs of treatment for ESRD had already been instituted. Nonetheless, it is clear that the members of Congress did not know how much money the ESRD Program would cost. The enormous increase in the size of the ESRD population had not been anticipated in 1972, nor had the dramatic escalation in expenditures. Original estimates of the first-year cost of the ESRD Program ranged from $35 million to $75 million, anticipating an increase to $250 million in the fourth year. Instead, the ESRD Program cost the federal government approximately $200 million a year in the first few years of the program (for about 15,000 patients); by 1976 the costs were already approximating $600 million (for about 35,000 patients); by the early 1980s, the annual costs to Medicare were around $2 billion (for about 75,000 patients); and the costs of the program today are over $5 billion (for more than 200,000 patients). Thus, approximately 0.08 percent of the population accounts for about 0.8 percent of the total health care expenditures.

Changes in demographics help to explain the increase in the numbers of patients with ESRD, but changes in patient selection criteria are relevant as well. ESRD patients who are very elderly and/or who are ill with other serious conditions are now often considered to be suitable candidates for treatment, whereas in the early stages of the ESRD Program they were not.

Although the ESRD Program is considered to be a success insofar as it pays for the medical care of a certain type of patient, the increasing medical and social costs involved have no doubt been an important ingredient in the reluctance of the federal government to include other catastrophic disease programs within Medicare, particularly those involving transplantation of other organs.

REFERENCES: Evans, R. W., et al. 1985. "The Quality of Life of Patients with End-Stage Renal Disease." *New England Journal of Medicine* 312: 553–559; Levinsky, N. G. 1993. "The Organization of Medical Care: Lessons from the Medicare End Stage Renal Disease Program." *New England Journal of Medicine* 329: 1395–1399; Rettig, R. A., and Lohr, K. N. 1994. "Measuring, Managing and Improving Quality in the End-Stage Renal Disease Treatment Setting." *American Journal of Kidney Diseases* 24: 228–234; Rettig, R. A., and Marks, E. 1983. *The Federal Government and Social Planning for End-Stage Renal Disease: Past, Present, and Future.* Santa Monica, CA: The Rand Corporation.

DEBORAH R. MATHIEU

ETHICAL, LEGAL, AND SOCIAL IMPLICATIONS (ELSI) PROGRAMS

These programs fund nonscientific but socially significant bioethical issues raised by the Human Genome Project, a multibillion dollar program designed to locate on the DNA all genes in the human body. The U.S. government has established two ELSI programs; one is funded by the Office of Health and Environmental Research within the Department of Energy (DOE); the other is funded by the National Center for Human Genome Research, which is at the National Institutes of Health (NIH) within the Department of Health and Human Services.

Both ELSI programs are overseen by the ELSI Working Group, which also establishes research priorities. The four priority areas initially identified by the Working Group are guidelines for the use of genetic tests in clinical practice; issues of privacy and confidentiality of genetic information; the use of genetic information by employers and insurers; and enhancing professional and public education regarding the ethical, legal, and social implications of genetics research. In addition, while the Working Group does not set policy, it does act as a resource for public policy analyses (it has played a role, for example, in federal policy analyses of cystic fibrosis carrier screening).

Funds for the ELSI programs derive from a federally mandated set-aside of 3 to 5 percent of federal appropriations for the year's genome initiative budget. In 1991, DOE-ELSI spent $1.44 million (3 percent) and NIH-ELSI spent $4.04 million (4.9 percent). Because no other area of bioethics rivals the funding resources of the ELSI programs, ELSI is influencing the world of bioethics by attracting philosophers, physicians, social scientists, and lawyers away from other bioethical issues to analyze issues in human genetics.

REFERENCES: Annas, G. J., and Elias, S., eds. 1992. *Gene Mapping: Using Law and Ethics as Guides.* New York: Oxford University Press; Langfelder, E. J., and Juengst, E. T. 1993. "Profile of ELSI Program, NIH." *Politics and the Life Sciences* 12(2): 273–

275; Yesley, Michael S., ed. 1993. *ELSI Bibliography: Ethical, Legal and Social Implications of the Human Genome Project.* Washington, D.C.: U.S. Department of Energy.

See also **HUMAN GENOME PROJECT; NATIONAL INSTITUTES OF HEALTH (NIH).**

DEBORAH R. MATHIEU

EUTHANASIA

Acts of euthanasia are commonly defined as either active or passive. What is commonly referred to as passive euthanasia has been sanctioned by many courts. Passive euthanasia is commonly understood to be the deliberate killing of a person who is medically dependent or disabled by acts of omission, such as the withholding or withdrawal of life-sustaining medical treatment (e.g., ventilation, tube feeding, resuscitation, dialysis, surgery, blood transfusions, or antibiotics). In contrast, active euthanasia is commonly understood to refer to deliberate killing of a person who is medically dependent or disabled by acts of commission (e.g., lethal injection, intentional overdose of pain control medication, carbon monoxide poisoning, or asphyxiation).

Those who oppose euthanasia do not deny the moral and legal right of competent persons to refuse useless or excessively burdensome treatments. The key issue is whether the purpose of the act of omission or commission is to terminate the life of the patient. For this reason, much opposition arises from the inclusion of tube feeding in the category of medical treatment that can be refused. With the exception of persons who have an imminent death expectation, or for whom nutrition and hydration are otherwise useless, the withdrawal of tube feeding is an act of killing by omission.

An important case in establishing the trend toward the sanctioning of voluntary passive euthanasia is *Bouvia v. Superior Court* in 1986. In that case a California court of appeals held that a competent person has the right to refuse treatment even when such treatment is "furnishing nutrition and hydration." The court also held that "quality of life" is a significant consideration in balancing the state interests in preserving life and the patient's right to refuse treatment. At the time, Elizabeth Bouvia was 28 years old and hospitalized with severe cerebral palsy. She was not terminally ill. Thus, the concept of medical treatment was broadened to include nutrition and hydration as subject to a patient's right to refuse treatment. Since then, passive euthanasia for competent patients has been widely sanctioned in the United States.

Much debate has arisen concerning passive euthanasia for patients who are not competent to make medical treatment decisions (i.e., nonvoluntary passive euthanasia). Two rationales are commonly used to justify passive euthanasia for persons who are incompetent: the best interest standard and the substituted judgment standard. These standards permit guardians or family members to make decisions constituting passive euthanasia for persons found to be incompetent to make decisions for themselves (e.g., persons in coma or persistent vegetative state, older persons with degenerative brain disease, persons with impaired cognition due to trauma or disease, and persons with mental retardation).

The most important case concerning nonvoluntary passive euthanasia, and the first one to reach the U.S. Supreme Court, is *Cruzan v. Missouri Dep't of Health* (1990). Nancy Cruzan, an adult, had been in a persistent vegetative state since she had been injured in an automobile accident several years before. She did not have a terminal condition. Nancy's parents, and coguardians, asked the Missouri State Hospital to terminate her tube feeding after it was determined that she would never regain cognitive ability. When the hospital refused this request, the guardians sought and obtained judicial authorization to withhold feeding by tube. The trial court ruled that Nancy had a fundamental right to refuse "death-prolonging procedures." The Missouri Supreme Court reversed, stating that the guardians could not order termination of Nancy's tube feeding without proving by clear and convincing evidence that Nancy had decided to terminate feeding by tube. The U.S. Supreme Court upheld the constitutionality of the clear and convincing standard established by the Missouri Supreme Court.

In *Cruzan* the U.S. Supreme Court held: (1) No fundamental right to refuse medical treatment can be asserted by a third party; (2) Nancy Cruzan had a fundamental right to life that was a personal interest that the state could protect; (3) in protecting Nancy Cruzan's fundamental right to life, the state was not required to take into account her quality of life; (4) guardians have an affirmative statutory duty to consent to the necessary care for their wards; (5) there are only two exceptions releasing guardians from this duty—the ward rejects the treatment in advance through a specific informed refusal, or the ward is burdened by extreme pain from the treatment; and (6) the existence of any of the exceptions must be proved by clear and convincing evidence.

Despite the Supreme Court's decision in *Cruzan,* passive euthanasia for incompetent patients has been widely sanctioned in the United States. Thus, the debate concerning euthanasia has important implications both for competent and incompetent patients.

In 1988 the *Journal of the American Medical Association (JAMA)* caused a storm of controversy by publishing an anonymous account of a gynecology resident who killed a patient by lethal injection. It was entitled "It's Over Debbie." Active euthanasia is now discussed freely in ethical, medical, and legal journals throughout the United States and the world. The articles appearing in these journals illustrate the controversial nature and complexity of the medical-legal-ethical issues inherent in the subject, and which attorneys and courts are called upon to struggle with.

The Netherlands is the first nation to permit active euthanasia. It offers the unique opportunity to assess the effects of active euthanasia upon law, medicine, and the health care of persons who are medically dependent and disabled. In essence, the practice of active euthanasia there constitutes a unique social experiment that is being analyzed by scholars native and foreign to that community of people. It is a living model that illustrates the advantages and disadvantages of sanctioned active euthanasia. In 1988, a scholarly journal, *Issues in Law & Medicine,* dedicated an entire issue to reporting the facts on the practice of euthanasia in the Netherlands. It gave a full accounting of the history and present practice of euthanasia in the Netherlands by utilizing firsthand accounts by Dutch scholars translated directly from the Dutch language. Since then, many articles and books have appeared dealing with euthanasia in the Netherlands.

The primary reasons that underlie the present press for sanctioning active voluntary euthanasia are (1) fear of pain and suffering; (2) pressure to reduce health care costs; and (3) prejudice and discrimination against persons who are older, ill, or disabled and whose quality of life is so poor that third persons decide that their lives are not worth saving. The persons whose lives are at stake in the practice of euthanasia are society's most vulnerable persons. Older persons and persons who are medically dependent and disabled deserve substantive and procedural safeguards to protect their rights to life, liberty, and property.

REFERENCES: Anonymous. 1988. "It's Over Debbie." *JAMA* 259:272; Bopp, Jr., James, and Avila, Daniel. 1991. "The Due Process 'Right to Life' in *Cruzan* and Its Impact on 'Right-to-Die' Law." *University of Pittsburgh Law Review* 53:193–233; Bopp, Jr., James, and Marzen, Thomas J. 1991. *"Cruzan:* Facing the Inevitable." *Law, Medicine & Health Care* 19:1–2, 37–51; Bostrom, Barry A., ed. 1988. "Euthanasia in the Netherlands." *Issues in Law & Medicine* 3:361–468; Bostrom, Barry A. 1989. "Euthanasia in the Netherlands: A Model for the United States?" *Issues in Law & Medicine* 4: 467–486; *Bouvia v. Superior Court,* 179 Cal. App. 3d 1127, 225 Cal. Rptr. 297 (1986); *Cruzan v. Missouri Dep't of Health,* 110 S. Ct. 2841 (1990); Hendin, Herbert. 1994. "Seduced by Death: Doctors, Patients, and the Dutch Cure." *Issues in Law & Medicine* 10:123–168; May, William E., et al. 1987. "Feeding and Hydrating the Permanently Unconscious and Other Vulnerable Persons." *Issues in Law & Medicine* 3:203–218.

BARRY A. BOSTROM

EUTHANASIA IN THE NETHERLANDS

Active euthanasia has been openly practiced in the Netherlands since 1972. The legal interdiction of euthanasia has never been abolished; however, a policy of nonprosecution has been adopted. It is assumed that doctors who carry out active euthanasia should conform to the rules of careful conduct established by the courts. The following list of rules is most often quoted:

1. Euthanasia can only be performed upon an explicit and emphatic request of the patient.

2. The patient should be informed about his condition and the possibilities of relieving his suffering.

3. Unless the patient objects, his family should be consulted.

4. The doctor should seek advice from a second, independently acting physician.

5. The case should be reported to the authorities.

6. The physician should claim having acted in a situation of higher necessity.

The public prosecutors are instructed not to start inquiries unless they have indications that the physician acted in disregard of the rules.

Some information on the Dutch health care and welfare system is needed for the correct understanding of Dutch euthanasia. The country has an excellent, comprehensive health service and a well-developed system of care for disabled persons and the elderly. Money matters play no role in a patient's decisions concerning medical treatment. Practically all of the country's residents have health insurance that covers all essential expenses including the costs of a prolonged or terminal illness. When some forms of medical help are refused to anybody because of a limited budget, the public vigorously oppose such policy. Economic considerations have sometimes been raised in the debate on medicoethical issues, but all available information indicates that the Dutch pro-euthanasia movement and the practice of euthanasia in the country have never been economically motivated.

Reliable information on the practice of euthanasia in the Netherlands has become available owing to the extensive study ordered by the Dutch government. The findings were published in the Report of the Governmental Committee (1991). Out of 130,000 people who died in 1990, 43,000 died suddenly, which precluded all medical decisions; 86,700 persons died while under medical care; and in 49,000 of these cases (56.5 percent), the physicians took decisions that could or did shorten the patients' lives. Sixty-two percent of the general practitioners and 54 percent of all doctors have at some time performed active euthanasia upon request of the patient or assisted a patient in committing suicide. Sixty-five percent of general practitioners think that in certain situations the doctor should propose euthanasia to a patient who has not asked for it himself. Ninety-eight percent of all doctors consider voluntariness of euthanasia a very important requirement. Nevertheless, 27 percent of doctors have terminated patients' lives without their request, and a further 32 percent think of such acts as "conceivable."

In the year of the government-ordered study (1990), active euthanasia upon the patients' request was carried out in 2,300 cases. Requests for euthanasia submitted by 6,700 patients were rejected. Physicians assisted 400 people in committing suicide. Doctors actively terminated the lives of 1,000 patients who did not request euthanasia (although some of them had discussed the subject in one way or another at some time in the past).

Some 22,500 patients who received morphine or morphinelike drugs for pain relief died of morphine overdose. In 36 percent of these cases (8,100), one of the physician's intentions, or his sole intention, was to terminate the patient's life. In 3,159 cases the intentional lethal overdose of morphine was administered with the patient's consent, and in 4,941 cases, this was done without the patient's knowledge.

The doctors also actively terminated the lives of some severely handicapped newborns, gravely ill children, psychiatric patients, and patients with acquired immunodeficiency syndrome (AIDS), but exact figures have not been obtained and these cases of euthanasia are not included in the above quoted totals.

In 5,800 cases the doctors, upon request of the patients, withheld or withdrew potentially effective life-prolonging treatment, and in 25,000 cases, this was done without the patient's request. Abstaining from medically futile treatment was not included in the study.

The majority of the patients, 83 percent of those who underwent active voluntary euthanasia, and 70 percent of patients whose lives were actively terminated without their explicit request, suffered from various forms of cancer. Other patients had cardiovascular disease, diseases of the nervous system (including stroke), lung disease, mental disorders, or other disease.

Many, but not all, patients who underwent active euthanasia were terminally ill. As estimated by the attending physicians, the life expectancy of 21 percent of the patients at the time of euthanasia was one to six months, and in 8 percent of the cases, it exceeded six months. Most patients whose lives were actively terminated without their request were incompetent; 14 percent of these patients were fully competent, and 11 percent partially competent; 27 percent of patients who died of an intentional overdose of morphine administered without their knowledge were fully competent.

Having studied the committee's report, the Dutch government proposed a bill that was passed by the two chambers of the Parliament on February 9 and November 30, 1993, as an amendment to the Act on Disposal of the Dead. The amendment does not legalize euthanasia (Art. 293 of the Penal Code, which makes euthanasia a crime punishable by up to 12 years' imprisonment, remains in force) but states that it is the duty of the physician who has carried out euthanasia upon request of the patient, or without such request, to report the case to the municipal coroner. The public prosecutor then decides whether to start an inquiry. In the last year before the introduction of the amendment the public prosecutors dismissed 1,318 reported cases of euthanasia and launched inquiries in 5.

Questions have been raised whether the "rules of careful conduct" are sufficient safeguards against abuse. The Report of the Governmental Committee showed that in 1990 the first rule of careful conduct, which states that active euthanasia can only be carried out upon request of the patient, was followed in 5,859 cases (2,300 cases of voluntary active euthanasia, 400 cases of physician-assisted suicide, and 3,159 patients who died of an intentional overdose of morphine administered with their consent). In 5,941 cases this rule was disregarded (1,000 cases in which the lives of the patients were actively terminated without their request, and 4,941 patients who died of intentional overdose of morphine administered without their consent). There was a varying compliance with the other rules. Eighty-four percent of doctors consult with another physician before performing euthanasia upon request of the patient. When patients' lives are terminated without their request, in 52 percent of the cases, the doctors omit consultations with other physicians. Ninety-four percent of doctors consult with the patients' families before carrying out voluntary euthanasia. When the life of a hospitalized patient is actively terminated without his request, in 45 percent of the cases, this is being done without the knowledge of the patient's family. In the death certificates, 72 percent of the doctors concealed the fact that the patient died by voluntary euthanasia. In cases of active termination of life without the patient's request, and in cases of intentional lethal overdose of morphine, the doctors, with a single exception, did not state the truth in the death certificates.

It has been pointed out that it is the doctors who inform the patient, decide on euthanasia, choose to follow or to disregard some of the rules, choose their own consultants, compose the reports on the basis of which their actions are to be judged, or decide not to report the case. Several observers came to the conclusion that when euthanasia is accepted by both the public and the medical profession, as is the case in the Netherlands, it cannot be controlled by the authorities. The ultimate safeguards against abuse reside not in the official rules but in the integrity, and the good judgment, of the members of the medical profession.

Euthanasia is now accepted by a large majority of Dutch people. However, the public debate continues, focusing on the still-controversial issues. The furthest-reaching argument has been put forward by the consistent advocates of autonomy who claim that by limiting euthanasia to sick people the society has violated the individual's right to self-determination; all people, not only the sick, have the right to choose death and should be entitled to medical assistance in committing suicide. Other issues still under discussion are the termination of life of persons unable to request euthanasia and the validity of requests for euthanasia submitted by children (if parents disagree) and by mentally ill persons.

REFERENCES: Jochemsen, Henk. 1994. "Grenzen verlegd, maar niet altijd duidelijk: Aktuele ontwikkelingen in de euthanasiediscussie in Nederland" [The limits have been moved further but are not always clear: Recent developments in the debate on euthanasia in the Netherlands]. *Perspectief* 7(7): 3–6; Keown, John. 1994. "Further Reflections on Euthanasia in the Netherlands in the Light of the Remmelink Report and the Van der Maas Survey." In *Euthanasia, Clinical Practice and the Law,* ed. Luke Gormally. London: The Linacre Centre; Ministerie van Justitie, Ministerie van Welzijn, Volksgezondheid en Cultuur. 1991. *Medische Beslissingen Rond Het Levenseinde. Rapport van de Commissie Onderzoek Medische Praktijk inzake Euthanasie* [Medical decisions concerning the end of life. Report of the Committee to Investigate Medical Practice Concerning Euthanasia]. The Hague: Sdu Uitgeverij; Royal Netherlands Society for the Promotion of Medicine. 1988. "Guidelines for Euthanasia." *Issues in Law & Medicine* 3: 429–37; Ten Have, Henk A. M. J., and Jos V. M. Welie. 1992. "Euthanasia: Normal Medical Practice?" *Hastings Center Report* 22:34–38; Tweede, Kamer. 1991–92. "Standpunt van het Kabinet inzake medische beslissingen rond het levenseinde. Concept voorstel wijziging van de Wet op de Lijkbezorging" [Government Statement on Medical Decisions Concerning the End of Life: Proposal to Amend the Law on the Disposal of the Dead]. *Handelingen van Tweede Kamer* 20:383; Van den Berg, Jan Hendrick. 1978. *Medical*

Power and Medical Ethics. New York: Norton; Van der Maas, P. J., J. J. M. Van Delden, and L. Pijnenborg. 1992. *Euthanasia and Other Medical Decisions Concerning the End of Life. An Investigation Performed upon Request of the Commission of Inquiry into the Medical Practice Concerning Euthanasia.* Amsterdam: Elsevier.

RICHARD FENIGSEN

F

FERTILITY CONTROL USE PATTERNS

The development of oral contraceptives (OCs) and intrauterine devices (IUDs) in the 1960s gave couples increased reproductive control. Initially, both the pill and the IUD were hailed as offering safe and effective means of fertility control. By 1968, however, the public was being warned by the government that the pill was not as safe as earlier suggested and that some users were at risk for a variety of diseases including breast cancer. Although oral contraceptives still enjoy the highest percentages of favorable opinion among women, concern over health risks are likely to decrease this gap. "Regardless of whether a link between OC use and breast cancer is proved, OC use will almost certainly decline if the public perceives a link" (Trussell and Vaughan, 1992, 1162).

The IUD suffered a similar fate in that initial enthusiasm was soon dampened by evidence of serious, and in some cases fatal, pelvic inflammatory disease (PID) infections in some IUD users. Ironically, in some cases these infections scarred the fallopian tubes, resulting in permanent sterility. Lawsuits and legal problems primarily directed at the Dalkon Shield IUD resulted in the near cessation of production of IUDs by American companies. As of 1989, there were only two types of IUDs available in the United States: the Progestasert and the new Copper T380A IUD (Sivin, Stern, and Diaz, 1992). These companies do not want to incur the legal costs of aggressive lawsuits against their products even though IUDs, other than the Dalkon Shield, appear to be of minimal risk to most women. In fact, one extensive study has concluded that the indictment of the Dalkon Shield itself was a mistake and that it, too, is a safe method of fertility control (Mumford and Kessel, 1992b).

Despite the approval of the injectable hormonal contraceptive Depo-Provera* by the U.S. Food and Drug Administration in October 1992 after 25 years of controversy over concerns of increased cancer risk and the development of many new OCs, the search for long-term fertility control continues. It is estimated that contraceptive failure alone led to 1.6 to 2.0 million accidental pregnancies in the United States in 1987 and that such pregnancies account for about half of the 1.5 million abortions performed each year (Kaeser, 1990, 131). With most couples electing to have small families, often while they are young, they are faced with up to 20 years of fertility control after completion of their family.

Rather than using a form of contraception that is at best inconvenient and not fully effective and is at worst a significant hazard to the woman's health, more couples have opted for sterilization as a permanent contraception solution. Almost 33 percent of the 30 million American women practicing contraception depend on sterilization (21.9 percent their own and 10.8 percent their partner), while 28 percent depend on birth control pills. "In the United States more than two-thirds of the couples who desire no more children have been sterilized; if current trends continue, the proportion will soon approach 80%" (Mumford and Kessel, 1992a, 1203).

Demographic trends indicate that demand for long-term methods of fertility control including sterilization is likely to intensify over the next several decades as the population ages. While oral contraceptives are the method of choice for large proportions of younger women, sterilization is the preferred option by age 30 and increases significantly after that point. As the cohorts of women over 35 increase in size during the 1990s, they will heighten the use of these long-term techniques.

Data demonstrate that, in terms of both attitude and practice, sterilization has become a widely accepted method of fertility control. One reason for this support is found in the comparison of failure rates of the various methods used. The very low failure rates of tubal ligation and vasectomy (0.4 percent and 0.15 percent, respectively) compare very favorably with the IUD (6.0 percent), the pill (6.2 percent), and especially condoms (14.2 percent) and diaphragms (15.6 percent).

Reinforcing this demand by couples for a failsafe, permanent method of contraception, a variety of organizations have expended considerable effort to make sterilization services available to individuals who desire them. The Association for Voluntary Surgical Contraception (AVSC) and the Planned Parenthood Federation of America spearhead these efforts. Both lobby for the elimination of statutory constraints on voluntary applications and the provision of such services as part of an overall population planning program. AVSC, through its nationwide education program, emphasizes an individual's right to know about and choose sterilization. Planned Parenthood presents sterilization as one aspect of an overall family planning program and has been a prime force behind the establishment of family planning clinics in the United States.

The increase in demand for long-term fertility control can also be traced to substantial refinements in sterilization and contraceptive techniques. This is most clear in female sterilization procedures. What once required inpatient surgery under general anesthesia and lengthy recovery periods is now available on an outpatient basis with local anesthesia and minimal inconvenience for the patient.

This not only has increased the acceptability of sterilization but also decreased its relative cost vis-à-vis the long-term costs of alternative contraceptive methods. Another advantage of sterilization or long-term implants for family planning clinics is administrative in that it requires reaching a client only once rather than on a continuing basis. This onetime-only factor and safety have made sterilization the most frequent means of fertility control in the world.

REFERENCES: Kaeser, Lisa. 1990. "Contraceptive Development: Why the Snail's Pace?" *Family Planning Perspectives* 22(3): 131–34; London, Robert S. 1992. "The New Era in Oral Contraception: Pills Containing Gestodene, Norgestimate, and Desogestrel." *Obstetrical and Gynecological Survey* 47(11): 777–82; Mumford, Stephen D., and Elton Kessel. 1992a. "Sterilization Needs in the 1990s: The Case for Quinacine Nonsurgical Female Sterilization." *American Journal of Obstetrics and Gynecology* 167(5): 1203–07; Mumford, Stephen D., and Elton Kessel. 1992b. "Was the Dalkon Shield a Safe and Effective Intrauterine Device?" *Fertility and Sterility* 57(6): 1151–76; Sivin, Irvin, Janet Stern, and Soledad Diaz. 1992. "Rates and Outcomes of Planned Pregnancy Use After Use of Norplant Capsules." *American Journal of Obstetrics and Gynecology* 166(4): 1208–13; Trussell, James, and Barbara Vaughan. 1992. "Contraceptive Use Projections: 1990 to 2010." *American Journal of Obstetrics and Gynecology* 167(4): 1160–64.

ROBERT H. BLANK

FETAL ALCOHOL SYNDROME

The emerging knowledge over the past two decades of the impact of maternally ingested alcohol on the developing fetus has led to universal acceptance of the fact that "alcohol is a teratogenic drug capable of producing lifelong disabilities after intrauterine exposure" (Streissguth et al., 1991).

If the pregnant woman is intoxicated at the time of delivery, the infant may experience a mild neonatal abstinence syndrome with usually neurological symptoms such as tremulousness and poor feeding. Onset of symptoms is often within the first day, peaks at three to five days, and lasts a total of five to seven days. If the infant has been exposed in utero to a sufficient dose of maternally ingested alcohol, physical and neurological evidence of fetal alcohol syndrome (FAS), or more broadly, alcohol-related birth defects (ARBD), may be found. The diagnosis of ARBD requires at least one feature from each of the following categories: (1) growth retardation, of prenatal origin; (2) characteristic facies, with short palpebral fissures, ptosis, microphthalmia, flat nasal bridge, long philtrum, thin and smooth upper lip, micrognathia, and hypoplastic maxilla; (3) central nervous system manifestations, with microcephaly, mental retardation, delayed development, hyperactivity, attention and learning deficits; and (4) a maternal history of alcohol use during pregnancy (Spohr, Willms, and Steinhausen, 1993; Streissguth et al., 1991). An increase in the risk of neoplasms such as neuroblastoma, hepatoblastoma, and adrenocortical carcinoma, as well as various cardiac anomalies, has also been reported with ARBD.

The risk of an infant being born with ARBD appears to be 30 to 40 percent in chronically alcoholic women, defined as more than 60 drinks per month or more than one ounce (30 ml) of absolute alcohol per day. Pregnant alcoholic women are also at an increased risk for placental abruption, spontaneous abortion, and stillbirth. Binge drinkers may place their infants at risk as lesser degrees of alcohol consumption have been associated with intrauterine growth retardation, behavioral and neurological difficulties (distractibility, poor social skills, lack of judgment, lowered academic achievement), and an increased risk of various congenital anomalies (Little and Wendt, 1991). There is evidence of decreased birth weight with an average daily consumption of one drink (15 ml of alcohol), and dose-dependent effects on mental performance have been reported in infants of women who drank in excess of 15 ml of alcohol per day during pregnancy (Jacobson, Jacobson, and Sokol, 1993; Little and Wendt, 1991). Thus, no "safe" level of alcohol consumption during pregnancy has been identified. However, there is no clear evidence of deleterious effects on a fetus of a well-nourished non-drug-abusing pregnant woman ingesting less than one alcoholic drink a day. This lack of data at lower levels of alcohol consumption has led to some controversy over professional recommendations of total abstention from alcohol during pregnancy, as in, for example, the position of the American Academy of Pediatrics.

FAS occurs in an average of 1.9 per 1,000 live births and can range from 6 (urban) to as high as 121 (Native American) per 1,000 live births (Little and Wendt, 1991). Some estimates are lower (0.5 to 1 per 1,000 live births), though recognition and reporting difficulties suggest that the true incidence of FAS is higher. Some estimate the overall incidence of ARBD as up to 3 per 1,000 live births, making FAS/ARBD the leading known cause of mental retardation (Streissguth et al., 1991). This fact is all the more tragic as it is also one of the few potentially preventable causes.

Alcohol crosses the placenta, resulting in similar blood alcohol levels in both mother and fetus. Decreased fetal metabolism of alcohol results in an increased susceptibility of the fetus to the effects of alcohol with, for example, a single drink by the pregnant woman, causing cessation of fetal breathing movements (Little and Wendt, 1991). The microcephaly reflects direct damage to fetal brain tissue from the in utero alcohol exposure. The observed variability in adverse effects is related to the gestational age at exposure, the amount of alcohol consumed, the presence of binge drinking, and the individual susceptibility of the fetus. The differences in study results reflect the difficulties in quantifying the above variables, as well as the presence of confounding variables such as smoking and other drug use such as marijuana and cocaine. As the mother may continue to use alcohol after birth, it is important to counsel her concerning the passage of alcohol in breast milk. Up to 25 percent of the maternal dose of alcohol is present in breast milk. The infant thus may exhibit drowsiness, diaphoresis, deep sleep, weakness, decrease in linear growth, and abnormal weight gain. There is also a suggestion of a decrease in motor skills at one year of age due to chronic alcohol exposure through breast feeding.

The characteristic facies become less distinctive with increasing age (Streissguth et al., 1991). The severity of the mental retardation appears to correlate with the degree of physical stigmata and reflects a persistent microcephaly. Postnatal growth deficiency remains prominent in infancy and early childhood. Speech and language problems are common in older children. In addition, severe behavioral problems contribute to characteristic learning disabilities, including hyperactivity and attention deficit disorders (compounded by continued maternal alcohol abuse), lack of impulse control, poor decision making, decreased ability to attain independence, decrements in short-term memory, and problems in quantitative functioning, perceptual motor skills and sustained attention (Brown et al., 1991; Coles et al., 1991; Streissguth et al., 1991). Unfortunately, fetal alcohol effects do not generally improve with time (Little and Wendt, 1991; Spohr, Willms, and Steinhausen, 1993). In a recent study of 61 patients with either FAS (70 percent) or ARBD (30 percent), none of the subjects were known to be independent in terms of both housing and income in spite of 42 percent having an IQ greater than 70. All of the individuals studied were unsuitable candidates for the usual job training programs, given the severe behavioral problems (Streissguth et al., 1991).

Therapy programs for disabled individuals with FAS/ARBD are of limited efficacy and problematic, given maladaptive behavioral problems (Streissguth et al., 1991). The dominant focus has thus been on prevention through programs aimed at either the prevention of alcohol abuse among women of childbearing age or prevention of pregnancy in alcoholic women. As there is no documented "safe" level of alcohol ingestion, professional and federal guidelines recommend abstinence from alcohol while pregnant. Alcoholic beverages now carry warning labels, and educational brochures, posters, and programs have been developed for communities and schools. Attention is being directed toward alcohol abuse treatment programs designed for women, with a heightened awareness of the family and social and cultural factors leading to alcohol abuse among women. Regardless of the above efforts, it is fair to say that the organized response to date in attempting to prevent the birth of an infant with FAS/ARBD has been inadequate relative to the magnitude of the problem.

REFERENCES: American Academy of Pediatrics: Committee on Substance Abuse and Committee on Children with Disabilities. 1993. "Fetal Alcohol Syndrome and Fetal Alcohol Effects." *Pediatrics* 91: 1004–1006; Brown, R. T., Coles, C. D., Smith, I. E., et al. 1991. "Effects of Prenatal Alcohol Exposure at School Age. II. Attention and Behavior." *Neurotoxicology and Teratology* 13: 369–376; Burd, L., and Moffatt, M. E. 1994. "Epidemiology of Fetal Alcohol Syndrome in North American Indians, Alaskan Natives, and Canadian Aboriginal Peoples: A Review of the Literature." *Public Health Reports* 109: 688–693; Coles, C. D., Brown, R. T., Smith, I. E., et al. 1991. "Effects of Prenatal Alcohol Exposure at School Age. I. Physical and Cognitive Development." *Neurotoxicology and Teratology* 13: 357–367; Jacobson, J. L., Jacobson, S. W., and Sokol, R. J. 1993. "Teratogenic Effects of Alcohol on Infant Development." *Alcoholism: Clinical and Experimental Research* 17: 174–183; Lewis, D. D., and Woods, S. E. 1994. "Fetal Alcohol Syndrome." *American Family Physician* 50: 1025–1032; Little, R. E., and Wendt, J. K. 1991. "The Effects of Maternal Drinking in the Reproductive Period:

An Epidemiologic Review." *Journal of Substance Abuse* 3: 187–204; Smitherman, C. H. 1994. "The Lasting Effect of Fetal Alcohol Syndrome and Fetal Alcohol Effect on Children and Adolescents." *Journal of Pediatric Health Care* 8: 121–126; Spohr, H., Willms, J., and Steinhausen, H. 1993. "Prenatal Alcohol Exposure and Long-term Developmental Consequences." *Lancet* 341: 907–910; Streissguth, A. P., Aase, J. M., Clarren, S. K., et al. 1991. "Fetal Alcohol Syndrome in Adolescents and Adults." *Journal of the American Medical Association* 265: 1961–1967.

ROBERT M. NELSON

FETAL/EMBRYO RESEARCH, TYPES

The broad array of research possibilities for fetal and embryo tissue complicates attempts to explicate the policy issues. One important distinction is that between investigational-type research that is not beneficial to the fetus and therapeutic research that is of potential benefit to the fetal subject but likely to be beneficial to future fetuses.

Another key distinction centers on the stage of development of the human organism where the research is conducted, from preimplantation to late fetal stages. The general sources of fetal material include tissue from dead fetuses; previable or nonviable fetuses in utero, generally prior to an elective abortion; nonviable living fetuses ex utero; fetal tissue transplantation research using tissue from dead fetuses; and embryos, in vitro and preimplantation. Although the variety of potential uses of fetal tissue is virtually unlimited, five areas are summarized here.

The first category of research deals with investigations of fetal development and physiology. The purpose of this research is to expand scientific knowledge about normal fetal development in order to provide a basis for identifying and understanding abnormal processes and, ultimately, curing birth deformities. These studies primarily involve autopsies of dead fetuses. However, studies of fetal physiology include the fetus in utero as well as organs and tissues removed from the dead fetus. In some instances, this research requires administration of a substance to the woman prior to abortion or delivery by cesarean section. That is followed by analysis to detect the presence of this substance or its metabolic effects in a sample of umbilical cord blood or in the fetal tissue. This research also focuses on the development of fetal behavior in utero by monitoring fetal breathing movements. Fetal hearing, vision, and taste capabilities have been documented by applying various stimuli to the live fetus in utero. Most controversial are the physiological studies that utilize observation of nonviable but live fetuses outside the uterus to test for response to touch and for the presence of swallowing movements.

The second type of research focuses on the development of techniques to diagnose fetal problems, such as amniocentesis.* The initial research was conducted primarily on amniotic samples withdrawn as a routine part of induced abortion to find the normal values for enzymes known to be defective in genetic disease. Once it was demonstrated that the particular enzyme was expressed in fetal cells and normal values were known, application to diagnosis of the abnormal condition in the fetus at risk was undertaken. Recent prenatal diagnostic research on fetuses involves extension of diagnostic capacities to additional diseases, development of chorionic villus sampling (CVS),* and attempts to detect fetal cells in the maternal circulation.

Research has also been directed at the identification of physical defects in the developing fetus. Ultrasound,* alpha-fetoprotein tests, amniography, tests for fetal lung capacity, and a variety of techniques for monitoring fetal well-being or distress are recent products of this category of fetal research. In each case, following animal studies that indicated the safety and efficacy of the procedure, human fetal research was conducted in a variety of settings. Fetoscopy,* for example, because of the potential risk to the fetus, was developed selectively in women undergoing elective abortion. The procedure was performed prior to abortion, and an autopsy was performed after to determine its technical success.

A third area of fetal research involves efforts to determine the effects of drugs on the developing fetus. These pharmacological studies are largely retrospective in design, involving the examination of the fetus or infant after an accidental exposure. For instance, all studies on the influence of oral contraceptives or other drugs on multiple births or congenital abnormalities were retrospective, as were most studies of the effects on the fetus of drugs administered to treat maternal illness during pregnancy. In these designs, no fetus was intentionally exposed to the drug for research purposes. However, some pharmacology research involves intentional administration of substances to pregnant women prior to abortion in order to compare quantitative movement of these agents across the placenta as well as absolute levels achieved in fetal tissues. These studies serve as guidelines for drug selection to treat intrauterine infections such as syphilis by examining the dead fetuses after abortion and demonstrating the superiority of one drug over another.

The availability of human embryos for research purposes followed the development of in vitro fertilization (IVF).* Embryos that remained untransferred for in vitro fertilization could be used for possible clinical or research purposes. Theoretically, these "spare" embryos could be augmented by the deliberate creation of embryos for research where donors consent to have their gametes or embryos used in this way. Other potential sources of human embryos for research could come from harvesting through embryo lavage. A move to the deliberate production of embryos for research is highly controversial even though that might be the only way to satisfy expanding research needs.

Although assisted reproduction technologies are all experimental at some stage and thus might be described as research, there are many nonclinical uses that more clearly fit the research paradigm. Among the many nonclinical uses of human embryos are to (1) develop and test contraceptives; (2) investigate abnormal cell growth; (3) study the development of chromosomal abnormalities; (4) implantation studies; and (5) cancer and acquired immunodeficiency syndrome (AIDS) research. Other potential genetic uses of the embryos include (1) attempts at altering gene structures; (2) preimplantational screening for chromosomal anomalies and genetic diseases; (3) preimplantation therapy for genetic defects; and (4) development of characteristic selection techniques including sex preselection. Furthermore, research on artificial placentas is dependent on the availability of human embryos at some stage.

A final area of fetal research involves the use of fetal cells for transplantation. Unlike other areas of fetal research where the tissue is used to develop a treatment that might help future fetuses, in fetal transplantation research the tissue is the treatment used to benefit an identifiable adult patient. Although some observers see no ethical difference between the transplantation of adult organs and that of tissues and fetal tissues to benefit individual recipients, others contend that the use of fetal tissue for this purpose is ethically questionable because there are no possible benefits to particular fetuses or to future fetuses.

REFERENCES: Fletcher, John C. 1993. "Human Fetal and Embryo Research: Lysenkoism in Reverse—How and Why?" In Robert H. Blank and Andrea L. Bonnicksen, eds., *Emerging Issues in Biomedical Policy.* Vol. 2. New York: Columbia University Press; Nelson, Robert M. 1993. "What Is the Purpose of Neonatal Drug Testing? Towards a Rational Social Policy." *Women and Politics* 13 (3–4): 83–98; Robinson, Bambi E. S. 1993. "The Moral Permissibility of *In Utero* Experimentation." *Woman and Politics* 13 (3–4): 19–30.

See also **FETAL RESEARCH REGULATIONS.**

ROBERT H. BLANK

FETAL RESEARCH REGULATIONS

Fetal research first appeared on the national policy agenda in the early 1970s after widely publicized exposés on several gruesome experiments conducted on still-living fetuses. In response, Congress passed the 1974 National Research Act (Public Law 93–345), which established the National Commission for the Protection of Human Subjects of Biomedical and Behavioral Research,* whose first charge was to investigate the scientific, legal, and ethical aspects of fetal research. The statute also prohibited all federally funded research on fetuses prior or subsequent to abortion until the commission made its recommendations and regulations were adopted.

In 1975 the commission issued its recommendations, which set a framework for the conduct of fetal research. In 1976, regulations for the federal funding of such research were promulgated (45 C.F.R. 46.201–211). Under the regulations, certain types of fetal research are fundable, with constraints based on parental consent and the principle of minimizing risk to the pregnant woman and the fetus. With respect to cadaver fetuses, the regulations defer to state and local laws in accordance with the provisions of the Uniform Anatomical Gift Act (UAGA).* The use of fetal cadaver tissue is to be treated the same as any other human cadaver.

With respect to research on live fetuses, the regulations provide that appropriate studies must first be done on animal fetuses. The consent of the pregnant woman and the prospective father (if reasonably possible) are required, and the research must not alter the pregnancy termination procedure in a way that would cause greater than "minimal risk" to either the pregnant woman or the fetus. Moreover, researchers must not have a role in determining either the abortion procedure or the assessment of fetal viability. Where it is unclear whether an ex utero fetus is viable, that fetus cannot be the subject of research unless the purpose of the research is to enhance its chances of survival *or* the research subjects the fetus to no additional risk and its purpose is to develop important, otherwise unobtainable, knowledge. Research on living, nonviable fetuses ex utero is allowed if the vital functions of the fetus are not artificially maintained. Finally, in utero fetal research is permissible if it is designed to be therapeutic to the particular fetus and places it at the minimal risk necessary to meet its health needs, or if it imposes minimal risks and produces important knowledge unobtainable through other means.

In 1985, Congress passed a law (42 U.S.C. 289) forbidding federal conduct or funding of research on viable ex utero fetuses with an exception for therapeutic research or research that poses no added risk of suffering, injury, or death to the fetus *and* leads to important knowledge unobtainable by other means. Research on living fetuses in utero is still permitted, but federal regulations require the standard of risk to be the same for fetuses to be aborted as for fetuses that will be carried to term.

In 1985, Congress also passed legislation (42 U.S.C. 275) creating a Biomedical Ethics Board whose first order of business was to be fetal research. In 1988, Congress suspended the secretary of Health and Human Services' (HHS) power to authorize waivers in cases of great need and great potential benefit until the Biomedical Ethics Advisory Committee conducted a study of the nature, advisability, and implications of exercising any waiver of the risk provisions of existing federal regulations. However, in 1989 the activities of the committee were suspended, leaving the question of waivers unresolved.

As with federal activity in fetal research, state regulation was largely a response to the broad expansion of research involving legally aborted fetuses after *Roe v. Wade** (1973). Many state statutes were enacted by conservative legislatures as an effort to foreclose social benefits that might be viewed as lending support to abortion. Of the 25 states with laws specifically regulating fetal research, 12 apply only to research with fetuses prior or subsequent to an elective abortion, and most of the statutes are either part of or attached to abortion legislation. Moreover, of the 13 statutes that apply to fetuses more generally, 5 impose more stringent restrictions of fetal research in conjunction with an elective abortion.

Under state law, research on fetal cadavers is regulated through the Uniform Anatomical Gift Act, which has been adopted by all 50 states. However, some states have excluded fetuses from the UAGA provisions, and others regulate it through fetal research statutes. Although a total of 45 states permit the use of tissues from elective abortions, 14 have provisions regulating research involving fetal cadaver tissue that deviate from the UAGA either in consent requirements or specific prohibitions on the uses of such tissue. Five states currently prohibit any research with fetal cadavers except for pathological examinations or autopsies. Of these, 4 apply exclusively to electively aborted fetuses.

State laws regulating research on live fetuses (in utero or ex utero) generally constrain research that is not therapeutic to the fetus itself. Because these state laws were adopted in the context of the abortion debate, the primary focus is on research performed on the ex utero fetus (Andrews, 1993). Twenty of the states regulate research on ex utero fetuses, while 14 regulate research on in utero fetuses. Although the specifics of the prohibitions and the sanctions designated differ by state, most would appear to prohibit research involving transplantation, nontherapeutic research, and preembryo research.

Another restriction imposed by some of the fetal research statutes addresses concerns over remuneration for fetal materials or participation in research. At present, at least 16 states prohibit the sale of fetal tissue, 7 for any purpose and 9 specifically for research purposes. Importantly, some of these apply only to elective abortions, not spontaneous abortions or ectopic pregnancies. In some states the penalties for violation are very stiff. For instance, selling a viable fetus for research in Wyoming is punishable by a fine of not less than $10,000 and imprisonment of 1 to 14 years (OTA, 1990, 135).

REFERENCES: Andrews, Lori B. 1993. "Regulation of Experimentation on the Unborn." *Journal of Legal Medicine* 14 (1): 25–56; Fletcher, John C. 1993. "Human Fetal and Embryo Research: Lysenkoism in Reverse—How and Why?" In Robert H. Blank and Andrea L. Bonnicksen, eds., *Emerging Issues in Biomedical Policy.* Vol. 2. New York: Columbia University Press; Office of Technology Assessment (OTA). 1990. *Neural Grafting: Regaining the Brain and Spinal Cord.* Washington, D.C.: U.S. Government Printing Office; Richard, Patricia Bayer. 1989. "Fetal Research Policy." In Robert H. Blank and Miriam K. Mills, eds., *Biomedical Technology and Public Policy.* Westport, CT: Greenwood Press.

See also **FETAL/EMBRYO RESEARCH, TYPES; NEURAL GRAFTING.**

ROBERT H. BLANK

FETAL SURGERY

There are three basic approaches to treating an endangered fetus. The first entails administering medication or other substances indirectly to the fetus through the mother's bloodstream (e.g., biotin, digitalis, cortisone, or related hormone drugs). Second, timely delivery can be induced so that the infant's problem can be treated immediately outside the womb. The third approach is direct surgical treatment of the fetus in the womb. Fetal surgery has been made possible by new developments in ultrasound,* amniocentesis,* and fetoscopy* and also by sophisticated surgical instrumentation designed specifically for these intricate procedures on fetuses.

The first reported fetal surgery was performed in April 1981 on a 31-week-old fetus twin suffering from a severe urinary tract obstruction. Doctors at several locales have implanted miniature shunting devices in the brains of fetuses that had been diagnosed as having hydrocephalus, a dangerous buildup of fluid in the brain. These shunts allow the fluid to be drained from the upper ventricles of the brain into the amniotic sac. In one case, surgeons also inserted a four-inch-long valve-control shunt to permit continued drainage during the remaining three months of pregnancy. Other applications of fetal surgery have drained a collapsed lung that became filled with fluid and drained excess fluid from the abdomen of another fetus. According to one source, in utero surgery is more practical than it might first appear. "First, *in utero* surgery takes place in a surgical field (the amniotic fluid) that is sterile at the onset. Second, the fetus responds in a fundamentally different way to injury than an adult. Fetal wounds heal without the scarring, inflammation, fibrosis, or contraction that affect adult wound healing" (Pergament, 1993, 141).

A more dramatic ex utero fetal surgery was conducted on a 24-week-old fetus to repair a diaphramatic hernia. After surgically opening the abdomen of the mother, the left side of the fetus was brought outside the uterus. After a 54-minute surgery, the uterus was closed in three layers with fibrin glue applied between them, and the amniotic fluid was replenished. At 32 weeks gestation, 7 weeks after surgery, a healthy baby boy was delivered via cesarean section.

Notwithstanding these successes, it must be stressed that all fetal surgeries are presently high-risk procedures limited in use to fetuses in danger of dying before or soon after birth without the surgery. Also, for many disorders it is improbable that effective treatment will be developed in the foreseeable future. Furthermore, the threat of precipitating preterm delivery or abortion remains a severe constraint on all but the most routine in utero interventions, despite great strides in prevention of those problems. Risk also confronts the mother any time fetal surgery is attempted. A dilemma of fetal surgery is that in "saving" a fetus who would otherwise die, a seriously disabled newborn may survive. Questions have also been raised as to whether the allocation of scarce resources to programs on ex utero fetal surgery is warranted.

The unique feature of fetal surgery is that it requires violation of the mother's right of personal autonomy if she does not consent to have the surgery. No new legal problems arise unless the mother refuses to consent, in which case the legal dilemma is agonizing, especially if she desires to carry the fetus to term. Of course *consent* is a subjective term. Although in theory it requires a free, informed choice, in practice, women might legally consent not out of free choice but instead under powerful cultural expectations of what constitutes a responsible decision. Although her "consent" obviates the legal problem, it raises severe ethical issues. In our society, the status of patient usually carries with it the notion of autonomy. But in these cases, whose rights take precedence, those of the fetus or those of the mother whose body must be "invaded" in order to facilitate the surgery?

REFERENCES: Evans, M. I., N. S. Adzick, M. P. Johnson, et al. 1994. "Fetal Therapy—1994." *Current Opinion in Obstetrics and Gynecology* 6(1): 58–64; Harrison, M. R., N. S. Adzick, M. Longaker, et al. 1990. "Successful Repair in Utero of a Fetal Diaphragmatic Hernia after Removal of Herniated Viscera from the Left Thorax." *New England Journal of Medicine* 322(22): 1582–1584; Johnson, M. P., T. P. Bukowski, C. Reitleman, et al. 1994. "In Utero Surgical Treatment of Fetal Obstructive Uropathy." *American Journal of Obstetrics and Gynecology* 170(6): 1770–1776; Kolder, V., J. Gallagher, and M. T. Parsons. 1987. "Court-Ordered Obstetrical Interventions." *New England Journal of Medicine* 316(19): 1192–1196; Pergament, E. 1993. "In Utero Treatment: Fetal Surgery." In R. H. Blank and A. L. Bonnickson, eds., *Emerging Issues in Biomedical Policy.* Vol. 2. New York: Columbia University Press.

See also **AMNIOCENTESIS; FETOSCOPY; PRENATAL DIAGNOSIS; ULTRASOUND/SONOGRAPHY.**

ROBERT H. BLANK

FETOSCOPY

Fetoscopy is the application of fiber optics technology that allows direct visualization of the fetus in utero. The fetoscope is inserted in an incision through the woman's abdomen, usually under the direction of ultrasound. Although only a very small area of fetal surface can be examined because of current limitation in instrumentation, the fetoscope can be maneuvered around in the uterus to examine the fetus, section by section. Fetoscopy is also used to sample fetal blood under direct observation from a fetal vessel on the surface of the placenta. This is accomplished by inserting a small tube into the uterus and aspirating a minute quantity of blood for diagnostic testing. Fetoscopy also has direct therapeutic use in the intrauterine transfusion of fetuses and considerable potential for introducing medicines, cell transplants, or genetic materials into fetal tissues in order to treat genetic diseases.

Despite substantial progress in fetoscopy and fetoscopic aspiration in the last decade, they are still considered applied research because of the hazards they pose for the fetus. Escalated rates of prematurity as well as a miscarriage rate of between 3 and 5 percent accompany these procedures and must be reduced considerably before fetoscopy can be considered routine medical practice. Also because of major advances in ultrasonography, some procedures such as fetal blood sampling that initially were performed by fetoscopy are now done via ultrasound. Fetoscopy, however, is a vanguard technology for future efforts at in utero treatment of genetic disease and for fetal surgery.

REFERENCES: D'Alton, Mary E., and Alan H. De Cherney. 1993. "Prenatal Diagnosis." *New England Journal of Medicine* 328(2): 114–120; Ghidini, Alessandro, W. Sepulveda, C. J. Lockwood, et al. 1993. "Complications of Fetal Blood Sampling." *American Journal of Obstetrics and Gynecology* 168(5): 1339–1344; Quintero, R. A., H. Reich, K. S. Puder, et al. 1994. "Umbilical-Cord Ligation of an Acardic Twin by Fetoscopy at 19 Weeks of Gestation." *New England Journal of Medicine* 330(7): 469–471;

Shulman, L. P., and S. Elias. 1990. "Percutaneous Umbilical Blood Sampling, Fetal Skin Sampling, and Fetal Liver Biopsy." *Seminars in Perinatology* 14:456–464.

See also **PRENATAL DIAGNOSIS.**

ROBERT H. BLANK

FOOD AND DRUG ADMINISTRATION

One of the oldest consumer protection agencies in the United States, the FDA has congressional authorization to test, approve, inspect, and set safety and efficacy standards for foods, food additives, drugs, chemicals, cosmetics, household devices, and medical devices involved in interstate commerce. Food and drugs for pets and farm animals also fall under the FDA's jurisdiction.

The FDA is part of the Public Health Service within the U.S. Department of Health and Human Services (DHHS). Its approximately 7,000 employees monitor the manufacture, import, transport, storage, and sale of products worth $570 billion annually, about one fourth of the U.S. national consumer dollar. The agency employs approximately 2,100 scientists who test to see if products are contaminated with illegal substances and review testing results submitted by companies seeking agency approval for drugs, vaccines, food additives, coloring agents, and medical devices.

The FDA has six centers responsible for issuing and enforcing regulations. The National Center for Toxicological Research is responsible for investigating the biological effects of widely used chemicals. The Engineering and Analytical Center tests medical devices, radiation emitting products, and radioactive drugs. The Center for Devices and Radiological Health collects and evaluates data on hazards to public health from medical devices and evaluates the safety, efficacy, and labeling of medical devices and diagnostic products. Its goals are to protect against unnecessary human exposure to radiation from electronic products in the home, industry, and medicine. This center also monitors the substances used to perform diagnostic tests on specimens taken from a body.

The Center for Drug Evaluation and Research regulates all testing, production, and labeling of drugs manufactured for interstate commerce. It is also responsible for reviewing and evaluating the new and investigational drug applications and regulating prescription drug advertising and promotional labeling. The Center for Food Safety and Applied Nutrition develops policies, standards, and regulations on foods (except for meats, which are under the jurisdiction of the Department of Agriculture), food additives, artificial colorings, and cosmetics. The center protects the food supply by testing samples, for example, ensuring that unacceptable pesticide levels are not present. The center also sees that medicated feeds and other drugs given to animals raised for food are not a threat to human health.

The Center for Biologics Evaluation and Research regulates biological products and conducts research related to the development, manufacture, testing, and use of biological products. This center also regulates all blood products and blood reagents, ensures the safety of the blood supply by inspecting blood bank operations, and safeguards the purity and effectiveness of biologics such as insulin and vaccines. The Center for Veterinary Medicine is responsible for the development of policies, standards, and regulations on the safety and efficacy of animal drugs, food additives, and veterinary devices.

The FDA is rooted in the efforts of one individual, Harvey W. Wiley, chief chemist of the Agriculture Department's Bureau of Chemistry during the early twentieth century. Responding to the publicity generated by Wiley's experiments on the safety of food additives and preservatives, Congress enacted the Food and Drug Act of 1906 (also known as the Wiley Act). Earlier legislation had set standards for the quality of biologic agents (e.g., serum and vaccines); the Wiley Act expanded this oversight activity to include the regulation of the food and drug industry. The Meat Inspection Act was passed the same day.

The Food, Drug and Insecticide Administration (FDIA) was created in 1927 within the Department of Agriculture. Also that year, Congress passed the Caustic Poison Act, requiring warning labels on poisonous substances as well as antidotes to protect children from being injured by lye and other dangerous chemicals normally found in the home. In 1930 the FDIA became the Food and Drug Administration (FDA). In 1938 the passage of the Food, Drug and Cosmetic (FDC) Act broadened the agency's regulatory power to cover cosmetics and medical devices, along with food and drugs. The FDA Act created purity and safety standards and authorized inspections of factories where regulated products are manufactured. This act is the most crucial piece of legislation in the food, drug, and cosmetic industries; it has been amended over 60 times. The act requires predistribution approval of new drugs, sets tolerance levels for unavoidable poisonous substances, and determines standards for food containers (identification, quality, and fill levels). The FDA Act added the power of court injunction to previous remedies of seizure and prosecution provided in the Wiley Act. In 1939 the first food standards under the FDA Act were issued for canned goods, and the FDA was transferred from the Department of Agriculture to the Federal Security Agency. The Public Health Service Act of 1944 gave the FDA authority to ensure the safety, purity, and potency of vaccines, serum, blood, and other biological products, to ensure the safety of milk and shellfish, and to oversee sanitary facilities for travelers on buses, trains, and planes.

In 1951 the Delaney Committee began a congressional investigation of the safety of chemicals in foods and cosmetics. This set the foundation for subsequent controls over pesticides, food additives, and certain coloring ingredients. The Durham-Humphrey Amendment to the FDA Act, passed in 1951, defined the types of drugs that must be used with medical supervision and restricted their sale to prescription by a licensed medical practitioner. In 1954 the Pesticides Amendments outlined procedures for setting safety limits of pesticide residues on raw agricultural commodities. The Food Additives Amendment, enacted in 1958, requires manufacturers of new food additives to establish safety; the Delaney Proviso prohibits the approval or continued sale of any foods containing additives shown to induce cancer in animals or humans.

In 1960, Congress enacted the Color Additive Amendments, which require manufacturers to establish the safety of color additives in foods, drugs, and cosmetics. The Federal Hazardous Substances Labeling Act, also passed in 1960, requires prominent warnings on dangerous household products.

In 1962, amidst the wake of the thalidomide tragedies, Congress responded to widespread public support for stronger drug regulation by passing the Kefauver-Harris Drug Amendments. For the first time, drug manufacturers were required to prove the efficacy of their products before marketing them. In 1966, the FDA contracted with the National Research Council to prove the efficacy of 4,000 drugs approved between 1938 and 1961. Also in 1966, the Fair Packaging and Labeling Act was added to the FDA Act. This act requires all consumer products in interstate commerce to be honestly and informatively labeled; the FDA is responsible for enforcing provisions pertaining to foods, drugs, cosmetics, and medical devices. The Fair Packaging and Labeling Act again broadened the FDA's powers by offering legal remedy.

The FDA began in 1972 to review over-the-counter drugs to enhance the safety, efficacy, and labeling of drugs sold without prescription. The Medical Device Amendments, passed in 1976, ensure the safety and efficacy of medical devices such as diagnostic equipment. The amendments require manufacturers to register with the FDA and follow quality control procedures; for example, some products must be tested before receiving premarket approval; others must meet performance standards before marketing.

In 1970 the Environmental Protection Agency was established and took over the regulation of pesticide tolerances previously controlled by the FDA. In 1973, Congress transferred oversight of poisonous substances to the newly created Consumer Product Safety Commission.

In 1983 the Orphan Drug Act enabled the FDA to promote research, approval, and marketing of drugs needed for treating rare diseases that would not otherwise be profitable. The Orphan Drug Act authorized financial incentives for companies to develop drugs for the treatment of illnesses having fewer than 200,000 U.S. citizens affected. The act was amended in 1985 to establish research grants, greater marketing protection to manufacturers of approved orphan drugs, and a National Commission on Orphan Diseases to evaluate government research activities on rare diseases. The Drug Price Competition and Patent Term Restoration Act, passed in 1984, permits the FDA to approve generic versions of brand-name drugs already proven effective. This act also allows manufacturers patent extensions of up to five years for the time lost due to the FDA's slower approval rate.

The AIDS (acquired immunodeficiency syndrome) Amendments to the Health Omnibus Programs Extension of 1988 require development of research and education programs, counseling, testing, and health care for AIDS patients, as well as a registry of experimental AIDS drugs. In May 1990, after pressure from the

AIDS lobby, the DHHS formally proposed the "parallel tract": a mechanism for approval of AIDS drugs that allows AIDS patients to receive the unapproved drug with minimal medical supervision while clinical trials are being conducted alongside.

The Nutrition Labeling and Education Act of 1990 requires all packaged foods to bear nutrition labeling and all health claims for foods to be consistent with guidelines from the secretary of Health and Human Services. The Safe Medical Devices Act of 1990 requires reporting from any facility using devices if failure is suspected in cases of injury or death.

The FDA authority is limited to interstate commerce. The FDA is empowered to prevent untested, harmful, and unsafe products from being sold; it may also seize products and prosecute persons or firms responsible for the legal violation. The agency cannot control prices but does regulate advertising or prescription drugs and medical devices.

The FDA can fulfill its statutory duties in three broad categories: analysis, surveillance, and correction. Most work conducted in analysis is preventive, occurring in the approval process before marketing. Surveillance duties are performed by field office inspectors with authorization to enter and inspect all factories and establishments producing drugs, medical devices, radiation-emitting products, as well as food and cosmetics. The FDA has many options under the heading of correction. If there is a possible law violation, the FDA sends a citation as an invitation, to an individual or firm, to prove that there is no violation. The regulatory letter is sent as an enforcement document to the head of the firm stating that unless apparent violative product conditions are corrected, legal action will be taken. A recall is conducted after release of a product, when either the manufacturer or the FDA decides to remove it from the marketplace. The entire recall process is overseen by the FDA and may include corrective actions. An injunction may be brought against an individual or firm to stop distribution or manufacture of a product in violation of the law. The FDA can initiate a seizure of goods by giving their location to a U.S. district court, which directs a U.S. marshal to take possession of the goods until the matter can be resolved. The U.S. attorney general may file a criminal action against an individual or firm upon recommendation of the FDA.

Annually, over 20,000 facilities are inspected to ensure that products are made correctly and labeled truthfully. As a part of the inspection process, over 70,000 domestic and imported product samples are collected for examination by FDA scientists, as well as checked for correct labeling. Some 3,000 products a year are found to be unfit for consumers and are withdrawn from the market, either by voluntary recall or by court-ordered seizure. In addition, more than 20,000 import shipments are detained annually at the port of entry because the goods appear to be unacceptable.

The FDA does not, itself, conduct research when deciding whether to approve new drugs but, rather, examines the results of studies performed by the manufacturer. The FDA must determine that the drug's benefits outweigh its negative side effects. The FDA's scrutiny does not end after approval and marketing; the agency collects tens of thousands of reports annually to monitor for any unexpected adverse reactions.

The FDA regulates the composition, quality, safety, efficacy, and labeling of all drugs for human use. All drugs meeting FDA qualifications go through premarket testing, which consists of both preclinical and clinical trials. In the preclinical trials, a chemical substance thought to be potentially useful is tested on animals. The goal of this testing is to establish the drug's therapeutic index (the ratio of a dose producing toxic effects to a dose producing desired effects). The effects on the animal as a whole are studied, as well as the drug's impact on individual organs and tissues. At this state, attempts are made to determine the drug's potential side effects and hazards. This ensures a drug's safety. An Investigational New Drug application must then be filed and approved before a manufacturer can begin testing a new drug on humans. The clinical testing of the drug on human subjects occurs in three phases. In phase I, tests on normal human volunteers are used to determine whether the drug produces any toxic effects. In phase II, the drug is administered to a small pool of patients who might benefit from it (e.g., cancer patients are given a promising cancer treatment). This stage is used to determine the drug's effectiveness, as well as safety for the indicated patient population. If the drug produces no serious side effects, and is shown to be effective, the drug moves into phase III testing. Now the drug is administered to a larger population. Success in phase III allows the manufacturer to submit the drug for FDA approval. A New Drug Application, which includes supporting evidence that the drug is both safe and effective, must be approved by the FDA before the manufacturer can market the new drug. Before marketing a copy (generic version) of an already approved drug, a manufacturer must submit to the FDA an Abbreviated New Drug Application, demonstrating the bioequivalence of the new drug to the approved drug.

REFERENCES: *Federal Regulatory Directory*, 6th ed. 1990. Washington, D.C.: Congressional Quarterly, 290–320; Janssen, W. F. 1992. "The U.S. Food and Drug Law: How It Came, How It Works." *FDA Consumer*. Washington, D.C.: DHHS Pub. No. (FDA) 92–1054; Kessler, D. A., R. B. Merkatz, R. Temple, et al. 1993. "Regulation of Somatic-Cell Therapy and Gene Therapy by the Food and Drug Administration." *New England Journal of Medicine* 329: 1169–1173; Merkatz, R. B., et al. 1993. "Women in Clinical Trials of New Drugs." *New England Journal of Medicine* 329: 292–296.

AMANDA LEWIS

G

GENENTECH V. WELLCOME FOUNDATION

Genentech accused the Burroughs Wellcome Foundation in 1990 of infringing two U.S. patents directed to tissue plasminogen activator (t-PA), a protein that facilitates the breakdown of blood clots. Wellcome made two variants of human t-PA: "met-t-PA," which differed from the natural molecule by a single methionine substitution, and "FE1X," wherein an 81 amino acid deletion had eliminated two of the five functional domains identified in the t-PA protein. Genentech argued that the recited "human t-PA" of the patent claims indicated any protein having the functional characteristics of human t-PA. In contrast, Wellcome urged that human t-PA should denote only a protein having all the properties *and* the structure of human t-PA. Siding with Wellcome, the trial court interpreted human t-PA as a structural prescription, implicating the amino acid sequence of human t-PA and "natural allelic variants" thereof, which did not cover met-t-PA or FE1X literally. Nevertheless, the jury determined that both t-PA analogues were de jure "equivalents" of the patented invention and, hence, fell within the scope of protection that the subject patent claims warranted *in fairness*. The jury verdict, which prompted Burroughs Wellcome to abandon its t-PA development program, was appealed in late 1992 to the U.S. Court of Appeals for the Federal Circuit. The Federal Circuit reversed the verdict, finding that the trial court should have granted Wellcome's motion for judgment as a matter of law.

REFERENCES: *Genentech Inc. v. The Wellcome Foundation Ltd.*, 14 USPQ2d 1363 (D.Del. 1990); *Genentech Inc. v. The Wellcome Foundation Ltd.*, 24 USPQ2d 1782 (D.Del. 1992); *Genentech Inc. v. The Wellcome Foundation Ltd.*, 31 USPQ2d 1161 (Fed. Cir. 1994).

MARY R. SCHLACHTENHAUFEN

GENE TECHNOLOGY AND THE RIGHT TO REFUSE TREATMENT

A competent person's right to refuse unwanted medical treatment is well established in the common law and likely has constitutional protection (see *Cruzan v. Director, Missouri Dept of Health* and the cases cited therein), although there may be exceptions in cases involving dependents or other special circumstances. Forced treatment has, however, been permitted where treatment is necessary to further a strong or compelling state interest. Although early cases typically involved epidemics and relatively minor interventions such as vaccination, the U.S. Supreme Court has gone so far as to uphold state mandated sterilization of the "feeble-minded" (*Buck v. Bell,* 274 U.S. 200 [1927]).

Within the field of genetics, questions concerning treatment refusal rights are often raised in the context of genetic testing. Mandatory testing is thought to be inconsistent with the high value we as a society accord to individual autonomy and self-determination, and bodily integrity, as reflected in laws requiring informed consent to many medical procedures. On the other hand, a "right not to know" is morally suspect when others may be harmed by an individual's ignorance, and mandatory screening of infants and minor children may be defended in terms of the state's *parens patriae* role. Of course, this argument is weakened if treatment is unavailable or available but beyond the financial means of the parent. In any event, adequate protection of individual and familial rights is particularly important, given the nature of the information that may result from testing and the risk of psychological and economic harm such information presents merely by its existence. Most commentators conclude that the burden of proof should be on advocates for mandatory testing; the President's Commission concluded that compulsion would only be justified to protect those unable to protect themselves and should only be justified in terms of benefit to those tested—not on grounds of social utility.

The trend is to make carrier and newborn screening programs voluntary, although testing of newborns for phenylketonuria (PKU) and other genetic diseases is still mandatory in many states. Susceptibility screening is extremely limited at present, and most of the ethical issues it raises will likely concern the interest that insurers, employers, and other third parties may have in this information. Mandatory prenatal testing would be especially problematic for at least two reasons. First, for some genetic diseases, the only "treatment" available to an affected fetus is abortion. Given the U.S. Supreme Court's strong endorsement of reproductive freedom in *Roe v. Wade,* it seems unlikely that forced abortion of an affected fetus—or forced sterilization of carriers of genetic defects, for that matter—would survive court scrutiny (but see the discussion of *Buck* above). Forced treatment in such circumstances would be troubling not only as a violation of principles of autonomy and bodily integrity—and a sign of the erosion of respect for life in general and the lives of the disabled in particular—but also as an indication that it is impossible to disentangle genetics from eugenics. Second, where the available treatment is fetal surgery, the logic that supports coerced testing also supports coerced surgery—performed, of course, on the woman carrying the fetus. If one has doubts about the propriety of the latter, one should also question the legitimacy of the former.

REFERENCES: Annas, George, and Sherman Elias, eds. 1992. *Gene Mapping: Using Law and Ethics as Guides.* New York: Oxford University Press; *Buck v. Bell* 274 U.S. 200 (1927); *Cruzan v. Director, Missouri Dept of Health,* 497 U.S. 261 (1990); Elias, Sherman, and George J. Annas. 1987. *Reproductive Genetics & the Law.* Chicago: Year Book Medical Publishers; Institute of Medicine. 1994. *Assessing Genetic Risks: Implications for Health and Social Policy.* Washington, D.C.: National Academy Press; President's Commission for the Study of Ethical Problems in Medicine and Biomedical Research. 1983. *Screening and Counseling for Genetic Conditions: A Report on the Ethical, Social and Legal Implications of Genetic Screening, Counseling and Education Programs.* Washington, D.C.: The Commission; *Roe v. Wade,* 410 U.S. 113 (1973).

MARY R. SCHLACHTENHAUFEN

GENETIC COUNSELING, TRAINING AND LICENSING OF COUNSELORS, LEGAL OBLIGATIONS, LIABILITY

Genetic counseling is a process of conveying complex genetic and medical information to individuals and/or families who have or are at risk of having birth defects and/or genetic disease. In general, the information that is given to these patients includes the etiology, natural history of a condition, current testing methods, prenatal diagnosis, and recurrence risks for future pregnancies. Genetic counselors are an essential link to genetic support groups, which may provide additional information, newsletters, support, and so on. The main goal of genetic counseling is to provide accurate information in a nondirective or nonpersuasive manner. It is the responsibility of genetic counselors to provide information about all legal reproductive options available to all individuals and families regardless of one's own values and beliefs. Genetic counselors acknowledge parental beliefs, values, and choices and hope to enable their clients to make an informed, independent decision (National Society of Genetic Counselors: Prenatal Genetic Counseling Fact Sheet, 1993).

Genetic counselors are professionals with master's degrees in medical genetics and counseling. The first master's degree genetic counseling training program was established in 1969 at Sarah Lawrence College in Bronxville, New York. Since this time, more than 1,000 genetic counselors have graduated from programs in the United States and Canada (Smith, 1993). Currently, there are 18 programs in the United States and 1 each in Canada, England, and South Africa and produce approximately 100 graduates annually. In addition, there are programs that offer a clinical genetics nurse specialty within a master's level nursing program. Applicants to these programs must have nursing degrees to be considered. The genetic counseling programs require a two-year curriculum with medical, genetic, and psychological course work and supervised clinical rotations. A minimum curriculum would require seven specific course work areas and involvement in at least 50 cases as the primary genetic counselor. These 50 cases should represent a variety of counseling situations (Smith, 1993). These recommendations have been outlined by the National Society of Genetic Counselors (NSGC), who sponsored a conference in 1989 to review all recommendations for genetic counseling training programs and reevaluate the existing programs. At this time the American Board of Genetic Counseling (ABGC) is in the process of reviewing the existing training programs for accreditation. By accrediting training programs this will allow the ABMG to set educational standards and guidelines for genetic counseling.

Currently, board certification of genetic counselors is provided by the ABGC. Prior to 1993, board certification was provided by the American Board of Medical Genetics (ABMG). In 1992, the ABMG was recognized by the American Board of Medical Specialties (ABMS), and board certification of genetic counselors could no longer be offered. Individuals who graduate from an accredited genetic counseling training program are board eligible upon graduation by the ABGC. National licensing of genetic counselors is not available at this time; however, this topic has been reviewed by the NSGC. In 1989, an NSGC ad hoc Committee on Licensure was formed to explore the advantages, disadvantages, and feasibility of professional licensure. Advantages included improved quality assurance, recognition of genetic counseling as a profession, identifying individuals who may not be practicing up to standards, and involving the consumer in the control process. Difficulties of licensure arise when considering that licensure is not available on a national level and is determined by each individual state. This presents a problem for states where there are inadequate numbers of genetic counselors to warrant licensure. This may also restrict interstate mobility. Other disadvantages include possible restriction of access to the field of genetic counseling, potential increased costs to the consumer, enforcement difficulties, and licensing fees for the practitioners. In general, the complex issues surrounding licensure in 1995 are very similar to the issues described by the ad hoc committee in 1989 (Doyle, 1995). At this time, there are a few states that are addressing the issue of licensure and other credentialing alternatives such as statewide registration or certification.

The NSGC, which was formed in 1979, is an organization composed of genetic counselors, geneticists, and other professionals who are providers of genetic services. The NSGC is the leading voice of genetic counselors by promoting a network for communication, furthering the professional interests of genetic counselors and dealing with issues regarding human genetics (National Society of Genetic Counselors: Code of Ethics, 1991). The NSGC has developed a Code of Ethics to provide a standard for the conduct of genetic counselors. The Code of Ethics deals primarily with relationships between the genetic counselor and their clients, their colleagues, and society. In addition, the NSGC has adopted numerous position statements and resolutions regarding issues such as access to care, nondiscrimination, confidentiality, disclosure and informed consent, cystic fibrosis screening, reproductive freedom, prenatal substance abuse, and fetal tissue research (National Society of Genetic Counselors: Position Statements, 1991–1993; National Society of Genetic Counselors: Resolutions, 1987–1992). With the discovery of the genetic contribution to common diseases such as cancer, diabetes, and heart disease, discrimination may become a major issue in the future regarding eligibility of medical and life insurance coverage or employment. An individual may be denied access to health care based on his or her genetic predisposition to genetic disease. The NSGC opposes discrimination against an individual based on the results of genetic testing. Consideration of this information is only appropriate when used to protect the individual's best interest (National Society of Genetic Counselors: Position Statements, 1991). The legal obligations of genetic counselors consist primarily of the duty to give accurate information and, if the information is not known by the counselor, to refer the patient to another professional who may be more knowledgeable in the particular area. Genetic counselors are liable only when these duties are not fulfilled.

In summary, the genetic counseling profession is composed of individuals specifically trained in the field of human genetics. Genetic counselors are part of a rapidly growing profession. With the onslaught of new genetic information and the undertaking of the Human Genome Project, there is a great demand for individuals who can convey this complex information to families and/or individuals who are seeking information regarding birth defects and genetic disease.
REFERENCES: Doyle, D. L. 1995. Personal communication; National Society of Genetic Counselors: Code of Ethics. 1991; National Society of Genetic Counselors: Position Statements. 1991–1993; National Society of Genetic Counselors: Prenatal Genetic Counseling Fact Sheet. 1993; National Society of Genetic Counselors: Resolutions. 1987–1992; Smith, A. C. M. 1993. "Update on Master's Genetic Counseling Training Programs: Survey of Curriculum Content and Graduate Analysis Summary." *Journal of Genetic Counseling* 2(3): 197–211.

CATHERINE WICKLUND and JACQUELINE T. HECHT

GENETIC DIAGNOSIS

Weatherall (1985) identifies the four categories of genetic disorders as the following: single-gene defects, chromosomal abnormalities, congenital malformations, and genes that contribute to other diseases. We find that the single-gene defects, or monogenetic diseases, are far easier to diagnose than the majority of diseases that are polygenetic, or caused by multiple genes, as is represented by the other three genetic categories. There are three types of monogenetic modes of inheritance: autosomal dominant, autosomal recessive, and X-linked disorders.

Of the 23 pairs of chromosomes, 22 pairs are considered autosomal. The sex chromosomes, indicated with an X and a Y chromosome for males and two X chromosomes for females, consist of the twenty-third chromosomal pair. Autosomal dominant diseases can appear in an offspring if only one parent carries the gene. For heterozygous (having dissimilar genes) parents, one half of the children can inherit the disease, whereas for homozygous (having identical genes) parents, all of the children can inherit the disease. Neurofibromatosis, Huntington's disease, polycystic kidney disease, and alpha$_1$-antitrypsin deficiency are examples of autosomal dominant diseases.

Autosomal recessive diseases occur only when the offspring inherits the gene from both parents. All of the children of two homozygous parents inherit and express the gene, whereas one fourth of the children of two unaffected heterozygous parents will inherit and express the gene. Thus, two unaffected heterozygous parents can have a child who is homozygous for the gene. In other words, two parents could be unknown carriers of a disease that could manifest itself in their offspring. Schulman and Black (1993) note that there are over 1,500 autosomal recessive Mendelian defects. Cystic fibrosis, sickle-cell anemia, thalassemia, and Tay-Sachs are examples of autosomal recessive diseases.

The third type of monogenetic disorders includes the X-linked diseases. X-linked diseases are identified by a recessive gene located on the X chromosome. Hence, while females can only be carriers of the X-linked disease, the gene is always expressed in the male. The following are a few of the common X-linked diseases: hemophilia, Duchenne and Becker muscular dystrophy, fragile X syndrome, and Lesch-Nyhan disease.

The second primary category of genetic disease includes the autosomal and sex chromosome abnormalities. Autosomal cytogenetic disorders include diseases caused by one extra chromosome. These include trisomy 21 or Down syndrome, trisomy 18, and trisomy 13. Sex chromosome abnormalities are associated with aberrations of the sex chromosomes, causing congenital malformations and mental retardation. Two examples include Klinefelter syndrome and Turner syndrome.

The third type of genetic disorder includes the most serious congenital malformations, including neural tube defects, which involve defects in the skull and spinal column. Two types of neural tube defects are anencephaly and spina bifida.

The final category of genetic disease involves the identification of the genetic contribution to other diseases. Weatherall (1985) lists the following four common diseases that are thought to have a genetic component: schizophrenia, manic-depressive disorders, epilepsy, and diabetes mellitus. These multifactorial diseases, along with coronary artery disease and cancer, while showing promising results within the new gene technology, still seem to remain a genetic mystery to researchers.

Schulman and Black (1993) note that about 3 percent of all newborns have a birth defect, and most birth defects are related to genetic disease. Other researchers place this estimate as high as 5 percent of all births. Of the approximately 100,000 genes, scientists have identified some 4,000 genetic disorders (Nightingale and Goodman, 1990). As the Human Genome Project evolves, hundreds of genes continue to be identified. For example, after a lengthy ten-year search, researchers identified different nucleotide patterns of repetition on chromosome 4 in those people with Huntington's disease by using recombinant

DNA analysis. This is a new technology that isolates DNA molecules into fragments for analysis.

Nightingale and Goodman (1990) explain that recombinant DNA is made by restriction enzymes that in essence cut the DNA into fragments. These DNA fragments can then be arranged and the nucleotide sequences studied. Nightingale and Goodman note that the most accurate form of recombinant DNA technology is via direct gene detection using a gene probe. However, there is a second, indirect method used that is based on analyzing restriction fragment–length polymorphisms, or RFLPs. By examining particular segments or markers of DNA, healthy nucleotide patterns can be discerned from the diseased patterns. Huntington's disease has been identified using RFLPs.

Recently, a marker for colon cancer was found on chromosome 2. Furthermore, scientists have recently developed a diagnostic test that can determine if a person carries the defective colon cancer gene. Those individuals identified with the defective gene can then be routinely examined for polyps before they become cancerous.

We must note that the recent explosion within the field of genetic diagnosis is primarily due to two major factors: (1) the rapid progress in the development of new reproductive technologies—beginning with the first in vitro fertilization (IVF)* 20 years ago; and during the same time period, (2) the wave of right-to-abortion laws passed during the early 1970s. The literature is replete with discussions linking reproductive technology advancement with abortion rights since therapeutic abortion is the one and only treatment available for most genetic diseases identified prenatally. Consequently, we see many ethical debates revolving around the limited treatment options and genetic testing.

As Langfelder and Juengst (1993) report, once a genetic disorder has been discovered, a genetic test can easily be developed before we even understand how the gene works or whether there is treatment available. Thus, "the development of genetic testing has raised numerous concerns about autonomy, confidentiality, privacy, and equity that are exacerbated by the range of contexts in which such tests are undertaken" (Andrews et al., 1994, 254). In short, the gene identification, and subsequent testing, is outpacing the treatment and policy options available, leading to controversial solutions that the federal government seems bent on ignoring. Indeed, major genetic disorders as diverse as Alzheimer's disease and amyotrophic lateral sclerosis (better known as Lou Gehrig's disease) continue to be identified at a bewildering pace. The speed of genetic identification is so bewildering, in fact, that this unbridled knowledge is leading us as a society to new genetic technological and ethical concerns—concerns that take time to unravel.

In spite of the lack of overarching policy guidelines, federal or otherwise, regarding genetic diagnosis, we have seen specific cases within various states begin to address these complicated and evolving legal issues. For example, Wright Clayton (1993) notes the voluminous body of statutory, regulatory, and case law that attends to these kinds of issues. As she notes, the regulatory information varies from state to state, with little consensus among the various states. For example, according to Wright Clayton's research, 25 states have either statutes and/or regulations concerning a general genetics program. These states include the following: Alabama, California, Colorado, Georgia, Illinois, Iowa, Louisiana, Maine, Maryland, Massachusetts, Michigan, Minnesota, Missouri, Montana, Nevada, New Jersey, New York, North Carolina, Ohio, Tennessee, Texas, Utah, Virginia, Washington, and Wisconsin. However, only 14 states have statutes and/or regulations regarding prenatal diagnosis and include the following: Alabama, California, Hawaii, Illinois, Maine, Maryland, Missouri, Nevada, Ohio, Oregon, Tennessee, Utah, Washington, and Wisconsin. Some of these states have explicit restrictions. For example, Missouri's statute disallows referral for an abortion unless the continuation of the pregnancy would threaten the life of the mother. Tennessee's statute is even more restrictive: Prenatal diagnosis of diseases is disallowed if there is no treatment available. As Wright Clayton (1993) points out, however, over 50 percent of the states remain silent with regard to the new gene technology and genetic diagnosis.

Langfelder and Juengst (1993) note that the ethical, legal, and social implications (ELSI) program of the National Institutes of Health (NIH)* has recently initiated a consortium of eight studies to "ascertain the appropriateness of population screening for cystic fibrosis carrier status, and the best methods of education and service delivery for those who wish to be tested." This is an important step forward, not only in ensuring less arbitrary and more consistent guidelines for genetic diagnosis in general but, perhaps, in serving as the beginning of the development of formal policy considerations as well. Thus, the genetic education and screening policies formulated for these monogenetic diseases can later serve as prototypes for the genetic diagnosis of the more complicated and least understood diseases.

REFERENCES: Andrews, Lori B., Jane E. Fullarton, Neil A. Holtzman, and Arno G. Motulsky, eds. 1994. *Assessing Genetic Risks: Implications for Health and Social Policy.* Washington, D.C.: National Academy Press; Langfelder, Elinor J., and Eric T. Juengst. 1993. "Ethical, Legal, and Social Implications (ELSI) Program, National Center for Human Genome Research, National Institutes of Health." *Politics and the Life Sciences* 12(2): 273–275; Nightingale, Elena O., and Melissa Goodman. 1990. *Before Birth: Prenatal Testing for Genetic Disease.* Cambridge: Harvard University Press; Schulman, J. D., and S. H. Black. 1993. "Genetics of Some Common Inherited Diseases." *Preconception and Preimplantation Diagnosis of Human Genetic Disease,* ed. Robert G. Edwards. Cambridge: University Press; Weatherall, D. J. 1985. *The New Genetics and Clinical Practice.* Oxford: Oxford University Press; Wright Clayton, Ellen. 1993. "Reproductive Genetic Testing: Regulatory and Liability Issues." *Fetal Diagnosis and Therapy* 8 (Suppl. 1): 39–59.

PATRICIA GAIL McVEY

GENETIC ENGINEERING

Genetic engineering is the ability to synthesize genetic material, to isolate and analyze genes of interest from different organisms, and to introduce new genetic material in a target "host" organism. Genetic material introduced into an organism may be additional or variant copies of genes native to that species of organism or genes from other species. The newly introduced genetic material is often referred to as recombinant DNA, which is synonymous with genetic engineering.

The rapid rise in the technological power and ease of genetic engineering has been accompanied by a number of significant legal developments. The first major issue to arise concerned the possible pathogenicity of genetically engineered, or recombinant, bacteria. In 1971, Stanford scientist Paul Berg proposed an experiment in which a phage (a virus that infects bacteria) would be used to transfer DNA from a virus that caused cancer in monkeys (SV-40 tumor virus) into a strain of E-coli (a bacteria that is quite common and a number of varieties of which are frequently found in the human intestinal tract). Concerns that the resulting bacterial strain would be a new human pathogen led to a meeting in January 1973 at Asilomar, California, which was the first scientific meeting to consider the hazards of genetic engineering research.

In February 1975, a second meeting was held at Asilomar, California, that has become famous as the beginning of the public oversight (rather than simply a debate among scientists) over recombinant DNA experimentation. It ultimately resulted in the formation of the National Institutes of Health Recombinant DNA Advisory Committee (NIH-RAC) and the promulgation of the NIH-RAC Guidelines for Research Involving Recombinant DNA Molecules. Compliance with the guidelines is mandatory for any research involving recombinant DNA that is conducted at an institution that receives any funds from the NIH. The NIH-RAC Guidelines have been frequently revised as additional experience has justified changes in the requirements for notification (of the Institutional Biosafety Committee or the NIH-RAC), preapproval, and conditions of containment for particular classes of experiments.

After the initial concerns about the hazards of experimentation with genetic engineering had been dealt with by the creation of the NIH-RAC, a more general debate arose as to whether the entire field of genetic engineering research and development required the creation of a new federal agency that would oversee the disparate applications of genetic engineering in pharmaceuticals and health care, agriculture, and industry. The creation of such an agency was rejected, and the field of regulation was left to existing agencies and their statutory authority, supplemented by additional agency regulations where needed.

A major controversy of a very different sort was the patentability of the resulting genetically engineered microorganisms. In *Diamond v. Chakrabarty,* the Supreme Court held that living organisms were patentable subject matter as compositions of matter, where the organisms were new and useful and the result of human invention. Although *Chakrabarty* was concerned with patent claims to bacteria, the United States Patent and Trademark Office (PTO) has subsequently interpreted *Chakrabarty* as authorizing the patenting of higher organisms. The first such patent for a novel mammalian species was for the Harvard

Oncomouse, a mouse strain that had been genetically engineered to express a human oncogene. The PTO issued a patent allowing the claim to the mouse (U.S. Pat. 4,736,866) and shortly thereafter issued a patent for a method for making transgenic mammals (U.S. Pat. 7,873,191). The PTO has, however, expressed the view in *In re Allen* that patentability is limited to nonhuman higher organisms subject matter.

While the basic issue of patentability of organisms has apparently been resolved, much of genetic engineering patent law is still developing, and serious controversies remain. The Human Genome Project,* a massive international effort to map and sequence all of the 23 pairs of human chromosomes, has raised anew the wisdom of granting patents to the first scientists to isolate and sequence a particular human gene. As of this writing, such patents are being issued. Even more controversy surrounded the NIH application to seek patent protection for more than 2,000 nucleotide sequences that were parts of genes, for which the remainder of the gene sequence and the function of the associated gene were unknown. The PTO issued a preliminary rejection of the NIH application, in part on the grounds that because the function of the associated gene and protein is unknown, the claimed nucleotide sequences lack utility. In February 1994, Harold Varmus, the director of the NIH (who succeeded Bernadine Healy, director at the time of the original application), decided to abandon efforts to pursue the patent application. However, the controversy continues for private sector efforts to generate and exploit large numbers of partial gene sequences. Craig Venter, the inventor behind the abandoned NIH patent application, continues his work in conjunction with a new biotech company, Human Genome Sciences, funded in part by a large investment from major pharmaceutical company SmithKline Beecham PLC. In response, Merck, the largest U.S.-based pharmaceutical company, funded a rival effort at Washington University in St. Louis, which would place all of its sequences into the public domain, potentially undermining the value of the SmithKline/Human Genome Sciences venture.

In the mid-1980s, a major focus of debate over genetic engineering was the dangers of the release into the environment of genetically engineered organisms. Although enough experience with genetic engineering had been gathered to provide a relatively high degree of assurance that such organisms would not be human pathogens, there was a great deal of concern over the possible environmental disruption that the introduction of such novel species might produce. The NIH-RAC Guidelines required prior approval for any release into the environment of an organism containing recombinant DNA, while the U.S. Department of Agriculture (USDA) and the Environmental Protection Agency (EPA) also asserted jurisdiction over various categories of environmental release and required prior agency approval for particular experiments. Thus, there was extraordinary scrutiny given to the first such experiment, which involved a bacteria (*Pseudomonas syringae*) genetically engineered to retard ice crystallization and thus to add protection against frost on treated crops. The experiment was finally begun in April 1987 and has been followed by numerous other such experiments, without known adverse effects to date.

The ultimate goal of much of genetic research is the treatment of diseases that have a genetic component. Such treatment can take the form of providing replacement proteins for the products of defective genes (as has long been done for hemophilia and diabetes) or can take the form of gene therapy, which is the genetic engineering of human cells, either ex vivo, followed by reimplantation, or in vivo, using some form of carrier to deliver the desired gene sequences to the target cells. Gene therapy that is aimed at cells that are not involved in sexual reproduction is termed *somatic cell therapy*, while gene therapy that would affect reproductive cells would potentially create inheritable changes and is termed *germ-line gene therapy*. The NIH-RAC has set up separate procedures for reviewing experiments in gene therapy and expressly limits approval to somatic cell gene therapy experiments that have adequate safeguards against inadvertent germ-line effects. Numerous gene therapy protocols have been undertaken, and the field of gene therapy has become the subject of corporate research and development as well as university research. The Food and Drug Administration (FDA),* which must approve any such experimental delivery of genetic material to human subjects, has also published a statement of its regulatory approach. The future development of human gene therapy is certain to engender debate over its proper application and scope, leading to additional statutory and regulatory controls.

REFERENCES: Day, Kathleen, 1994. "Merck to Reveal Findings on Human Genetic Code; Move Stirs Debate over Research Secrecy." *The Washington Post*, p. b11, September 29, 1994; *Diamond v. Chakrabarty*, 100 S. Ct. 2204 (1980); FDA. "Application of Current Statutory Authorities to Human Somatic Cell Therapy Products and Gene Therapy Products." 58 FR 53248–01, October 14, 1993; *In re Allen*, 2 U.S.P.Q.2d 1425, Bd. Pat. App. (1987); National Research Council. 1988. *Mapping and Sequencing The Human Genome*. Washington, D.C.: National Academy Press; "New Startups Move in as Gene Therapy Goes Commercial." *Science* 260:914, May 14, 1993; NIH. "Points to Consider in the Design and Submission of Protocols for the Transfer of Recombinant DNA into Human Subjects." 54 FR 36698–02, August 31, 1989; NIH-RAC. "Guidelines." 52 FR 16976, May 7, 1986; Office of Science and Technology Policy "Coordinated Framework for the Regulation of Biotechnology." 51 FR 23302, June 26, 1986; Swazey, Judith P., Sorenson, James R., and Wong, Cynthia B. 1978. "Risks and Benefits, Rights, and Responsibilities: A History of the Recombinant DNA Research Controversy." S. Cal. L. Rev. 51:1019; Weis, Rick. 1994. "NIH Abandons Bid to Patent DNA Fragments Exclusivity; Could Impede Important Genetic Research, Director Says." *The Washington Post*, p. a01, February 11, 1994.

ROBERT A. BOHRER

GENETIC MONITORING AND PROFILING FOR THE WORKPLACE

The Human Genome Project* and the remarkable advances in genetic technologies for mapping and identifying human genes have accelerated interest in the ethical, legal, and social implications (ELSI) of this work and their ramifications for biomedical policy. A major policy decision of the Congress has been the commitment of (now) 5 percent of the funding for the Genome Project for its ELSI program.

For many years, there has been a nascent interest in the potential usefulness of genetic testing of workers and job applicants, as well as the potential for misuse, misunderstanding, and discrimination. The Occupational Safety and Health Act of 1970 instructs the Occupational Safety and Health Administration (OSHA) to set health standards so that, within technological feasibility, no worker, even if exposed at the level of the standard for a full working lifetime, would suffer any adverse effect.

The origin of the concept of genetic testing for susceptibility of workers to workplace hazards is generally attributed to J.B.S. Haldane. His 1938 book *Heredity and Politics* postulated that prevention of potter's bronchitis might be achieved by excluding from such work those at special risk to develop the condition. In 1980, there were prominent newspaper stories about sickle-cell screening programs at large companies, alleging restriction of jobs based on the results; the companies claimed that they were responding to explicit employee requests for on-site, company-sponsored screening, for the convenience of the employees.

Congressional hearings and an Office of Technology Assessment (OTA) study soon followed. OTA surveys reported in 1983 and 1990 showed very little use and relatively low expectation of use of genetic testing among Fortune 500 companies, utilities, and unions. In fact, there has been very little scientific effort to date in identifying and validating tests appropriate for workplace applications.

Genetic testing might be undertaken in the work setting for several quite distinguishable reasons. The first is to diagnose the underlying cause of a specific medical problem. The ethical imperative for such testing is similar to testing in the differential diagnosis of any other condition.

The second reason for testing is better termed monitoring of biomarkers of early effects, or genetic toxicology, the study of effects on the genes of various exposures. Chromosomal aberrations and sister chromatid exchanges have been monitored in persons exposed to ionizing irradiation or such chemicals as arsenic, benzene, epichlorohydrin, ethylene oxide, lead, cadmium, zinc, and vinyl chloride monomer. Complementary studies have measured mutation rates for marker genes in blood lymphocytes or sperm. This type of testing is only as good as the reliability and validity of the test and its appropriateness to the setting; these features are shared with many nongenetic tests. These tests are not widely used, nor are they proposed for routine use.

The third type of genetic testing is properly called screening of asymptomatic persons, to detect inherited predispositions to disease or other adverse responses from otherwise well-tolerated exposures related to the job. We call this field of genetics ecogenetics, reflecting the common interaction of inherited and environmental factors in disease. There are numerous relevant examples of traits that directly affect the biotransformation or the site of action of chemicals prescribed as pharmaceutical agents, pesticides, air pollutants, food additives, food contaminants, and infectious agents, like malaria organisms. The test may detect variants in the gene itself or measure protein products of the gene, namely, specific enzymes, receptors, binding proteins, or hemoglobin. The DNA test genotypes the person for that trait and should need to be performed only once, since the genes do not change and are the same in all (nucleated) cells. The protein tests determine the expression of the gene (the phenotype), which may change over time, depending on the pattern of gene expression in various tissues and the role of chemical inducers and modifiers—in the diet, for example.

Finally, genetic screening might be directed at predisposition not to effects from chemical exposures specific to the job but to common diseases, like coronary heart disease, cancers, kidney disease, neurobehavioral disorders, or breast cancer. As long as the United States lacks universal health insurance with protection against exclusions for preexisting conditions or traits, employers bear most of the high and rapidly rising cost of employment-based health insurance; they have a strong incentive to reduce their risks of financing catastrophic illnesses. Employers may do so by helping workers practice disease prevention and health promotion, by not hiring or retaining workers with high-risk profiles for such illnesses, or by both approaches. It is certain that the identification of numerous gene markers for predisposition to common diseases from spin-offs of the Human Genome Project will have the greatest application in this fourth type of testing.

As long as employers or individuals are risk rated for health insurance premiums, employers and insurance companies will logically seek lower-cost people to employ or insure. Physicians and genetic counselors are all too familiar with cases in which insurance companies have cancelled, restricted, or denied life, health, disability, mortgage, or auto insurance coverage for patients or family members. Many of these decisions were ill informed, based on carrier status, rather than homozygous inheritance of a recessive gene; based on textbook descriptions of the most severe manifestations of quite variable autosomal dominant conditions; or based on confusing genetic and nongenetic causes of similar-sounding diagnoses. The insurer has little incentive to take the risk of any uncertainties.

If employer-sponsored health promotion programs expand, workers and their representatives may negotiate through collective bargaining voluntary access to services provided by third parties. Credible protection of confidentiality against disclosure to the employer or an insurer is essential. Such voluntary services could be compatible with ethical principles of autonomy, beneficence, nonmaleficence, and justice. The employers and their contractors must comply with legal precepts of a safe and healthful workplace under the Occupational Safety and Health Act and of protections against discrimination based on race or handicap under Title VII of the Civil Rights Act of 1964, the Rehabilitation Act of 1973, and the Americans with Disabilities Act of 1990* (see references). At least ten states (Louisiana, Florida, New Jersey, North Carolina, Maryland, Missouri, California, Illinois, Iowa, Virginia) have enacted statutes to prohibit discrimination based on particular genetic traits or hereditary disorders in general (see Gostin, 1991, 141; AAAS/ABA, 1992, 97).

It is common for genetic traits to occur with different frequency in different racial or ethnic groups; therefore, testing might affect specific racial groups disproportionately, making the Civil Rights Act relevant. Title VII protects both against racially disparate treatment and racially neutral treatment that has a racially disparate impact. The Americans with Disabilities Act expressly forbids the use of medical tests to detect disabilities in employees unless the testing provides information about the individual's capability to perform the functions of the specific job. The scope of this act remains to be established, since it is silent on asymptomatic genetic traits that represent a probability of future risk of impairment.

Development and validation of genetic tests for job-related exposures must be carried out in the context of full compliance with engineering and process controls on exposures, so as to protect all workers, including those who may have various predispositions for which no tests have been conceived. Research must precede routine screening. Research can be planned and undertaken only with full participation of all parties to determine what will be done, what might be learned, who will have access to the results and who will not, and what criteria will be applied if screening were later to be considered (Omenn, 1982). A report from the Institute of Medicine (Andrews et al., 1994) recommended that legislation be enacted to prevent medical risks, including genetic risks, from being considered in decisions on whether to issue or how to price health care insurance and to forbid employers from collecting genetic information not clearly job related on prospective or current employees.

REFERENCES: American Association for the Advancement of Science/American Bar Association (AAAS/ABA) National Conference of Lawyers and Scientists. 1992. *The Genome, Ethics and the Law: Issues in Genetic Testing.* Washington, D.C.: AAAS; American Society of Human Genetics. 1994. "Statement on Genetic Testing for Breast and Ovarian Cancer Predisposition." *American Journal of Human Genetics* 55:i–iv; Andrews, Lori B., Jane E. Fullarton, Neil A. Holtzman, and Arno G. Motulsky, eds. 1994. *Assessing Genetic Risks: Implications for Health and Social Policy.* Washington, D.C.: National Academy Press; Gostin, Larry. 1991. "Genetic Discrimination: The Use of Genetically Based Diagnostic and Prognostic Tests by Employers and Insurers." *American Journal of Law and Medicine* 17: 110–144; Haldane, J. B. S. 1938. *Heredity and Politics.* London: Allen and Unwin, 179; Holtzman, Neil A. 1989. *Proceed with Caution: Predicting Genetic Risks in the Recombinant DNA Era.* Baltimore: Johns Hopkins Press; Lappe, Marc. 1983. "Ethical Issues in Testing for Differential Sensitivity to Occupational Hazards." *Journal of Occupational Medicine* 25: 797–808; Omenn, Gilbert S. 1982. "Predictive Identification of Hypersusceptible Individuals." *Journal of Occupational Medicine* 24: 369–374; Omenn, Gilbert S., Curtis J. Omiecinski, and David L. Eaton. 1990. "Eco-genetics of Chemical Carcinogens." In *Biotechnology and Human Genetic Predisposition to Disease,* ed. Charles R. Cantor, C. Thomas Caskey, Leroy E. Hood,

Daphne Kamely, and Gilbert S. Omenn. New York: Wiley-Liss, 81–93. U.S., Congress, Office of Technology Assessment. 1990. *Genetic Monitoring and Screening in the Workplace.* Washington, D.C.: Government Printing Office.

GILBERT S. OMENN

GENETIC SCREENING

In the United States, advances in genetic testing technology have frequently stimulated the enactment of state and federal laws. The interplay of scientific advance and legislative response is most apparent in newborn screening programs.

In 1962 Massachusetts became the first state to mandate newborn screening for phenylketonuria, a hereditary inborn error of metabolism that may be averted through the prompt introduction of a low phenylalanine diet. By the end of 1964, more than 30 states had enacted similar legislation. In most jurisdictions, screening was compulsory but did permit exemptions, should parents object on religious grounds. Of the 43 states that had enacted phenylketonuria screening laws by 1968, 22 authorized state agencies (usually the departments of public health) to screen for other inborn errors of metabolism as new tests became available, 9 states made explicit provision to cover the costs of dietary treatment, and the same number provided funds for public education about newborn screening (Reilly, 1975).

For three decades, newborn screening technology has steadily expanded, as have state laws and regulations intended to implement the new screening tests. Until recently, newborn screening focused exclusively on disorders that caused mental retardation but that could be averted with a specific, timely intervention (e.g., phenylketonuria [PKU] and hypothyroidism). The determination in the mid-1980s that the early use of prophylactic penicillin in infants with sickle-cell anemia could significantly reduce morbidity and mortality (Brown et al., 1989) led many states to include this disorder on the screening menu. There are active newborn screening programs in every state, the District of Columbia, and Puerto Rico. Depending on the particular jurisdiction, children may be screened for between three and eight disorders. For example, in 1990, Massachusetts screened 94,444 children for phenylketonuria, hypothyroidism, galactosemia, maple syrup urine disease, homocystinuria, adrenal hyperplasia, toxoplasmosis (an infectious disease), and the hemoglobinopathies. In the United States in 1990, all states screened children for phenylketonuria and hypothyroidism, 38 screened for galactosemia, 22 screened for maple syrup urine disease, and 42 screened for sickle-cell anemia and other hemoglobin disorders (CORN, 1992). This screening effort generated more than 15 million genetic tests. During 1990, at least 16 states did not bill families for testing; in other states, charges ranged from $5 to $30. Newborn screening programs actively follow up children with positive results suggestive of disease. They do not rigorously follow children who are identified as carriers of sickle-cell anemia, nor do they routinely provide counseling to their mothers concerning the possibility that a subsequent pregnancy could lead to the birth of a child with sickle-cell disease (CORN, 1992).

The most recent disease to be added to the roles of newborn screening is adrenal hyperplasia, a potentially fatal disorder of steroid biosynthesis that is responsive to treatment once the diagnosis is made. Authority to add to the panoply of disorders targeted by newborn screening is usually found in state regulations.

The advent of phenylketonuria screening programs created significant controversy within the medical community. Concerns about test sensitivity and specificity and fears that healthy infants with false-positive results could be harmed by being placed inappropriately on a low phenylalanine diet were paramount (Rouse, 1966). Critics also argued that screening should be conducted only after obtaining the informed consent of the mother and that programs must provide genetic counseling to the families of affected children and develop programs of public education (Bessman, 1966). In 1967 the American Academy of Pediatrics warned that premature and injudicious legislation threatened to do irreparable harm to the orderly development of mass screening. In 1975 the National Research Council (NRC) Committee for the Study of Inborn Errors of Metabolism issued a detailed report that criticized PKU screening in this country, especially when compared with programs in other nations (NRC Committee, 1975). In 1973, Maryland created a Commission on Hereditary Disorders that embraced voluntary testing, informed consent, and public and professional education. To this day, however, largely for reasons of cost, most states continue to operate mandatory testing programs.

The tremendous growth of newborn screening has created the expectation that state-run programs will succeed in promptly identifying affected children. Yet one study identified 43 children with PKU and 33 with congenital hypothyroidism who had been missed by state screening programs since their inception (Holtzman et al., 1986). Many of these children became plaintiffs in lawsuits. Despite imperfections, newborn screening has been highly successful in averting mental retardation. In 1990 the state programs identified 337 infants with PKU, 1,190 with hypothyroidism, and 86 with galactosemia in time to provide them with preventive therapy (CORN, 1992).

Carrier screening is intended to identify otherwise healthy persons who may, depending on whom they marry, be at high risk for having children with a severe genetic disorder. In the United States, population-based screening programs have been undertaken to identify carriers for sickle-cell anemia and Tay-Sachs disease. Since its start in the mid-1970s, Tay-Sachs screening has been community based, conducted largely without government intervention, and highly utilized by the Ashkenazi Jewish population, in which the disease allele is relatively common. In contrast, sickle-cell screening programs, which were introduced about 1970, were often implemented by law. Between 1970 and 1972, 12 states and the District of Columbia enacted statutes that essentially mandated carrier screening of black persons, usually by tying it to entry into the public schools or to obtaining a marriage license. Most state laws failed to provide access to genetic counseling. Concerns about privacy and genetic discrimination evoked a strong backlash against the programs (Reilly, 1975).

In 1972 the United States enacted the National Sickle Cell Anemia Control Act, which made $115 million available to state-based screening programs that were voluntary in nature and provided access to appropriate genetic counseling. The federal law quickly reduced concerns about poorly drafted compulsory state laws. The enactment of the National Sickle Cell Anemia Control Act stimulated a wave of interest in disease-specific legislation. In 1973 the National Cooley's Anemia Control Act appropriated $11 million to foster screening programs for beta-thalassemia. The then–Department of Health, Education and Welfare actively opposed disease-specific legislation and worked to develop a more comprehensive approach (Reilly, 1975).

The most significant federal legislation pertaining to genetic screening is the National Genetic Disease Act (Title XI of the Public Health Service Act), which was enacted in 1976 but not funded until 1978. The funds were used by the Maternal and Child Health (MCH) Bureau to build and improve genetic services at the state level. By 1990 all 50 states, the District of Columbia, Puerto Rico, and the Virgin Islands had enjoyed at least four years of federal support. Since then the states have undertaken some financial responsibility for these programs. In 1983, MCH began using Title XI dollars to support what is today ten multistate regional genetic networks that operate under the aegis of a Council of Regional Networks (CORN) for Genetic Services. Since 1985 the MCH genetic service program has supported the development of statewide newborn sickle-cell screening programs (MCHB, 1992).

Rapid advances in molecular biology and the advent of DNA-based diagnostics in the 1980s promise explosive growth in genetic screening. In 1983 the President's Commission for the Study of Ethical Problems in Medicine and Biomedical and Behavioral Research* issued a report on genetic screening that supported the expansion of genetic screening services as long as new tests had been properly validated and the benefits of population screening had been demonstrated in pilot studies (President's Commission, 1983).

Advances in prenatal screening have had a significant impact on the standard of care expected of obstetricians. Although there has been some state legislative activity, the major changes have occurred in response to policies adopted by professional medical groups and as a result of malpractice litigation. The age-related risk of bearing a child with Down syndrome and advances in amniocentesis and fetal chromosome analysis have created a legal duty on the part of obstetricians to inform older women about this risk and about the existence of a relevant diagnostic test. In many states during the later 1970s and 1980s, women who gave birth to children with Down syndrome, but who had not been apprised of their age-related risks, successfully sued their physicians, actions that have been called ''wrongful birth'' lawsuits (Capron, 1979). In 1992, about 300,000 women underwent amniocentesis, the vast majority to assess the fetus for chromosomal abnormalities. In about 98 percent of these tests, there was no discernible cytogenetic defect.

The rapid expansion of prenatal diagnosis in the 1970s gave birth to commercial genetic testing laboratories. In most states these have been licensed pursuant to general rules for diagnostic testing laboratories promulgated by the departments of public health. Two states, California and New York, have subjected genetic testing companies to a significantly higher level of regulatory oversight. For example, California has published comprehensive regulations that must be satisfied to operate a cytogenetics laboratory, and New York has rigorously scrutinized and at times rejected the proposed use of novel genetic testing technologies.

Even more far reaching than the advent of amniocentesis and fetal chromosome analysis has been the rise of biochemical testing to identify pregnant women who are at increased risk for bearing children with spina bifida. First utilized in England in the mid-1970s (U.K. Collaborative Study, 1977), maternal serum alpha-fetoprotein (MSAFP) testing (which measures the concentration of a chemical made by the fetus that crosses the placenta into the maternal circulation) spread rapidly to the United States. In 1986, California enacted a law that requires physicians to inform women about the availability and purpose of MSAFP testing, but most states have not become so directly involved in promoting this test (Cunningham and Kizer, 1990). About 70 percent of pregnant women in California choose to be tested. Use of MSAFP testing increased significantly in 1985 after legal counsel to the American College of Obstetricians and Gynecologists (ACOG) published a bulletin alerting physicians to a possible malpractice liability for failure to tell women about the test (ACOG, 1985). The rapid growth of MSAFP testing stimulated the American Society of Human Genetics (ASHG) to develop a policy statement on laboratory practices (ASHG, 1987). So far, only a few lawsuits have been brought against physicians for failure to inform women about this test.

During the 1990s, there has again been extensive state-based legislation concerning genetic testing (McEwen and Reilly, 1992). These laws, which have been enacted in response to fears expressed by consumers, generally limit the use that insurance companies and/or employers can make of genetic data to evaluate persons who apply for coverage or employment. In 1989 Representative Conyers (D–Mich) introduced The Human Genome Privacy Act (H.R. 1888), a bill intended to safeguard the privacy of genetic data derived through federally funded research or clinical activities. Hearings were held on an amended version of the bill in 1991 (H.R. 2045), but it was not reported out of committee. It is uncertain whether the Americans with Disabilities Act of 1990 (P.L. 101–336) extends protection from workplace discrimination to otherwise healthy persons who are predisposed to or likely later to develop a genetic disorder.

Several professional groups have contributed to policy discussions on the regulation of genetic screening. During 1990–1992 the American Society of Human Genetics cautioned that it was premature to deploy population-based screening to identify carriers of the gene for cystic fibrosis (Caskey et al., 1990). There has been relatively little research on population-based screening, especially screening intended to apprise persons about reproductive risks or to predict late-onset disease. Research is needed concerning how most effectively to provide pretest education and posttest counseling. Of special importance is the need to study the impact of genetic data on individuals and families. Recognizing the need for such activity, the National Institutes of Health (NIH) Office for Protection from Research Risks (OPRR) in 1993 issued new guidelines for conducting human genetic research, material that is relevant to the conduct of pilot screening studies (NIH, Office of Extramural Research, OPRR, 1993). Also in 1993 the Institute of Medicine (IOM) completed a major study of genetic screening and concluded that population-wide screening should be introduced only after careful technical assessment of new tests, planned provision of pretest education and posttest counseling, and consideration of related costs and benefits (IOM, 1994).

REFERENCES: American College of Obstetricians and Gynecologists (ACOG). 1985. *Professional Liability Implication of AFP Tests: Department of Professional Liability Alert.* Washington, D.C.: American College of Obstetricians and Gynecologists; American Society of Human Genetics (ASHG). 1987. "Policy Statement for Maternal Serum Alpha-Fetoprotein Screening Programs and Quality Control for Laboratories Performing Maternal Serum and Amniotic Fluid Alpha-Fetoprotein Assays." *American Journal of Human Genetics* 40: 75–82; Bessman, Samuel P. 1966. "Legislation and Advances in Medical Knowledge—Acceleration or Inhibition?" *Journal of Pediatrics* 69: 334–38. Brown, Audrey K., et al. 1989. "Care of Infants with Sickle Cell Disease." *Pediatrics* (Supp.): 897–900; Capron, Alex M. 1979. "Tort Liability in Genetic Counseling." *Columbia Law Review* 79: 618–96; Caskey, C. Thomas, et al. 1990. "The American Society of Human Genetics Statement on Cystic Fibrosis Screening." *American Journal of Human Genetics* 46: 393; Council of Regional Networks (CORN) for Genetic Services. 1992. *Newborn Screening Report: 1990.* New York: CORN Central Office; Cunningham, George C., and Kizer, Kenneth W. 1990. "Maternal Serum Alpha-Fetoprotein Screening Activities of State Health Agencies: A Survey." *American Journal of Human Genetics* 47: 899–903; Holtzman, Carol S., et al. 1986. "Descriptive Epidemiology of Missed Cases of Phenylketonuria and Congenital Hypothyroidism." *Pediatrics* 78: 553–58; Institute of Medicine (IOM) Committee on Assessing Genetic Risks. 1994. *Assessing Genetic Risks: Implications for Health and Social Policy.* Washington, D.C.: National Academy of Sciences; Maternal and Child Health Bureau (MCHB). 1992. *Fact Sheet: Genetic Services Program.* Washington, D.C.: U.S. Department of Health and Human Services; McEwen, Jean E., and Reilly, Philip R. 1992. "State Legislative Efforts to Regulate Use and Potential Misuse of Genetic Information." *American Journal of Human Genetics* 51: 637–47; National Institutes of Health, Office of Extramural Research, Office for Protection from Research Risks. 1993. *Protecting Human Research Subjects: Institutional Review Board Guidebook.* Bethesda: NIH; NRC Committee for the Study of Inborn Errors of Metabolism. 1975. *Genetic Screening: Programs, Principles, and Research.* Washington, D.C.: National Academy of Sciences; President's Commission for the Study of Ethical Problems in Medicine and Biomedical and Behavioral Research. 1983. *Screening and Counseling for Genetic Conditions.* Washington, D.C.: U.S. Government Printing Office; Reilly, Philip R. 1975. "Genetic Screening Legislation." In *Advances in Human Genetics,* ed. Harry Harris and Kurt Hirschhorn. New York: Plenum; Rouse, Bruce M. 1966. "Phenylalanine Deficiency Syndrome." *Journal of Pediatrics* 69: 246–49. U.K. Collaborative Study of Alpha-Fetoprotein in Relation to Neural Tube Defects. 1977. "Maternal Serum Alpha-Fetoprotein Measurement in Antinatal Screening for Anencephaly and Spina Bifida in Early Pregnancy." *Lancet* 1: 1323–32.

PHILIP R. REILLY

GRISWOLD V. CONNECTICUT

In November 1961, the executive director and medical director of Planned Parenthood League of Connecticut were arrested for violating a state statute that made it a crime to use "any drug, medicinal article or instrument for the purpose of preventing conception" or to "assist, abet, counsel, cause, hire or command another" to do so. The Circuit Court for the Sixth Circuit in New Haven found the two health care providers guilty and fined them $100 each. After their convictions were affirmed on appeal by the appellate division and the Connecticut Supreme Court of Errors, the defendants sought review by the U.S. Supreme Court. In a 7–2 decision issued on June 7, 1965 (381 U.S. 479), the U.S. Supreme Court reversed the convictions, finding that the Connecticut law violated a married couple's constitutional right to privacy, derived from the "penumbras" and "emanations" of the Bill of Rights. The majority opinion cited a number of cases recognizing a "zone of privacy" protected by the First, Third, Fourth, Fifth, and Ninth Amendments and asserted that marriage is "a relationship lying within the zone."

Seven years later, in *Eisenstadt v. Baird,* 405 U.S. 438 (1972), the Supreme Court extended the *Griswold* holding to all individuals when it struck down a Massachusetts law making it a felony for anyone except a physician or pharmacist to sell, lend, or give away any contraceptive to an unmarried couple or individual, or to offer to do so. The 6–1 opinion held, "If the right of privacy means anything, it is the right of the individual, married or single, to be free from unwarranted governmental intrusion into matters so fundamentally affecting a person as the decision whether to bear or beget a child." Subsequently, in 1977, in *Carey v. Population Services,* 431 U.S. 678 (1977), the Supreme Court further extended that right to young people, striking down a New York statute severely limiting the sale and distribution of contraceptives to minors. In a 7–2 decision, the Supreme Court struck down a law criminalizing the sale or distribution of contraceptives to minors under age 16 or to advertise or display contraceptives. In its ruling, the Supreme Court upheld a district court finding that the law violated the First Amendment as well as the right to privacy found in *Griswold, Roe,* and their progeny.

REFERENCES: Chesler, Ellen. 1992. *Woman of Valor: Margaret Sanger and the Birth Control Movement in America.* New York: Simon & Schuster; Gordon, Linda. 1990. *Woman's Body, Woman's Right, Birth Control in America.* New York: Penguin Books;

Hatcher, Robert, et al. 1990. *Contraceptive Technology 1990–1992.* New York: Irvington; Potts, M. 1988. ''Birth Control Methods in the United States.'' 20 *Fam. Plan. Persp.* 288.

ANDREA MILLER

H

HARRIS V. McRAE

In September 1976, Cora McRae, a low-income pregnant woman—joined by the New York City Health and Hospitals Corporation, Planned Parenthood, and a private physician—filed suit in federal district court against the "Hyde Amendment," a limitation on the use of federal Medicaid funds for abortions first enacted by Congress that year. An amendment to the fiscal year 1977 appropriation for the Department of Health, Education, and Welfare, the measure barred the use of federal Medicaid funds for abortions except "when the life of the mother would be endangered if the fetus were carried to term." Medicaid, Title XIX of the Social Security Act, is a joint federal/state program established by Congress in 1965 to provide health care to low-income individuals. Plaintiffs argued that by limiting federal Medicaid reimbursement to cases of life endangerment while covering the costs of childbirth, the Hyde Amendment violated the First, Fourth, Fifth, and Ninth Amendments of the U.S. Constitution. The U.S. District Court for the Eastern District of New York issued a preliminary injunction against enforcement of the Hyde Amendment in October 1976. Although not a final judgment on the measure's constitutionality, the order implied that the district court would ultimately strike down the Hyde Amendment. The secretary of Health, Education, and Welfare appealed the granting of the preliminary injunction to the U.S. Supreme Court.

Before the justices could review the challenge to the Hyde Amendment, three decisions were issued on June 20, 1977, concerning state laws and regulations limiting abortion coverage in the Medicaid program or abortion services in public facilities. In *Maher v. Roe,* 432 U.S. 464 (1977), two Medicaid-eligible women challenged Connecticut's regulations concerning state Medicaid benefits for first-trimester abortions, including preauthorization for the procedure, certification that an abortion is "medically necessary," and a requirement that the procedure be performed in an accredited hospital or clinic. In their lawsuit, the low-income women noted that similar restrictions did not apply to other medical procedures, particularly those associated with childbirth. In a 6–3 ruling, the U.S. Supreme Court held that the stringent level of constitutional protection afforded to the right to privacy in the context of a criminal abortion statute does not extend to a state benefits scheme. Holding that a state may constitutionally promote childbirth over abortion in its Medicaid program, the Court stated that "[t]he indigency that may make it difficult—and in some cases, perhaps, impossible—for some women to have abortions is neither created nor in any way affected by the Connecticut regulation." In *Beal v. Doe*, 432 U.S. 438 (1977), a 7–2 majority of the Supreme Court also rejected a challenge by several Medicaid-eligible women to Pennsylvania's limitation of coverage for abortions to those certified as "medically necessary" by two physicians in addition to the attending physician. Although upholding the challenged provisions, including a requirement that the procedure be performed in an accredited hospital, the majority sent the case back to the lower courts for a review of the two-physician certification requirement. Finally, in *Poelker v. Doe*, 432 U.S. 519 (1977), the Court issued a per curiam opinion expressing the views of six justices, which relied on the reasoning in *Maher v. Doe* to uphold a St. Louis policy prohibiting the performance of abortions in city-owned hospitals unless continued pregnancy would result in a woman's physiological injury or death. The Court held that, "as a policy choice," the city may "provide publicly financed hospital services for childbirth without providing corresponding services for nontherapeutic abortions."

Rather than hearing the appeal in *McRae*, on June 29, 1977, the Supreme Court vacated the preliminary judgment and ordered the district court to further consider the case in light of the Supreme Court's June 20 decisions. On remand, additional plaintiffs were allowed to intervene in the case, including four Medicaid-eligible women, additional physicians, and the Women's Division of the Board of Global Ministries of the United Methodist Church as well as two of its officers. In an amended complaint, the women, health care providers, and religious plaintiffs argued that the court could avoid ruling on the constitutionality of the Hyde Amendment because Title XIX requires state Medicaid programs to cover medically necessary abortions even when federal reimbursement is not available. Plaintiffs further asserted that the Hyde Amendment violates the due process clause of the Fifth Amendment and the establishment and free exercise clauses of the First Amendment. The district court conducted a trial between August 1977 and September 1978, issuing an opinion in January 1980 finding that the Hyde Amendment was a violation of the constitutional guarantees of equal protection and free exercise of religion. Plaintiffs then appealed to the U.S. Supreme Court.

In a 5–4 decision on June 30, 1980 (4481 U.S. 297), the U.S. Supreme Court upheld the funding restriction, finding that "the Hyde Amendment . . . places no governmental obstacle in the path of a woman who chooses to terminate her pregnancy, but rather, by means of unequal subsidization of abortion and other medical services, encourages alternative activity deemed in the public interest.'' The Court further found that ''the financial constraints that restrict an indigent woman's ability to enjoy the full range of constitutionally protected freedom of choice are the product not of governmental restrictions on access to abortions, but rather of her own indigency.'' The majority found that the establishment clause was not violated by a governmental policy that ''may coincide with the religious tenets of the Roman Catholic Church'' and refused to rule on the free exercise of religion arguments after finding that the plaintiffs did not have standing to raise such constitutional claims. Before reaching the constitutional issues, the Court also rejected plaintiffs' argument that states participating in the Medicaid program are required by Title XIX of the Social Security Act to fund ''medically necessary'' abortions for which federal funds are not available. In *Williams v. Zbaraz,* 448 U.S. 358 (1980), which was issued with *Harris v. McRae,* a 5–4 majority of the Court also upheld an Illinois statute prohibiting the use of state medical assistance funds for abortions not necessary to save a woman's life.

Every year since 1976, the Hyde Amendment has been reenacted, barring federal reimbursement for low-income women's abortions except in extremely limited circumstances. Similar restrictions have been attached to numerous other federal programs, at times affecting millions of U.S. citizens, including government employees, members of the armed services and the Peace Corps, Native Americans on reservations, and women in federal prisons. Following the cutoff of federal coverage for abortion services, more than two thirds of the state legislatures adopted similar limitations on state Medicaid funds. As a result, low-income women who obtain safe and legal procedures must often postpone terminating their pregnancies, using resources earmarked for family necessities, and exposing themselves to the risks associated with later abortions; others endanger their lives and health trying to self-abort. Studies estimate that between 18 and 23 percent of Medicaid-eligible women living in states that do not fund abortions carry unwanted pregnancies to term because they cannot afford to pay for the procedure.

REFERENCES: Donovan, Patricia. 1995. *The Politics of Blame: Family Planning, Abortion and the Poor.* New York: Alan Guttmacher Institute; Frankfort, Ellen, with Kissling, Frances. 1978. *Rosie, the Investigation of a Wrongful Death.* New York: Dial Press; Henshaw, Stanley K., and Wallisch, Lynn S. 1984. ''The Medicaid Cutoff and Abortion Services for the Poor.'' 16 *Family Planning Perspective* 170; Trussel, James, et al. 1980. ''The Impact of Restricting Medicaid Financing for Abortion.'' 12 *Family Planning Perspective* 120.

ANDREA MILLER

THE HASTINGS CENTER

The Hastings Center was established in 1969, in Hastings-on-Hudson, New York, to carry out research and educational programs on ethics and the life sciences. The center was very much a child of its times. The 1960s had seen an unprecedented number of important clinical developments, which taken together came to transform American medicine and that of other countries as well. They included kidney dialysis, organ transplantation, oral contraception, the widespread use of high-technology neonatal and adult intensive care units, the common use of respirators and advanced forms of artificial hydration and nutrition, and a wide range of problems concerning the care of terminal patients, including that of the legal determination of death.

Simultaneously with those technological developments, posing moral problems of a kind unknown to traditional medical ethics, came a number of cultural changes. They centered on the rights of women and minorities, a new concern for the environment, and the changing relationship between medicine and the wider society, one that moved sharply in the direction of wider public oversight and participation. Revelations about the abuse of human subjects in medical research, concern about the doctor-patient relationship, and the growing cost of health care added additional impetus to the newly emerging field of bioethics.

Beginning in 1968, Daniel Callahan, a philosopher by training, became interested in starting a research organization devoted to these problems. At that time, no such organization wholly devoted to these issues existed, and most medical schools did not offer a course or even much time to ethical problems. In the winter of 1969, Callahan talked with a Hastings neighbor, Willard Gaylin, a psychiatrist, who liked the idea and thereafter worked with him to organize the center. The center began with the name of the "Institute of Society, Ethics and the Life Sciences," a name that was descriptive, if cumbersome. The center was organized as a nonprofit, nonpartisan organization, and in 1969 and early 1970, it was legally established and a board of directors chosen.

By the fall of 1970, Callahan and Gaylin had raised enough money to open a small office and hire its first staff members. Early support for the center came from the National Endowment for the Humanities, John D. Rockefeller III, the Rockefeller Foundation, and some small gifts. The center from the outset established a number of ideals for its work: that it would genuinely be nonpartisan, open to a variety of viewpoints; that it would be interdisciplinary, giving no discipline intellectual primacy (though physicians, lawyers, philosophers, and theologians have been its most frequent staff members); that it would try to balance research and educational work; and that it would aim to blend a mix of theoretical and practical issues. In 1971, the *Hastings Center Report* was first published, now widely considered the preeminent journal in the field of bioethics with a circulation of 12,000. In 1978, another journal was started, *IRB: A Review of Human Subjects Research.*

During its first decade, The Hastings Center (as it came to be called informally until its name was legally changed) focused on four major areas of inquiry: the problem of death and the termination of treatment; developments in the field of genetics; behavior control (by which was meant the use of medical means to control or manipulate behavior); and issues of population and sexual reproduction. Continuing work was also carried out on the doctor-patient relationship and human subject research. Efforts were made to work on the foundations of bioethics as well, particularly with a major project on the foundations of bioethics and its relationship to the sciences. Additional theoretical projects looked at the relationship between individual good and common good (and Callahan and Gaylin became known as skeptical of, and resistant to, the heavy focus on autonomy that had come to mark the field in the 1970s; their own bias was in a more communitarian direction, though that was by no means shared by all staff members over the years).

By the 1980s, the staff and budget of the center had grown significantly, and by the early 1990s, the staff consisted of 30 full-time employees and an annual budget near $2.5 million. As time went on, moreover, the center engaged in an increasingly wide range of activities, particularly of an educational kind. Through workshops, a visiting scholars program, and frequent consultations, the center undertook to provide an introduction to the field or particular issues to a large number of people. Beginning in the mid-1980s, its educational work was extended to an international context.

As the mid-1990s approached, the center was working on a wide range of research issues, which had now come to include environmental ethics as well as its traditional interest in bioethics. Its international educational work was complemented by two long-term international projects, one on the goals of medicine, the other on the allocation of resources to the elderly. Other research projects at the center looked at technology assessment, the moral issues occasioned by long-term contraceptives, ethical issues in the care of Alzheimer's patients, and a number of projects touching on the allocation of health care resources. With the help of some special grants, the center has taken a particular interest in central Europe, developing a relationship with the Charles University Medical School in Prague and bringing a steady stream of scholars from that part of the world to the center.

The Hastings Center is governed by a 24-person board of directors. Its annual budget is sustained by individual and corporate gifts, by a membership program, by government and private grants, and by a small endowment. The center is now located on the campus of Pace University (though not affiliated with the university) in Briarcliff Manor, New York, about 25 miles north of New York City.

REFERENCES: "Hastings Center, Institute of Society, Ethics and the Life Sciences." 1982. In *The Greenwood Encyclopedia of American Institutions.* Vol. 5: *Research Institutions and Learned Societies.* Westport, CT: Greenwood Press.

DANIEL CALLAHAN

HEALTH CARE ETHICS

The term *health care ethics* is used in preference to *bioethics* to indicate the relation to the health of human subjects and in preference to *medical ethics* to include topics related to the promotion of human health that are not directly the responsibility of medical professionals, such as the environmental and spiritual relationships of the human person.

Thus, an ethics of health care needs to concern itself with the following principal areas. First, it must deal with establishing an adequate view of human health as the optimum functioning of the human person as a whole, since this is the goal of health care. Since there are a variety of different views current on the nature and dignity of the human person, a critique of these views and an attempt to synthesize them in a balanced and unified model are indispensable in order to adequately ground ethical judgments about the means to this goal.

Second, this model of the healthy human person must be related to the wider community and the issues of the public organization of institutions and policies for the promotion of health. None of us can achieve health or maintain it in isolation from the community in which we live, and we all have ethical responsibilities to protect and promote the rights of others to health.

Third, since within the community the primary responsibility for understanding the effective means to health is assigned to the learned profession of medicine, it is necessary to understand the ethical traditions and duties of this major profession. The heart of all the learned professions is the relation of trust and confidentiality that is required between the professional who guides a client in matters of the gravest, intimate, and personal importance. The health care professional must respect the human dignity of the person seeking healing and guidance in healthy living, avoiding any tendency to "paternalism" or to treat the patient as a mere object of technical manipulation and experimentation.

Fourth, the foregoing understanding of the goals of health care and the responsibilities of those who promote it also needs to be correlated with ethical theories that provide principles and procedures by which ethically sound decisions may be achieved. In our society, ethical principles derived from many religious traditions compete with others of a secular type, and these secular ethics derive from a variety of philosophies. All these different ethical systems also suffer distortion from special interests and advocacies that render them more ideologies than honest efforts to achieve realistic moral truth. Consequently, health care ethics must be a critical and discriminating discipline that exposes unethical positions on ethical issues and seeks to establish principles that have a rational and objective foundation that can really contribute to public debate and consensus.

In the light of such objective principles, insofar as we are able to arrive at them in the present state of knowledge, a health care ethics will proceed to identify the chief ethical issues that arise in our social and personal efforts toward human health, from the very beginning of human life to its earthly end. Today these chiefly include the ethical issues involved in the management of the environment, in natural and artificial reproduction and genetic therapy and control, in the prevention of disease, in the surgical and chemical manipulation and reconstruction of the body, in the relation of psychological and somatic health, and in the care of the aging and the dying. Because ethics deals with the whole person, health care ethics also must discuss the spiritual meaning of the experiences of suffering, the transmission of life, the life struggle, and the dying process as they transcend human control in both their positive and negative effects on human health.

The development of a discipline of health care ethics is, of course, a part of the history of bioethics and medical ethics in general; but this special discipline has differentiated itself as a distinctive study only in the last half a century. In the United States, which in many ways has pioneered in this development, two factors have been paramount. The first has been that the advance of ''high-tech'' medicine and professional specialization has caused a breakdown of the relationship between the physician and the patient, so many patients feel they are neither known nor respected as persons but have become the victims of a medical machine. Consequently, they resort to malpractice litigation and to alternative forms of healing. A second factor is the breakdown of an ethical consensus in American culture as the result of rapid social change and secularization. Hence, both professionals and patients turn to ethicists and ethical committees to resolve ethical disagreements.

These two factors have led to an enormous literature and the development of a distinct discipline dealing with the topics just mentioned. In some areas, wide agreement has been reached, for example, on the question of the need for free and informed consent by persons to any medical intervention. In other areas, however, such as abortion or prolongation of life, debate continues to rage. Such debate cannot be profitable unless it is grounded in a critical discipline.

REFERENCES: Ashley, Benedict M., and Kevin D. O'Rourke. 1994. *Ethics of Health Care.* Washington, D.C.: Georgetown University Press; Beauchamp, Tom L., and James Childress. 1989. *Principles of Biomedical Ethics.* New York: Oxford University Press; Kelly, David F. 1979. *The Emergence of Roman Catholic Medical Ethics in North America.* New York: Edwin Mellen Press; Pellegrino, Edmund D., and David C. Thomasma. 1988. *For the Patient's Good: The Restoration of Beneficence in Health Care.* New York: Oxford University Press; Pellegrino, Edmund D., and David C. Thomasma. 1993. *The Virtues in Medical Practice.* New York: Oxford University Press; Veatch, Robert M. 1991. *The Patient-Physician Relation.* Bloomington: Indiana University Press.

BENEDICT M. ASHLEY

THE HEMLOCK SOCIETY USA

The Hemlock Society USA is the voice of a grassroots movement for Americans who want control over their end-of-life decisions, including the option of physician aid-in-dying. The society empowers patients through its promotion of patients' rights and acts as an information clearinghouse for those involved in legislative action and court cases dealing with physician aid-in-dying.

Since its inception in 1980, Hemlock initiated a national conference on voluntary euthanasia, was instrumental in laying the groundwork for living will laws, drafted the Humane and Dignified Death Act (the first piece of right-to-die legislation), published the best-selling *Final Exit,* and was a major force in the passage of Oregon's Measure 16, the first law in the United States to legalize physician aid-in-dying. The society's 85 chapters in 40 states attest to the grass-roots nature of this right-to-die organization.

The Hemlock Society USA is a nonprofit educational and research organization and depends on membership fees, donations, and the sale of books and literature for its existence. It is headquartered in Eugene, Oregon.

REFERENCES: Burnell, George M. 1993. *Final Choices: To Live or Die in an Age of Medical Technology.* New York: Insight Books, Dworkin, Ronald. 1993. *Life's Dominion: An Argument About Abortion, Euthanasia and Individual Freedom.* New York: Alfred A. Knopf; Humphry, Derek. 1991. *Final Exit: The Practicalities of Self-Deliverance and Assisted Suicide for the Dying.* Eugene, OR: The Hemlock Society USA; Humphry, Derek, and Ann Wickett. 1986. *The Right to Die: Understanding Euthanasia.* New York: Harper and Row; Quill, Timothy. 1993. *Death and Dignity: Making Choices and Taking Charge.* New York: Norton; *TimeLines, Newsletter of The Hemlock Society USA.* 1980–1995. Kris Larson and Scott Judd, eds. Eugene, OR: The Hemlock Society USA.

KRIS A. LARSON

HIV TESTING

The development in 1982 of an enzyme-linked immunosorbent assay (ELISA) to detect antibodies to human immunodeficiency virus (HIV) provided the means to easily and inexpensively test individuals and screen populations. Although it does not test for HIV directly, ELISA can identify those persons who have been exposed to it. Because of problems with false positives if a person tests positive, ELISA is repeated. If that test is positive, another form, the Western blot, is used. If the person tests positive on all three, the chance of HIV infection approaches 100 percent. On the other hand, because of the lag time of three to six months in the body's production of antibodies, a negative test can never be interpreted as the absence of HIV. This can lead to a false assurance that one is not infected, but more important, it means that testing is no panacea to be used indiscriminately.

Testing for HIV has been carried out to protect the blood supply, to ensure that infected patients obtain appropriate medical treatment, and to promote behavior changes to reduce HIV transmission. "Knowledge of HIV infection status can be beneficial in assisting individuals to adopt behavior that will reduce their chances of becoming infected or infecting others" (Anderson et al., 1992, 1535).

The presence of an accurate, inexpensive test creates policy issues concerning its proper use. Because acquired immunodeficiency syndrome (AIDS) to date is concentrated in identifiable high-risk groups, any screening efforts targeted at those groups threatens further stigmatization. When insurance companies, employers, or other third parties gain access to such information, discrimination is possible despite being prohibited by the Americans with Disabilities Act.*

In the mind of the public, the distinction between testing positive for HIV and having AIDS is not clearly understood. Affected children have had to obtain court orders to attend school, and in some cases, physical intimidation was used against their parents. This near hysteria about AIDS among some segments of the population should not be surprising in light of the rapidity and sensational way in which AIDS has become a top mass media story. The early ambivalence of the experts concerning modes of transmission, incubation period, and most recently, the effectiveness of preventive measures does not instill confidence in a public that has been told that AIDS represents an epidemic rivaling the black plague.

Testing has therefore become a difficult policy issue, with strong feelings on both sides about its use. Although there is little opposition to voluntary testing, the possibility of mandatory screening programs of various target groups has been most controversial. Opponents argue that because of the stigmatization surrounding AIDS and the lack of a cure, once a person is identified, the issue centers on the question of privacy. Moreover, mandatory screening of any groups makes little sense if it fails to produce changes in behavior needed to impede the spread of AIDS, and this raises other questions concerning notification of sexual partners of infected persons, employers of infected workers, or coworkers. In other words, once the screening is done, what we do with the information becomes problematic. Opponents fear pressures to further isolate, stigmatize, or potentially quarantine persons identified as HIV positive.

In contrast, proponents of mandatory screening for HIV argue that the health of the public takes precedence over individual privacy, particularly when the disease is fatal. As a result, mandatory screening programs have been initiated by the U.S. military, the Department of State, and the Department of Labor. Furthermore, there are currently laws in several states and proposals in others to require screening in prisons, hospitals, or drug-dependence clinics and surveillance and contact testing. Often these proposals (and laws) have been advocated (and passed) despite opposition from the medical profession and health professionals.

One of the major issues in testing policy, then, is how to operationalize a policy that is effective yet not counterproductive. Because HIV is not distributed equally throughout the population, any testing program, voluntary or mandatory, must target particularly high-risk groups. Intravenous drug users, gay males, and hemophiliacs have been obvious target populations. Other groups have been selected often either because they were readily available (i.e., prisoners, immigrants, hospital patients, members of the armed forces, persons applying for marriage licenses) or because they were in occupations where public health concerns were high (i.e., prostitutes, health care workers, food workers). In each of these instances, however, the critical questions were: How will the data collected be used? Who will get the results of testing? What will be done to persons who test positive?

One reason to test persons who are at high risk is so that early therapy can be initiated. Although fully effective treatment is not yet available, antiretroviral drugs can delay the progression of HIV disease and increase survival for some patients. Evidence suggests that early access to such care is critical and even more likely to be so in the future when earlier therapy interventions become available. Evidence also demonstrates that most HIV-infected persons are unaware of their status. Too often they learn of their HIV infection only after the onset of an opportunistic infection or other serious HIV-related disease. One result is that only about 20 percent of eligible persons are receiving therapy or needed counseling.

The dilemma in such testing is clear. On the one hand, it is in the patient's interest to know his or her status so that therapy can be initiated and for intensive counseling that might alter behavior and reduce transmission of HIV. On the other hand, HIV testing in hospitals raises questions of confidentiality and discrimination found in all testing programs. Although it could be more efficient to test only those patients from high-risk categories, many persons deny high-risk behavior. Moreover, the compliance rate for voluntary testing when sensitively presented is high. In one study at Johns Hopkins Hospital, 96 percent of 351 patients agreed to be tested, and 15 percent of those were found to be seropositive (Quinn, 1992, 487).

Testing of patients has become even more critical due to outbreaks of drug-resistant tuberculosis (TB) among hospitalized HIV-positive patients. According to Stoeckle and Douglas (1993, 223), the risk of active TB among persons with HIV is "exceedingly high," and increased susceptibility of HIV-positive persons has contributed to outbreaks not only in hospitals but in other institutional settings including prisons and residential facilities for drug treatment. Although Quinn (1992, 488) argues that testing will benefit not only the health workers and other patients but also the HIV patient who can be given a reliable tuberculin skin test and needed treatment, others see a danger that the resulting need for increased protection of the public health will create a climate in which the rights of individuals with TB and HIV may be disregarded (Bayer, Dubler, and Landesman, 1993, 649).

There has been considerable debate over the testing of patients in order to protect health care workers who are vulnerable especially when drawing blood or performing invasive procedures. As of March 1993, at least 36 health workers had been infected in occupational exposures according to the Centers for Disease Control (CDC). Of the 36, 14 were laboratory technicians, 12 were nurses, and 4 were nonsurgical M.D.s, and almost all were infected by needlesticks. Of the 36, 8 have developed AIDS. In addition, 75 other cases of suspected infection of health workers on the job have been reported but not fully verified.

Although the initial concern over health care workers focused on the threat of transmission of HIV from infected patients to the workers, the verified transmission from an infected Florida dentist to five of his patients in the late 1980s heightened public awareness and generated considerable controversy. Moreover, because there were no identifiable breaches from standard infection control practices in the dentist's office to explain the transmissions, the reliability of these practices was called into question. In response, calls for restrictions on the professional activities of some health care workers were intensified, congressional hearings were held, and the Centers for Disease Control was under pressure to modify its guidelines.

REFERENCES: Anderson, John E., Ann M. Hardy, Kathy Cahill, and Sevgi Aral. 1992. "HIV Antibody Testing and Posttest Counselling in the United States." *American Journal of Public Health* 82(11): 1533–35; Bayer, Ronald, Nancy Neveloff Dubler, and Sheldon Landesman. 1993. "The Dual Epidemics of Tuberculosis and AIDS: Ethical and Policy Issues in Screening and Treatment." *American Journal of Public Health* 83(5): 649–54; Mishu, Ben, and William Schaffner. 1993. "HIV-Infected Surgeons and Dentists: Looking Backward and Looking Forward." *Journal of the American Medical Association* 269(14): 1843–44; Quinn, Thomas C. 1992. "Screening for HIV Infection: Benefits and Costs." *New England Journal of Medicine* 327(7): 486–88; Stoeckle, Mark Y., and R. Gordon Douglas, Jr. 1993. "Infectious Diseases." *Journal of the American Medical Association* 270(2): 223–24.

See also **AIDS VACCINE AND TREATMENT RESEARCH.**

ROBERT H. BLANK

HODGSON V. MINNESOTA

In July 1981, pregnant young women and mothers of pregnant minors, four women's health clinics, and two physicians filed suit in the U.S. District Court for the District of Minnesota seeking to prevent enforcement of the state's two-part statute concerning parental notification prior to a young woman's abortion. The law required written notice to both biological parents of an unemancipated minor at least 48 hours prior to the procedure, except in extremely limited circumstances; a second portion of the law provided that should this requirement be found unconstitutional, it would be enforced with the addition of a judicial bypass proceeding during which a young woman could seek to convince a judge that she is "mature and capable of giving informed consent" to an abortion or that the procedure without notice to both parents would serve her "best interests." Plaintiffs argued that the measure violated the Fourteenth Amendment's guarantees of due process and equal protection. The district court immediately granted a temporary restraining order preventing only the provision without a bypass option from taking effect and subsequently issued a preliminary injunction against that measure in March 1982. The two-parent notification requirement with a judicial bypass option was enforced for four and a half years before the district court began holding a trial on the constitutionality of both provisions in February 1986. Nine months later, the court issued a permanent injunction blocking enforcement of the entire statute, finding that the lack of a bypass rendered the first section unconstitutional, while the second provision was invalid due to the mandated waiting period even in the context of a bypass option; the court further indicated that the consent requirement with a bypass failed to serve the state's interests. The state of Minnesota appealed to the U.S. Court of Appeals for the Eighth Circuit.

Although an August 1987 decision by a three-judge panel of the appellate court affirmed the lower court's opinion, Minnesota was granted a rehearing, and the appeals court vacated and withdrew its prior opinion three months later. In August 1988, a full panel of the appeals court issued an opinion agreeing with the district court and the three-judge panel that Minnesota could not constitutionally require a minor to notify her parents of her intention to have an abortion without providing a judicial bypass option. Nonetheless, the court reversed the previous panel and the district court, holding that the notification requirement with a bypass alternative was constitutional and that the mandatory waiting period of 48 hours was not a significant burden on young women. The U.S. Court of Appeals for the Eighth Circuit then granted a stay of its ruling pending U.S. Supreme Court review, which was sought by both parties.

In a 5–4 opinion on June 25, 1990 (497 U.S. 417), the Court struck down the first portion of the statute, asserting that "the requirement that *both* parents be notified, whether or not both wish to be notified or have assumed responsibility for the upbringing of the child, does not reasonably further any legitimate state interest." Although unable to agree on specific reasoning, five justices found constitutional the parental notification provision that provided for a judicial bypass. The Court's decision in *Hodgson* was issued along with a ruling in *Ohio v. Akron Reproductive Health Center,* 497 U.S. 502 (1990), finding constitutional a requirement that a physician notify or obtain the written consent of one parent at least 24 hours prior to performing an abortion on an unmarried and unemancipated minor; should the woman and an adult sibling, step-, or grandparent each certify that the minor fears physical, sexual, or severe emotional abuse from one of her parents, notification can be given to that adult relative. The statute also contained a bypass mechanism through which a court could either grant a minor the right to consent or provide constructive authorization through its inaction. A 6–3 majority found that the bypass mechanism in the Ohio law satisfied the Court's previously announced requirements and that the statute was therefore constitutional.

The decisions in *Hodgson* and *Akron* were consistent with a series of decisions beginning in the mid-1970s. During that decade, the U.S. Supreme Court upheld state laws mandating parental consent or notification prior to a young woman's abortion, as long as there was an "alternative" for waiving the requirement. In its first ruling on minors and abortion, in *Planned Parenthood of Central Missouri v. Danforth,* 428 U.S. 52 (1976), a 5–4 majority of the Court struck down a requirement that an unmarried minor obtain one parent's written consent prior to an abortion, reasoning that the law provided an unconstitutional veto power to a third party. A unanimous decision issued on the same day, however, in *Bellotti v. Baird,* 428 U.S. 132 (1976) (*Bellotti I*), held that a Massachusetts law requiring a woman under the age of 18 to obtain the consent of both parents or a judge prior to an abortion could be interpreted in a manner that did not conflict with *Planned Parenthood v. Danforth.* Specifically, the Court noted that the statute could be construed to allow either a "mature minor" or a minor whose "best interests" would be served by obtaining an abortion to seek a court order allowing the procedure without first consulting her parents. When the Massachusetts law came before the Supreme Court three years later, in *Bellotti v. Baird,* 443 U.S. 622 (1979) (*Bellotti II*), eight justices voted to strike down the law, which the Massachusetts Supreme Judicial Court interpreted to (1) require consent from available parents for any nonemergency procedure, (2) require notice to an available parent of a court proceeding, or (3) allow a court to withhold consent even if "the minor is capable of making, and has made, an informed and reasonable decision." Four justices found fault with the "judicial bypass" procedure because it required parental consultation in every case and allowed the court to override the decision of a "mature minor." In contrast, the other four justices found the statute unconstitutional because it provided either a parent or a judge with an absolute veto over the decision to have an abortion.

The right of a minor woman to obtain an abortion continued to come before the Supreme Court in the early 1980s. In *H.L. v. Matheson,* 450 U.S. 4398 (1981), a 6–3 majority upheld on narrow grounds a Utah statute requiring notice to the parents of a dependent, unmarried woman under the age of 18. The Court distinguished the Utah law from the ones at issue in *Bellotti II* and *Danforth,* finding that parental notice is not equivalent to consent and that the Utah law did not give parents or a judge veto power over a young woman's decision to obtain an abortion. The Court did not reach the constitutionality of the law as applied to mature or emancipated minors. Three years later, the Supreme Court issued rulings in companion cases, *City of Akron v. Akron Center for Reproductive Health,* 462 U.S. 416 (1983), and *Planned Parenthood v. Ashcroft,* 462 U.S. 476 (1983). A 6–3 majority struck down the Akron ordinance, which required a woman under the age of 15 to obtain the "informed" written consent of one parent 24 hours prior to an abortion. However, five members of the Court upheld a Missouri mandate that a woman under age 18 obtain the "informed" written consent of one parent or a court prior to an abortion.

In effect, in half of the states by the mid-1990s, parental consent and notification requirements force more young women to delay their abortions even when involving their parents or seeking court approval or leaving the state for the procedure. Some young women risk parental retaliation, which can include physical and psychological abuse, while others seek illegal or self-induced abortions.

ANDREA MILLER

HORMONE RESEARCH FOUNDATION V. GENENTECH

Hormone Research Foundation (HRF) asserted that U.S. Patent No. 3,853,833 ("the '833 patent"), directed to synthetically derived human growth hormone (hGH), was infringed by Genentech's recombinantly derived hGH products, Protropin and Protropin II. The '833 patent disclosed solid-phase peptide synthesis of a 190-residue sequence thought, at the time of filing, to be the correct sequence of hGH. That sequence later was found, however, to be off by

one amino acid from the actual 191-residue sequence for hGH. Genentech moved for summary judgment on the grounds that its Protropin products did not infringe claims of the '833 patent that prescribed an amino acid sequence "corresponding" to the variant 190-residue sequence. The trial court concluded that "corresponding" meant "identical" in this context and, hence, that the Genetech products did not literally infringe the HRF patent claims. Informed by the prosecution history of the '833 patent, the U.S. Court of Appeals for the Federal Circuit affirmed the grant of Genentech's summary judgment motion.
REFERENCES: Greenfield, Michael S. 1993. "Recombinant DNA Technology: A Science Struggling with the Patent Law." *Intellectual Property L. Rev.* 25:135–178; *Hormone Research Foundation v. Genentech,* 708 F. Supp. 1096, 8 USPQ2d 1377 (N.D. Calif. 1988), *reversed in part,* 904 F.2d 1558 (Fed. Cir. 1990).

STEPHEN A. BENT

HUMAN GENOME PROJECT

DNA, deoxyribonucleic acid, holds the very key to our understanding of genetic disease. This double-helical molecule, composed of two long, twisted strands of chemical compounds called nucleotides, is the primary component of the 46 chromosomes found in humans.

Human genes, nested inside the DNA chains, are sequences of nucleotides, and it is these sequences that scientists involved in the Human Genome Project have been feverishly identifying or mapping and sequencing. Mapping is the first phase of the project, which involves dividing, characterizing, and ordering the chromosomes into small fragments (DOE, 1992). The second phase involves the more complicated task of gene sequencing, which is the determination of the estimated 3 billion nucleotide sequences of the ordered DNA fragments (DOE, 1992). While the immediate goal of the Human Genome Project is to map and sequence all of the genes in the human genome, the ultimate goal of the project is to develop a global scientific tool, within 15 years, to be used for the identification and eventual treatment of genetic disease (McCrary and Allen, 1994).

The $3 billion Human Genome Project, initiated in 1990, is jointly funded by the Department of Energy (DOE) and the National Institutes of Health (NIH).* The primary agencies involved with the genetic mapping and DNA sequencing are the Office of Health and Environmental Research in the Office of Energy Research from DOE and the National Institute of General Medical Sciences,* the National Cancer Institute,* the National Institute of Allergy and Infectious Diseases,* the National Institute of Child Health and Human Development,* and the National Institute of Neurological Disorders and Stroke from NIH (Office of Technology Assessment, 1988).

McKusick (1992) reports that 5,000 of the estimated 50,000 to 100,000 expressed genes of the human genome have been either partially or completely characterized and recorded in the *Mendelian Inheritance in Man,* an online encyclopedic gene database, named after the father of genetics, Gregor Mendel.

Additionally, another online database, the GDB or genome database, is supported by DOE and NIH and maintained at Johns Hopkins University. GDB is the official database of the Human Genome Project and is accessible through Telenet and Internet (McKusick, 1992, 35).

Five percent of the overall budget ($5.1 million for fiscal year 1992) for the Human Genome Project is allocated for research into the ethical, legal, and social implications (ELSI) of genetic research (Durfy, 1993). The most often-cited ethical problem related to genetic research is the general fear of abuse or misuse of the genetic information obtained from the Human Genome Project. Allegations reminiscent of Huxley's *Brave New World* or Hitler's experimentation with eugenics cast an ominous shadow over the new gene technology. As the DOE (1992, 28) report suggests, "[W]hile human genome research itself does not pose any new ethical dilemmas, the use of data arising from these studies presents challenges that need to be addressed before the data accumulate significantly."

However, the call for consistent policy guidelines, while being discussed by policymakers and scientists alike, has not seen substantive action either at the federal or the state level. Policies regarding prenatal and preimplantation genetic screening and diagnosing vary among the states, with no consistent or overarching theme. Questions of reproductive freedom and the manipulation of human embryos via gene therapy are seemingly being decided on a case-by-case basis. As Andrews et al. (1994, 260) note, "The expansion of available tests fostered by the Human Genome Project will present complicated issues with respect to the testing of newborns and other children." Additionally, cries of genetic discrimination are being assaulted on the insurance industry, as well as on certain employers. However, we have seen a handful of progressive statutes passed in several states to prevent genetic discrimination, especially with regard to those circumstances not protected by the Americans with Disabilities Act of 1990.*

As technology improves the speed of mapping and sequencing the genes, fundamental questions regarding the Human Genome Project arise concerning whether or not this is "bad science" or "big science." Furthermore, as Mc-Kusick (1992) notes, other salient arguments continue to be debated, such as whether the Human Genome Project provides proper scientific doctoral training or whether we should allocate funding to other areas of scientific research. Hilgartner (1995, 303) reports the general concern regarding the Human Genome Project's impact on "international and interlaboratory collaboration, on the bureaucratization of research, and on the ethos of science."

With these thoughts in mind, the following nine specific areas of ELSI research are currently under way (Durfy, 1993, 467):

1. Fairness in the use of genetic information;
2. The impact of knowledge of genetic information on the individual;
3. Privacy and confidentiality of genetic information;

4. The impact of the Human Genome Initiative on genetic counseling;
5. Reproductive decisions influenced by genetic information;
6. Issues raised by the introduction of genetics into mainstream medical practice;
7. Uses and misuses of genetic information in the past and the relevance to the current situation;
8. Questions raised by the commercialization of the products from the Human Genome Initiative;
9. Conceptual and philosophical implications of the Human Genome Initiative.

As the results from these multifaceted studies begin to be assessed, perhaps we will see more directive and less arbitrary policies suggested from within the ELSI component of the Human Genome Project.

REFERENCES: Andrews, Lori B., Jane E. Fullarton, Neil A. Holtzman, and Arno G. Motulsky, eds. 1994. *Assessing Genetic Risks: Implications for Health and Social Policy.* Washington, D.C.: National Academy Press; Department of Energy (DOE), Office of Energy Research, and Office of Health and Environmental Research. 1992. *Human Genome Program: Primer on Molecular Genetics.* Washington, D.C.: U.S. Department of Energy; Durfy, Sharon J. 1993. "Ethics and the Human Genome Project." *Arch. Pathol. Lab. Med.* 117:466–69; Hilgartner, Stephen. 1995. "The Human Genome Project." In *Handbook of Science and Technology Studies,* ed. Sheila Jasanoff, Gerald E. Markle, James C. Petersen, and Trevor Pinch. Thousand Oaks: Sage Publications; McCrary, S. Van, and William L. Allen. 1994. "The Human Genome Initiative and Primary Care." In *Health Care Ethics: Critical Issues,* ed. John F. Monagle and David C. Thomasma. Gaithersburg, MD: Aspen Publishers; McKusick, Victor A. 1992. "The Human Genome Project: Plans, Status, and Applications in Biology and Medicine." In *Gene Mapping: Using Law and Ethics as Guides,* ed. George J. Annas and Sherman Elias. New York: Oxford University Press; Office of Technology Assessment. 1988. *Mapping Our Genes: Genome Projects: How Big, How Fast?* Baltimore: Johns Hopkins University Press.

See also **GENETIC DIAGNOSIS; PREIMPLANTATION GENETIC DIAGNOSIS; PRENATAL GENETIC DIAGNOSIS; PRESYMPTOMATIC GENETIC DIAGNOSIS.**

PATRICIA GAIL McVEY

HUMAN SUBJECTS OF BIOMEDICAL RESEARCH

In fiscal year (FY) 1993, over $30 billion was invested in the United States in support of biomedical research and development; of that, the U.S. government invested $12 billion (39 percent), private industries invested $15.5 billion (over 50 percent), and private foundations invested $1.5 billion (about 5 percent). Consequently, the U.S. federal government is the largest single supporter of biomedical research in the world. Within the U.S. government, the National Institutes of Health (NIH)* is the largest biomedical research agency. In FY 1993 the NIH invested almost $10 billion, or 70 percent of the total federal expenditure; the remaining $2.2 billion was invested by 15 other federal departments and agencies.

A considerable portion of this research activity involves the use of human subjects. The wide scope of federal investment in research involving human subjects called for a regulatory framework that is effective in adequately protecting subjects, is consistent across the entire federal spectrum, is bureaucratically efficient, and is acceptable to the research community. Such a regulatory structure—known as the Common Federal Rule for the Protection of Human Subjects—was promulgated in 1991 (56 *Federal Register,* June 18, 1991).

The rule governs all research on human subjects funded by the U.S. government. By requiring that local Institutional Review Boards (IRBs) evaluate all human subject research in the light of three moral principles—respect for persons, beneficence, and justice—the rule seeks to ensure that virtually all human subjects participating in research in the United States enjoy consistently strong protections of their rights and welfare. Research projects that have not met policy guidelines are prohibited from receiving federal funding. This regulatory structure, which took many years to construct, was spearheaded by NIH, the largest biomedical research agency in the federal system.

In February 1966 the Public Health Service (PHS), urged by the NIH, issued its first policy concerning the protection of human subjects; that policy was revised three times in the late 1960s, and in 1971, it was rewritten by the NIH to include all research involving human subjects supported by the Department of Health, Education, and Welfare (DHEW; later to become the Department of Health and Human Services [DHHS]). Extension of the policy to the entire DHEW meant not only that all of the agencies within the Public Health Service (Centers for Disease Control,* Health Resources and Services Administration, Indian Health Service, NIH, Food and Drug Administration,* etc.) were subject to the same set of regulations but that even such agencies as the Social Security Administration and the Health Care Financing Administration (agencies within DHEW but outside the PHS) were required to follow the Policy for the Protection of Human Subjects whenever they conducted research involving human subjects.

In 1974 the NIH upgraded its efforts to protect human subjects. It created the Office for Protection from Research Risks (OPRR) within the Office of the Director. On behalf of the Public Health Service and the entire DHEW, the OPRR coordinated efforts to develop and promulgate regulations for the protection of human research subjects. These efforts extended to the private sector because virtually every institution subject to the regulations elected to apply the federal regulations to all research involving human subjects conducted within their institutions, irrespective of the source of funding.

Congress also acted on behalf of research subjects in 1974 by passing the National Research Act (P.L. 93–348), which established the National Commission for the Protection of Human Subjects of Biomedical and Behavioral Research* (National Commission). The National Commission issued 17 reports and appendixes, most of which dealt with mechanisms to improve the protections for the rights and welfare of human subjects of biomedical and behavioral research. When the National Commission completed its work, the NIH, operating through the OPRR, initiated efforts to upgrade federal regulations for the protection of human subjects, this time in the light of the reports and recommendations of the National Commission. Basic DHHS Regulations for the Protection of Human Subjects were thoroughly revised, updated, and reissued in January 1981 (45 CFR 46).

In the process of updating its regulations governing research involving humans funded by agencies within DHHS, the NIH persuaded the Food and Drug Administration (FDA) to do the same. The FDA regulations, which cover drugs, devices, and biologics involved in interstate commerce, pertain to most of the research involving human subjects conducted in the private sector. The NIH regulations, on the other hand, pertain to the lion's share of government-supported research involving human subjects. The two agencies coordinated their efforts to revise their respective regulations for the protection of human subjects and published the revised regulations in January 1981 (45 CFR 46; 21 CFR 50 & 56). FDA regulations were, so far as the law permitted, congruent with NIH regulations. Since 1981, then, DHHS-funded research and FDA-regulated research sponsored by pharmaceutical houses and medical device manufacturers have been governed by regulations that are virtually identical. In this way, uniform regulatory protections for the rights and welfare of human subjects gradually expanded to cover most human research subjects in the United States. One major obstacle to uniform regulations remained, however: protection of subjects involved in research supported by federal agencies outside of DHHS.

In 1981, the President's Commission for the Study of Ethical Problems in Medicine and Biomedical and Behavioral Research* (President's Commission) issued a report on the systems utilized to protect the rights and welfare of human subjects involved in research conducted or supported by all federal departments and agencies. It found that federal departments and agencies (other than agencies within DHHS) involved in research used a variety of policies and procedures to protect human research subjects, and in some cases, subjects were offered no governmental protection of any kind. To promote protections for human subjects and to reduce the burdens on research institutions required to comply with multiple federal regulatory systems, the President's Commission recommended that all federal departments and agencies adopt the DHHS regulations for the protection of human subjects (45 CFR 46).

In response to these recommendations, the chairman of the Federal Coordinating Council for Science Engineering and Technology (FCCSET) appointed in 1982 an *Ad Hoc* Committee for the Protection of Human Subjects; in 1983, the *Ad Hoc* Committee was succeeded by a standing Interagency Human Subjects Coordinating Committee (Interagency Committee) chartered by FCCSET and chaired by the director, OPRR. The creation of the Interagency Committee, which is advisory to heads of departments and agencies that support research involving human subjects, is one of the most productive accomplishments of the process to create the Common Rule. In consultation with the White House Office of Science and Technology Policy (OSTP) and the Office of Management and Budget, the Interagency Committee proposed a Model Federal Policy based on the DHHS regulations (45 CFR 46) and on public comments. All relevant federal departments and agencies concurred on the Model Federal Policy in March 1985. This important step was the first of many that had to be taken to create a Common Federal Rule. In June 1986, OSTP published for public comment in the *Federal Register* the Proposed Model Federal Policy for Protection of Human Subjects, and after reviewing the resulting comments, the Interagency Coordinating Committee proposed revising the Model Policy in the form of a Common Federal Rule to be adopted by each of the 16 federal departments and agencies that support research involving human subjects. In June 1991, a Common Federal Rule for the Protection of Human Subjects was promulgated when each of the relevant agencies published identical regulations for the protection of human subjects in a single issue of the *Federal Register* (56 *Federal Register,* June 18, 1991). This complex procedure was necessary because there is no central regulatory authority grounded in statute that oversees the entire executive branch of the government. For this reason, each agency published, under its own authority, a regulation that was identical to that published by all of the other agencies.

The entire effort was coordinated by the OPRR with the strong assistance of the OSTP. Nearly ten years had elapsed between the issuance of the initial recommendation and the fulfillment of the recommendation by the U.S. government. The time was spent in educating each agency concerning the responsibilities that it would be assuming when the Common Federal Rule came into existence, preparing the research community to receive and implement the rule, obtaining clearances from Offices of General Counsel in each department and agency, and persuading agency heads throughout the government to give final approval.

The only exception to the uniformity of the rule pertains to FDA regulations. By law, the FDA has authority over test articles involved in interstate commerce, and so it could not, strictly speaking, be party to a rule that exercises authority over awardee institutions. Nevertheless, the FDA modified its regulations pertaining to drugs, devices, and biologics to make research involving these items congruent with the requirements imposed by all of the other federal agencies. The differences between FDA requirements for protecting human subjects when regulated articles are being tested in research and those that govern all other federal departments and agencies in conducting, supporting, or regulating research involving human subjects are so minor that they are unlikely, except in rare instances, to inconvenience regulated institutions.

The Common Federal Rule went into effect on August 19, 1991. It requires an approved written assurance of compliance between the research institution and the federal agency or department, including certification that the proposed research has been approved by the appropriate IRB, which must be submitted to OPRR. The IRBs evaluate research proposals as well as research in progress, requiring compliance with certain protections: The risks to subjects are minimized; the risks to subjects are reasonable in relation to the benefits of the research; selection of subjects is equitable; informed and voluntary consent is obtained and documented; research data are monitored to ensure the safety of the subjects; adequate provisions are taken to protect the privacy of the subjects; and adequate provisions are taken to protect especially vulnerable groups (such as children and the mentally retarded).

Some human subject research is exempted from the policy. This type of research examines, for example, common educational practices; educational tests, surveys, interviews, or observation of public behavior; publicly available existing data, documents, records, pathological and diagnostic specimens; public service programs; and taste and food quality evaluations.

The Common Federal Rule is unique. No other regulation or set of regulations is promulgated by all relevant departments and agencies of the federal government and provides uniform regulation. Surely, though, there are other candidates for cross-cutting regulations that standardize behavior; a widely endorsed common rule governing misconduct in science, for instance, would no doubt be welcomed by federal regulators and by the research community that is slowly learning how to cope with misconduct.

REFERENCES: Federal Policy for the Protection of Human Subjects. 56 *Federal Register*, June 18, 1991; Grodin, M. A., and Glantz, L. H., eds. 1994. *Children as Research Subjects*. New York: Oxford University Press; National Commission for the Protection of Human Subjects of Biomedical and Behavioral Research. 1979. *Ethical Principles and Guidelines for the Protection of Human Subjects of Research*. Washington, D.C.: Government Printing Office; Porter, Joan P., and Dustira, Alicia K. 1993. "Policy Development Lessons from Two Federal Initiatives." *Academic Medicine* 68: S51–S55; President's Commission for the Study of Ethical Problems in Medicine and Biomedical and Behavioral Research. 1981. *Protecting Human Subjects*. Washington, D.C.: Government Printing Office.

CHARLES R. McCARTHY and ERIC M. MESLIN

I

INFANT CARE REVIEW COMMITTEE (ICRC)

One of the several types of health care ethics committees (cf. Institutional Ethics Committee*), the ICRC is distinctive for U.S. biomedical policy as an instrument of the legislative intent of a federal law, the Child Abuse Amendments of 1984. This law (cf. infra.) defined neonates imperiled by extreme prematurity, birth trauma, or congenital defects as "disabled infants with life threatening conditions." As such, withholding medically indicated treatment from them constitutes both discrimination against a disabled person and child abuse. Three conditions under which it is permissible to withhold treatment are (1) if the infant is "irreversibly comatose," (2) if the provision of treatment would be "futile in terms of the survival of the infant," or (3) if the treatment would be "virtually futile" under circumstances that "the treatment itself . . . would be inhumane."

Acceptance of these standards for withholding medically indicated treatments in these cases has been controversial. The substantive criteria contained in the law are ambiguous. Decision making and prognosis for each neonate is inherently unique, difficult, and uncertain. Rapid advances in the technology of the neonatal intensive care unit compounds the problem because of variant experiences. Finally, we have attained neither an ethical nor a societal consensus on quality-of-life issues that are the consequences of many of these decisions.

For all these reasons, the Department of Health and Human Services (DHHS) regulations implementing this law turned to the procedural convenience of the committee model and strongly encouraged the establishment of ICRCs, providing guidelines for their activities. According to these guidelines regarding protection of "disabled infants with life threatening conditions," the roles of an ICRC will be (1) to educate their families and health care providers, (2) to develop and recommend polices and guidelines to provider institutions preventing the withholding of medically indicated treatment from them, and (3) to provide prospective and retrospective review of their cases with the intent of providing counsel to providers and institution administrators.

The composition of the ICRC, according to these guidelines, is multidisciplinary, including a physician, nurse, hospital administrator, social worker, representative of a disability group, and lay community member, with leadership provided by a member of the hospital's medical staff. It is advisory in nature but is responsible for keeping the institution informed on all provisions of state law requiring the report of suspected neglect of seriously ill newborns to the state child protective services agency. (Federal funding for these state agencies is contingent upon their provision of programs and procedures to address reports of medical neglect of "disabled infants with life threatening conditions.")

Efforts to help assess the value and appropriate level of neonatal technology in the care of infants, however, were not limited to the DHHS approach. The American Academy of Pediatrics (AAP), following the recommendations of the President's Commission for the Study of Ethical and Legal Problems in Medicine and Biomedical and Behavioral Research (1983), provided guidelines for "infant *Bioethics* committees" (1984), signaling a broadening of the "infant *care* review" committee scope of activity.

By following HHS regulations that call for the continued treatment, and therefore the prolongation of the life, of all noncomatose, nondying infants, the ICRC responds to a mandate to render an exceedingly narrow medical and legal judgment on prognosis and treatment. The AAP alternative allows procedural consideration of broader ethical issues. In addition to addressing the principles of beneficence (protection of the disabled infant) and substitute judgment (deciding for the infant), the AAP guidelines permit consideration of additional bioethical principles including patient (family) autonomy, quality of life of the infant and/or the family, and the calculus of the benefits and burdens of proposed therapies and procedures to maintain life. While both the ICRC and the infant bioethics committee are envisioned as interdisciplinary, the American Academy of Pediatrics guidelines differ from the ICRC in that it provides for the inclusion of clergy and a "person trained in ethics or philosophy." In addition, although the AAP infant bioethics committee calls for a mandatory *review* of all cases proposing forgoing life-sustaining treatment for an infant, their guidelines do not categorically foreclose on nontreatment decisions.

The differences between these two approaches to assessing the value and appropriate level of neonatal technology define the current legal and ethical controversy in the care of imperiled newborns. The case made by the AAP that ICRCs are concerned with medical rather than ethical decision making cannot be ignored. ICRC guidelines, moreover, directly provide for an agency implementing the substance of the Federal Child Abuse Amendments. This is a role that is not consistent with the original impulse to seek a procedural resolution of infant care decision.

The prevalence of the committee approach is uncertain. A 1986 national survey of hospitals with neonatal intensive care units and/or 1,500 or more births per year concluded that 52 percent of these hospitals had established ICRCs. Other studies have shown that where there is broader hospital ethics activity in general, dense population, pediatric teaching services, and/or a Level III neonatal intensive care service, there is more likely to be a pediatrics bioethics function. Whether this function is performed by an ICRC following DHHS guidelines, by an AAP-style infant bioethics committee, or by the general Hospital Ethics Committee (HEC) is difficult to ascertain.

Resolving such questions is a task not only for future research, which might probe more finely into the functioning of these committees, but for a resolution among health professionals as to which of these approaches is most appropriate and responsive to the bioethical aspect of these difficult patient care decisions. REFERENCES: American Academy of Pediatrics. 1984. ''Guidelines for Infant Bioethics Committees.'' *Pediatrics* 74: 306–310; American Academy of Pediatrics. 1994. ''Guidelines on Foregoing Life-Sustaining Medical Treatment.'' *Pediatrics* 93: 532–536; *Federal Register.* January 12, 1984. 49: 1622–1654; Fleming, G. V., S. S. Hudd, S. A. LeBailly, and R. M. Greenstein. 1990. ''Infant Care Review Committees: The Response to Federal Guidelines.'' *American Journal of Diseases of Children* 144: 778–781; Fost, Norman. 1986. ''Infant Care Review Committees in the Aftermath of Baby Doe.'' In *Compelled Compassion: Government Intervention in the Treatment of Critically Ill Newborns,* ed. Arthur L. Caplan, Robert H. Blank, and Janna C. Merrick. Totowa, NJ: Humana; Rothenberg, Karen H. 1989. ''Medical Decision Making for Children.'' In *BioLaw,* Vol. 1, ed. James F. Childress, and Ruth D. Gaare. Bethesda, MD: University Publications of America; Weir, Robert F. 1987. ''Pediatric Ethics Committees: Ethical Advisers or Legal Watchdogs?'' *Law, Medicine and Health Care* 15: 99–109.

JOSEPH C. d'ORONZIO

INFORMED CONSENT AND NEW GENE TECHNOLOGY

Informed consent in medicine is based on the Fourteenth Amendment right to privacy and the common-law doctrine of due process. The legal doctrine of informed consent imposes on the physician two general duties: to disclose information about treatment to patients and to obtain their consent before proceeding with treatment. The doctrine consists of three elements, which are voluntariness, competency, and information.

Voluntariness refers to consent being given willingly by the patient. *Competency* refers to the patient's mental and/or emotional ability to give a consent. At the time of an emergency, the patient is typically not viewed as competent to make an informed consent as to a course of treatment.

The last element, *information,* refers to the adequacy of the information given the patient. In general, the patient must receive information as to the known hazards (risks) of the proposed procedure, the benefit of the proposed procedure, and alternative procedures that may be available. In theory, this information should be conveyed to the patient in language the patient can understand.

Justifications for a ''less than adequate disclosure'' include an emergency situation, the incompetency of the patient, patient waiver, and therapeutic privilege. The patient under the stress of an emergency is viewed as not being able to give an informed consent, especially as regards withholding a treatment that threatens the patient's life. The emergency does not permit evaluation of competency, time for information exchange, or even personalized assessment of likely future outcomes.

In the clinical setting, competency to accept or reject medical treatment requires, at a minimum, that the patient possess the ability to understand and communicate the information related to his or her care and treatment, the ability to reason and deliberate about one's goals, and the ability to choose in light of some goals and values.

Some patients may prefer not to be told anything about their proposed course of treatment. In those situations, the physician is still required to offer an informed consent. There is no requirement, however, to force the patient into responding to the information offered. Some patients may elect to leave the decision of a course of treatment entirely to the physician (Wadlington, Waltz, and Dworkin, 1980).

Therapeutic privilege is a controversial exception to the informed consent doctrine. If, in the opinion of the physician, disclosure of a pending procedure would frighten or otherwise compromise the good of the patient, then limited information or no information may be provided (Roth, Meisel, and Lidz, 1977). The exception has been formulated by courts and legislatures in a variety of ways.

A physician's failure to give informed consent is not a legal wrong in itself. A "standard of causation" must be applied. For there to be a legal wrong, the risk that the physician failed to disclose must actually befall the patient.

Informed consent for minors typically focuses on the competency element. Other special considerations involving children as research subjects is discussed by Grodin and Glantz (1994). Genetic research on children or their parents inevitably leads to disclosure of information about both (Murray, 1994). Informed consent for experimental procedures and devices that are last-ditch efforts to save a patient typically focuses on the information element of informed consent. While well established in the United States, informed consent is not yet the doctrine among all modern medical systems (Pincus, 1993). In the case of biomedical experiments, informed consent policy is guided by the Nuremberg Code.*

Informed consent may require a full financial disclosure from the physician because failure to make a financial disclosure is a violation of trust that undermines patient autonomy. The goal is to protect patients from physicians whose judgment might be influenced by profit and who might thus be in a conflict-of-interest position with their own patients (Annas, 1990).

REFERENCES: Annas, G. J. 1990. "Symposium on *Moore v. Regents of the University of California.*" *Biotechnology Law Report* 239 (4); Grodin, M. A., and L. H. Glantz, eds. 1994. *Children as Research Subjects: Science, Ethics, and Law.* New York: Oxford University Press; Murray, T. H. 1994. "Assessing Genetic Technologies: Two Ethical Issues." *International Journal of Technology Assessment in Health Care* 10: 573–582;

Pincus, R. C. 1993. "Has Informed Consent Finally Arrived in Australia?" *Medical Journal of Australia* 159: 25–27; Roth, L. H., A. Meisel, and C. W. Lidz. 1977. "Tests of Competency to Consent to Treatment." *American Journal of Psychiatry* 134: 3; Wadlington, W., J. R. Waltz, and R. B. Dworkin. 1980. *Cases and Materials on Law and Medicine.* Mineola, N.Y.: Foundation Press, 484–502.

GERALD GOODMAN

INFORMED CONSENT IN EXPERIMENTAL PROCEDURES

At the conclusion of World War II, the Allied governments brought legal action against physicians and certain other professional and government officials of Nazi Germany for their performance of medical experiments on unwilling human subjects. An outcome of those legal processes was the Nuremberg Code* for the conduct of medical experiments using human subjects. The Nuremberg Code has as its basis the requirement that medical experiments that will involve human subjects yield results that are unprocurable by any other methods or means of study. Specifically, the code requires:

• The voluntary consent of the human subject.
• The experiment should procure results not obtainable by any other method or means of study.
• The results should be based on initial animal studies.
• The experiment should avoid all physical and mental suffering.
• The experiment should not anticipate the death of the subject.
• The degree of risk should be in proportion to the humanitarian importance of the problem to be solved.
• Planning and facilities should be designed to facilitate the safe conduct of the experiment.
• The experiment should be conducted by qualified persons.
• The study subject should be free to leave the experiment at any time.
• The scientist in charge should be prepared to terminate the experiment at any time the experiment is judged to be a hazard to the subject.

Paramount to ethical considerations for medical experiments involving humans is the test of social good—that experiments yield results for the good of society (*Nuremberg Military Tribunals*), 1949. Technologies such as genetic technology bring into focus the question of whether what can be improved should be improved (Murray, 1994). Gender issues may present unique requirements for an informed consent (Mastroianni, Faden, and Federman, 1994). The duty and responsibility for ascertaining the quality of the informed consent rest upon each individual who initiates, directs, or engages in the experiment. It is a personal duty and responsibility that may not be delegated to another with impunity. Throughout, the Nuremberg Code stresses the individual as the most important factor in the conduct of human experimentation. In studies on human subjects, the cooperation of the subjects is practically always essential (Ivy, 1947).

As to the question of who is conscriptable to serve as a subject for human experimentation, least and last of all should be the sick (Jonas, 1969). The afflicted should not be called upon to bear additional burden and risk. They are society's special trust and the physician's trust in particular. Jonas states that the physician is obligated to the patient and to no one else. He is not the agent of society or the interests of medical science, the patient's family, his cosufferers, or future sufferers from the same disease.

Informed consent for human subjects in medical experiments has been codified in the Code of Federal Regulations, 1983, Title 45, Part 46, Protection of Human Subjects (revised March 8, 1983).

REFERENCES: Ivy, A. C. 1947. "Nazi War Crimes of a Medical Nature." *Federal Bulletin* 33: 133–146; Jonas, H. 1969. "Philosophical Reflections on Experimenting with Human Subjects." *Experimentation with Human Subjects,* 1–31; Mastroianni, A. C., R. Faden, and D. Federman, eds. 1994. "Women and Health Research." In *Ethical and Legal Issues of Including Women in Clinical Studies.* Washington, D.C.: National Academy Press; Murray, T. H. 1994. "Assessing Genetic Technologies: Two Ethical Issues." *International Journal of Technology Assessment in Health Care* 10: 573–582; *Trials of War Criminals Before the Nuremberg Military Tribunals Under Control Council Law No. 10.* 1949. Washington, D.C.: U.S. Government Printing Office, 2:181–182.

                                                            GERALD GOODMAN

INFORMED CONSENT IN HUMAN EXPERIMENTATION

Obtaining the informed consent of a potential human subject of research is one of the primary ethical requirements universally agreed necessary when humans are to be involved as research subjects. It is a process of communication leading to full disclosure of the purposes, benefits, and hazards of a specific research project, thus ensuring that each potential subject understands the fundamental requirements of the research and can make an informed decision to participate voluntarily.

Since the fifth-century B.C. Oath of Hippocrates, both the public and biomedical/behavioral scientists have shown their concern with appropriate ethical safeguards for human subjects utilized in research. These concerns were general in nature and lacked focus or consistency until the infamous Nazi medical research atrocities were disclosed during the Nuremberg Trials following World War II. The resulting Nuremberg Code,* emphasizing the requirement to obtain the subject's voluntary participation and informed consent, became an unofficial standard to judge research with human subjects. In 1964 the Declaration of Helsinki made similar recommendations, and the requirement for fair and realistic informed consent has remained a central ethical principle for research with human subjects.

Obtaining the informed and voluntary consent of each research subject is a requirement of all human subjects research funded by the U.S. government (see the Common Federal Rule for the Protection of Human Subjects), based on regulations promulgated by the U.S. Department of Health and Human Services (45 CFR 46, 21 CFR 50, 21 CFR 56). These regulations are administered, enforced, and monitored by local committees called Institutional Review Boards (IRBs).

In the consent process, information is communicated clearly by the investigator to the subject and involves discussion of the procedures involved, a realistic description of the possible benefits, and a frank review of any possible harm that might result from participation. Other elements of the informed consent process include an explanation and rationale for the research project, an invitation to participate, a review of selection and exclusion criteria, and a review of what alternatives to the research are available. It is important that the investigator clearly review standard or other treatment options available, should the potential subject elect not to participate in the research study. The researcher must also disclose any financial risks or compensation as a result of participation, as well as the availability of compensation in the event of research-related injury. It must be very clear that participation is voluntary with no element of coercion to participate, and that the subject may withdraw without penalty. An explicit pledge must be made to provide any new information that may relate to a subject's willingness to participate and a description provided of all circumstances allowing the investigator or sponsor to end the subject's participation in the research.

A written consent form must be used to allow the subject to read and understand these elements. This consent form must be signed by the subject and must contain the investigator's signed affidavit attesting that he/she has obtained the research subject's voluntary and informed consent. The consent form must be written in language easily understood by the average subject without excessive scientific terms. It must include specific contact sources for information regarding the research, emergency needs, or questions regarding the rights of the research subject and must document the methods of assuring confidentiality. The informed consent form may not include language that would cause the subject to waive or appear to waive any of his/her legal rights, nor may the consent release or appear to release the investigator, the sponsor, or the institution from liability for negligence. A copy of the signed consent form must be provided to the subject. Obtaining the subject's informed consent to participate in the research is an ongoing process, however, not just a form signed at one discrete time.

When the research involves vulnerable subjects (children, institutionalized subjects, the cognitively impaired, etc.), or the research design involves incomplete disclosure or deception, the IRB may require special protections. Consent for research may be given by a proxy for the subject when the subject is unable to give consent. This proxy must be legally empowered to make medical decisions, for example, a parent for children. Proxy authority may vary with legal jurisdictions and is usually established at the state level. The permission of a parent to enroll a child as a research subject is not enough, however; the child must also assent. The child's willingness to participate in the research must be documented and may not be inferred from the child's failure to object.

The informed consent regulations are not meant to preempt any applicable federal, state, or local law that requires additional information to be disclosed for the informed consent process to be legally effective. Under prescribed circumstances and when the research involves minimal risk or less, the IRB may waive the requirement for written consent documentation or the requirement for informed consent entirely (21 CFR 50.23). Any decision to alter or waive normal consent procedures must be clearly documented in the IRB committee minutes.
REFERENCES: Beecher, H. K. 1966. "Ethics and Clinical Research." *New England Journal of Medicine* 274: 1354–60; Faden, Ruth R., and Beauchamp, Tom L. 1986. *A History and Theory of Informed Consent.* New York: Oxford University Press; Katz, Jay. 1984. *The Silent World of Doctor and Patient.* New York: Free Press; Rothman, K. J., and Michels, K. B. 1994. "The Continuing Unethical Use of Placebo Controls." *New England Journal of Medicine* 331: 394–98.

WILLIAM F. DENNY

IN RE A.C.

In re A.C. is one of a series of cases in which the courts have been asked to order a cesarean section on a pregnant woman with a viable fetus. The case is unusual because the cesarean section was ordered over the objections of all of her physicians. It is also unique because it is the only case of a compelled cesarean section to have been litigated on a full record with the participation of knowledgeable and informed amici.

Angela Carder (A.C.) was first diagnosed with Ewing's sarcoma of the left thigh at age 13 years. Her therapy included experimental chemotherapy and radiation therapy at the National Cancer Institute* (NCI). She was one of the first survivors of this oncological illness. At age 24, she was diagnosed with a second malignancy, an osteosarcoma of the femur bone of the same leg. She was treated again at NCI. This treatment included chemotherapy and a hemipelvectomy (amputation of the left leg and part of the left pelvis) (Dr. Jeffrey Moscow, affidavit, November 5, 1987).

At age 27, while in remission, A.C. married and became pregnant. She was referred by Dr. Jeffrey Moscow at the NCI to the George Washington University (GWU) high-risk-pregnancy clinic. She had biweekly prenatal visits beginning at 15 weeks gestation (*In re A.C.,* 1990, 1239).

On June 9, 1987, A.C. went for her routine 25-week prenatal visit and complained of right shoulder pain and shortness of breath. An X ray was indicative of tumor metastasis (*id* at 1238). A.C. was hospitalized at GWU on June 11 for diagnostic and therapeutic purposes. Although A.C. had made it clear throughout the pregnancy that she wanted to be pregnant and have a child, she emphasized that her medical needs were primary, even if it meant some risk to the fetus (Dr. Lewis Hamner III, trial court testimony). Despite this, her physicians at

GWU were hesitant to institute treatment that would harm the fetus (Dr. Lawrence Lessin, trial court testimony). As a result, no medical regimen was begun, and A.C. deteriorated rapidly. On June 15, she was told her illness was terminal. A.C., her family, and her physicians discussed the goal of getting her to 28 weeks gestation for the sake of the fetus. She agreed to palliative treatment. They discussed a possible need to perform a cesarean section at that time to maximize the chances of the fetus. It was not discussed what should be done if she deteriorated before the twenty-eighth week. However, when now asked whether she still wanted to have the baby, A.C. was somewhat ambivalent: "I don't know, I think so" (trial court testimony of Dr. Lessin, *In re A.C.*, 1990, 1239).

Despite the plan to institute palliative treatment, A.C. received no cancer treatment on June 15, and overnight her prognosis became imminently terminal. She was transferred to the intensive care unit (ICU) for mechanical ventilation. Her attendings at GWU believed that she would die in less than 48 hours. The family and all her attending physicians at GWU agreed that no intervention should be undertaken for the fetus and that the fetus should be allowed to die with A.C. (*id* at 1239–40). Upon learning about this decision, the hospital administration sought judicial declaratory relief.

A hearing was conducted by the Honorable Emmet Sullivan at GWU Hospital. No attempt was made to involve A.C. Dr. Hamner, her primary obstetrician, stated that she was too sedated to make an informed decision and that decreasing her sedation would further compromise the well-being of the woman and the fetus. The court also made no attempt to determine A.C.'s own intent. Her family testified that A.C. would not have wanted to undergo a cesarean at this time. Her GWU obstetricians concurred and unanimously stated that they would not perform the procedure if it were ordered (*id* at 1239–40).

Court testimony concentrated on the issue of fetal viability. Dr. Maureen Edwards, a neonatologist, stated that a 26½-week fetus has a 50 to 60 percent chance of survival with less than a 20 percent risk of significant neurological morbidity (trial court testimony of Dr. Maureen Edwards, *id* at 1239). (The testimony is controversial. See data cited by Tuohey, 1991.) Although others questioned the applicability of this general data to this particular pregnant woman–fetal dyad, all the physicians agreed that the fetus's best chance was to operate immediately.

Lawyers for the fetus and the district argued that the court needed to balance the potential life of the fetus against the short, sedated life span of a terminally ill patient. A.C.'s lawyer held that A.C. would have refused a cesarean section and that the state should only intervene when there is compelling reason to overrule a patient's refusal, which did not exist in this case. He cited *Colautti v. Franklin* (1979) in which the Supreme Court struck down a statute that required a woman to undergo a procedure that involved a trade-off between her health and fetal survival.

In his decision, Judge Sullivan stated that the court did not know A.C.'s present view whether or not she wanted the child to live. He cited *In re Maydun* (1986), a case in which a cesarean section was ordered over a competent woman's objections. In *Maydun,* the court used a balancing analysis. Although Judge Sullivan noted that *Maydun*'s health was only minimally threatened by a cesarean section and that A.C. might not survive the surgery, Judge Sullivan further noted that A.C.'s death was imminent regardless of whether the cesarean section was performed. He concluded that "the state has [an] important and legitimate interest in protecting the potentiality of human life" (*In re Maydun,* 1986: 1240).

Justice Sullivan refused to give a stay. In the two hours it took to find an obstetrician who would agree to perform the surgery and the preparation of the operating room, Dr. Hamner went to see A.C., whom he found capable of communicating. He did not tell her explicitly that a hearing was in progress but explained that "it's been deemed that we should intervene on behalf of the baby by cesarean section." He then asked whether she would consent to an emergency cesarean section. She said she would, and he reported this to the court (trial court testimony of Dr. Hamner, *In re A.C.,* 1990, 1240). Dr. Hamner discouraged the court from moving to her bedside, but he, Dr. Weingold, A.C.'s mother, and husband went to A.C.'s room to confirm her consent to the procedure. At this meeting, Dr. Hamner explained that a judge had ordered a cesarean section but that her physicians would not perform it without her consent. A.C. mouthed, "I don't want it. I don't want it" (*id* at 1240–41). The trial court reconsidered its ruling in light of A.C.'s two statements and reaffirmed its original order indicating that her intent was unclear (*id* at 1241). Her attorney requested a stay from the appeals court. A three-judge panel denied the stay after a short conference call (*In re A.C.,* 1987, 613). A baby girl was delivered by cesarean section and died within 2½ hours, A.C. died two days later.

On November 10, 1987, the court of appeals gave an opinion in which they elaborated upon their rationale. They recognized considerations of bodily integrity and the right of an adult to refuse medical treatment but stated that "they should not have been dispositive here." Rather, they believed that the appropriate consideration was a balance of potential life of the unborn child with the terminal condition of its mother:

The Caesarean section would not significantly affect A.C.'s condition because she had, at best, two days left of sedated life; the complications arising from the surgery would not significantly alter that prognosis. The child, on the other hand, had a chance of surviving delivery, despite the possibility that it would be born handicapped. Accordingly, we conclude that the trial judge did not err in subordinating A.C.'s right against bodily intrusion to the interests of the unborn child and the state, and hence we denied the motion for stay. (*id* at 613)

On November 24, 39 organizations asked the D.C. Court of Appeals to reconsider its rulings. A.C.'s attorneys petitioned for a rehearing en banc because the ruling "involves questions of exceptional importance" that would likely present themselves in the future (Petition for Rehearing and Suggestion That Rehearing Be *En Banc,* submitted by Robert E. Sylvester, Esq., and Lynn M. Paltrow, Esq., November 24, 1987). The court of appeals agreed (*Matter of A.C.,* 1988, 203.) The case was argued on September 22, 1988, and a decision was reported on April 26, 1990 (*In re A.C.,* 1990).

The court of appeals vacated the trial court's ruling because its use of a balancing analysis was in error (*id* at 1247). The court stated that the proper question was: "[W]ho has the right to decide the course of medical treatment for a patient, who although near death, is pregnant with a viable fetus?" (*id* at 1237). Their answer was that the decision should be made by the pregnant woman. If she is incompetent, "then the decision must be ascertained through the procedure known as substituted judgement" (*id*). Since the trial court did not follow these procedures, its decision was vacated.

The appellate decision reaffirmed the right to bodily integrity and the right to refuse treatment. The court explicitly rejected the notion that these rights are held any less strongly by the terminally ill, incompetent persons, or pregnant women (*id* at 1247). Its ultimate holding is quite broad: "We hold that in virtually all cases the question of what is to be done is to be decided by the patient—the pregnant woman—on behalf of herself and the fetus" (*id* at 1237). Although the court denied that its decision was meant to "foreclose the possibility that a conflicting state interest may be so compelling that the patient's wishes must yield," it noted that "we anticipate that such cases will be *extremely rare and exceptional*" (*id* at 1252, italics added).

However, despite such broad language, the appellate decision is also notable for what it did not do. The decision did not rule on the legality of the preceding compelled cesarean decisions. Instead, it denied that its opinion should be read as approving or disapproving of its holding in *Maydun* because the facts were significantly different (*id* at 1252, fn 23). It also distinguished itself from *Jefferson v. Griffin Spalding County Hospital Authority* (1981), the only other appellate court ruling on a compelled cesarean section. Again the court stated that the facts were too different: In *Jefferson,* the surgery was recommended to promote both the woman's and the fetus's health (*id* at 1243, fn 7). This omission may limit the impact that this case will have on future judicial action regarding a pregnant woman's right to refuse a cesarean section.

REFERENCES: Annas, George. 1982. "Forced Caesareans: The Most Unkindest Cut of All." *Hastings Center Report* 12 (3): 16–17, 45; Annas, George. 1988. "She's Going to Die: The Case of Angela C." *Hastings Center Report* 18 (1): 23, 25; Annas, George. 1990. "Foreclosing the Use of Force: A.C. Reversed." *Hastings Center Report* 20 (4): 27–29; Colautti v. Franklin, 439 U.S. 379, 99 S. Ct. 675, 58 L.Ed.2d 596 (1979); Diamond, Margaret. 1990. "Comment: Echoes from Darkness: The Case of Angela C." *University of Pittsburgh Law Review* 51 (4): 1061–96; *In re A.C.,* 533 A.2d 611 (D.C. 1987); *In re A.C.,* 539 A.2d 203 (D.C. 1988); *In re A.C.,* 573 A.2d 1235 (D.C. 1990); *In re Maydun,* 114 Daily Wash. L. Rptr 2233 (D.C. Super Ct. July 26, 1986); *Jefferson v. Griffin Spalding County Hospital Authority,* 247 Ga. 86, 274 S.E.2d 457 (1981); *Matter of A.C.,* 539 A.2d 203 (D.C. App. March 17,

1988); Tuohey, John F. 1991. "Terminal Care and the Pregnant Woman: Ethical Reflections on *In re A.C.*" *Pediatrics* 88 (6): 1268–73.

LAINIE FRIEDMAN ROSS

IN RE CONROY

In 1985 the New Jersey Supreme Court issued an opinion that has become one of the most influential contributions to the debate over when, if ever, life-sustaining treatment can be removed from incapacitated persons by surrogate decision. The nephew for Claire Conroy, acting as her legally appointed guardian, petitioned the New Jersey courts for authority to withdraw her tube feeding. Conroy was an 84-year-old woman with organic brain syndrome and other physical disabilities. She resided in a nursing home and could interact with her environment only to a limited, rudimentary degree. Her severe dementia was not expected to improve.

Although Conroy died before the case reached the New Jersey Supreme Court, the court decided to resolve the issues presented to it because of their public importance. The court recognized that at stake was not only Conroy's potential interest in dying a "natural death without undue dependence on medical technology or unnecessarily protracted agony" but also her "fundamental right to expect that [her life] will not be foreshortened against [her] will." While the court considered the erroneous impingement of either interest to be "deeply unfortunate," it concluded that "it is best to err, if at all, in favor of preserving life." The challenge for the court was to create substantive and procedural guidelines for surrogate decision making that protected the interest in life enjoyed by incapacitated patients while giving due regard to their right to refuse unwanted treatment.

The guidelines adopted by the court combined elements of the "substituted judgment" and "best interests" approaches then extant in "right to die" jurisprudence. The court established a three-prong test for determining whether treatment could be withheld that focused first on the patient's subjective intent, if any, to accept or refuse treatment. Thus, the surrogate should examine all evidence indicating that the patient had already exercised his or her judgment for or against treatment, and if the evidence is sufficiently clear, this judgment should be substituted in place of any judgment that might be reached by the "reasonable or average person."

The court recognized, however, that this subjective inquiry often would fail to yield sufficient evidence of the patient's intent. According to the court, the substituted judgment approach then would be inappropriate because "in the absence of adequate proof of the patient's wishes, it is naive to pretend that the right to self-determination serves as the basis for substituted decision-making." Instead, an objective basis for removing treatment must be evident before treatment can be withheld or withdrawn. This stage of the inquiry focused on the patient's objectively discernible best interests.

The court rejected a best-interests approach that required the administration of treatment irrespective of its impact on the patient and instead considered pain and suffering to be potential factors justifying the removal of treatment even absent a clear refusal by the patient. Thus, if there was some "trustworthy" evidence of a general attitude by the patient disfavoring treatment that nevertheless fell short of proving the existence of a specific and informed advance refusal by the patient, then treatment could be withheld if the patient was experiencing unavoidable physical pain that outweighed any pleasure derived from living. If evidence of the patient's intent was lacking altogether, then treatment could be withheld or removed only when the patient was experiencing "recurring, unavoidable and severe pain" and any benefits to survival were "clearly and markedly" outweighed by the painful burdens of treatment.

The court declined to permit considerations other than pain and suffering to be evaluated as bases for removing treatment. Incorporating such factors as "dependency," "quality of life," or "social utility," the court concluded, "would create an intolerable risk for socially isolated and defenseless people suffering from physical or mental handicaps." The court acknowledged that very few nontreatment decisions could be justified on the basis of patient suffering, given medicine's ability to manage pain, and the difficulties of measuring suffering and comparing it to the patient's quantum of pleasurable experience. Nevertheless, the court preferred the "safer, known way" of counterposing against the benefit of life only the objectively discernible burden of physical suffering, and not more nebulous considerations, because "there was a lot to lose by being wrong."

Had Conroy still been living, the court would have returned the case to the lower courts to determine whether her situation met any of the newly developed tests. In a 1987 ruling, *In re Peter,* the court declined to apply the best-interests aspect of this approach to surrogate decisions for patients diagnosed as persistently unconscious because (1) a majority of the court believed that "most people" would not want to be kept alive in a persistent unconscious condition and (2) persons in this condition cannot feel pain and are not aware, thus foreclosing any surrogate attempt to balance the benefits of awareness against the burdens of pain. Instead, according to the court, the prolonged lack of consciousness itself would render death to be in a patient's best interests.

REFERENCES: *In re Conroy,* 486 A.2d 1209 (N.J. 1985); *In re Peter,* 529 A.2d 419 (N.J. 1987).

DANIEL AVILA

IN RE QUINLAN

In 1976, the New Jersey Supreme Court issued its landmark decision establishing in principle the right of a guardian to refuse life-sustaining medical treatment on a ward's behalf. The case involved a 21-year-old woman, Karen Ann Quinlan, diagnosed as persistently unconscious. She required a respirator, a nasogastric feeding tube, and around-the-clock nursing care. Her family asked Karen's physicians to remove the respirator, based on the family's belief that under the circumstances mechanically assisted respiration was extraordinary. The physicians believed that such a decision would be based on Karen's quality of life and therefore would not conform with accepted medical practice and ethics.

The New Jersey Supreme Court ruled that persons with or without the capacity to refuse life-sustaining treatment had a constitutionally protected right to "abandon specialized technological procedures." This right would prevail in cases involving patients who could not be restored to "long life and vibrant health." The court noted that with treatment Karen Quinlan was expected to die within a year "with no potential for resumption or continuance of other than a 'vegetative' existence." Her right to refuse treatment could be exercised by a surrogate even absent clear proof of a prior directive by Karen since, in the court's opinion, "an overwhelming majority" of society's members in the same circumstances would make the same choice for themselves or others.

According to the court, neither the state's interest in preserving life nor the attending physicians' ethical objections would outweigh Karen's putative interest in refusing treatment. The court created a sliding-scale approach to balancing these competing interests by holding that "the State's interest *contra* weakens and the individual's right to privacy grows as the degree of bodily invasion increases and the prognosis dims." The court concluded that given Karen's "hopeless loss of cognitive or sapient life[,]" the state (i.e., the judiciary) had no basis for compelling treatment. The court ruled, in addition, that law enforcement officials could not prosecute a surrogate decision to remove Karen's treatment as homicide or assisted suicide since in the court's view Karen's subsequent death would result from "existing natural causes." The court thus found "a real and in this case determinative distinction between the unlawful taking of life of another and the ending of artificial life support systems as a matter of self-determination."

Similarly, the court ruled that Karen's attending physicians had no compelling ethical basis for opposing the guardian's request because "Karen's present treatment serves only a maintenance function [and] cannot cure or improve her condition but at best can only prolong her inevitable slow deterioration and death[.]" According to the court, "it is perfectly apparent from the testimony [below] that humane decisions against resuscitative or maintenance therapy are frequently a recognized *de facto* response in the medical world to the irreversible, terminal, pain ridden patient[.]" The court concluded that it would be irrational and inconsistent to require Karen to be treated when accepted medical ethics would support the removal of treatment from "a competent patient terminally ill, riddled by cancer and suffering great pain."

The court ruled that a family member—in this case, Karen's father—could be appointed as legal guardian for the purpose of effectuating the removal of Karen's life-sustaining care. Acting as guardian, the father could consult with the attending physicians to see whether Karen's circumstances had worsened to the point that the physicians now would support the removal of treatment or transfer Karen to the care of new physicians willing to comply with his nontreatment request. The court recommended that an ethics committee or like body in the hospital where Karen resided examine the case. If the physicians and the committee agreed that Karen would not regain consciousness, then her life support could be withdrawn without incurring civil or criminal liability.

Several aspects of this case and its aftermath are worth noting. First, the prognosis of Karen's life expectancy as presented to the court proved to be erroneous. After her respirator was removed, and without further mechanical respiration, Karen survived for another nine years, far exceeding expectations of her survival *with* a respirator. She died on June 11, 1985. Second, during this period, Karen continued to receive nourishment and fluids through a gastrostomy tube because her family opposed its removal (Quinlan and Quinlan, 1977). Third, the court created an influential though troublesome test for gauging the strength of a state's interest in preserving life based on a patient's mental condition and prospect for regaining mental functions. By holding that New Jersey had no compelling justification for maintaining the lives of those who permanently lacked cognition, the court ratified a disability-based criterion for deciding who lives and who dies.

REFERENCES: *In re Quinlan*, 355 A.2d 647 (N.J. 1976); Quinlan, Joseph, and Julia Quinlan. 1977. *Karen Ann: The Quinlans Tell Their Story*. Garden City, NY: Doubleday; United Press International. June 12, 1985. "Karen Ann Quinlan, 31, Dies 9 Years After Coma Decision." *New York Times*, p. 1 col. 2.

DANIEL AVILA

IN RE WANGLIE

Oliver Wanglie had been married to Helga Wanglie for 53 years. On their wedding day he had promised to cherish her in sickness and in health, "until death do us part." In May of 1990, sickness had come, Helga Wanglie was near death, and her husband was determined to keep his vow. Helga's doctors could not cure her body and believed it was time for the sickness to end and for Helga Wanglie to die.

Right-to-die cases usually involve gravely ill, unconscious patients who have not left any advance directive as to the kind of health care they should receive if they become incapacitated. In such cases a surrogate decision-maker, usually a family member or close friend, petitions the court for the right to terminate the life-sustaining treatment keeping the patient alive. Often such petitions are unopposed, but sometimes the matter is contested by overly cautious hospital officials and doctors who are afraid of a lawsuit or aggressive pro-life advocates who oppose the taking of innocent human life. In most of the reported cases the petitions are granted and the patient dies once the life-sustaining treatment is terminated.

In re Wanglie was unique and captured the public's attention because it was a "right-to-live" case. Helga Wanglie's treating physicians wanted to disconnect their patient's ventilator so she could "die with dignity" while her husband, hoping for a miracle, wanted to keep the ventilator in place.

Wanglie presented a different perspective on the ethical questions usually presented in right-to-die cases. When medical science can no longer help a comatose patient, should the patient's doctor or the family have the final authority to make life-and-death decisions? If the patient's religious philosophy differs from the physician's medical philosophy, how should the decision be made? Where a doctor institutes life-sustaining treatment but later concludes such medical treatment is futile, does the doctor have the right to terminate the procedure? What duties does a physician have to a terminally ill patient who does not want to follow the doctor's advice to terminate the life-sustaining treatment?

Both parties lined up prominent ethicists to testify on the issues presented, but in the end, the case was decided on less esoteric grounds. Minnesota law requires the guardian to be the individual whose appointment is in the "best interest of the incapacitated person," (M.S.A. § 525.552 Subdt. 5 [1990]), and it also lists a number of relevant factors for the court to consider and evaluate in nominating a guardian (M.S.A. § 525.539 Subdt. 7 [1990]). While the newspapers and the experts debated whether it was in Mrs. Wanglie's best interest to stay alive, hoping for a miracle, or to die with dignity, the court conducted a very ordinary evidentiary hearing on the issue of who should be appointed as Mrs. Wanglie's guardian. The hospital had nominated a professional conservator who had approximately 80 clients but who had never met Mrs. Wanglie. Mr. Wanglie nominated himself.

During the hearing, the hospital's witnesses admitted that Oliver Wanglie was well qualified to oversee Mrs. Wanglie's social, religious, and emotional needs, but they argued strenuously that the court should find Mr. Wanglie incompetent to make any additional decisions about his wife's medical care. The hospital's position was interesting, since the same physicians were arguing that further medical treatment for Mrs. Wanglie would be futile, and on cross-examination, Mr. Wanglie's lawyer also pointed out that except with regard to the issue of removing the ventilator, Wanglie had thoughtfully agreed with the treating physicians about every major decision in his wife's case. Now those same physicians were attacking his capacity to make good medical decisions.

Oliver Wanglie took the stand and was aggressively cross-examined. The hospital's attorney asked Mr. Wanglie if he would follow the court's order to disconnect his wife's ventilator if he were appointed guardian. Mr. Wanglie stated that he did not think the court would order him to do that but that he would even oppose the court in an effort to keep his wife alive. The hospital's attorney arqued that this response should be the deathblow for Wanglie's petition, but the court determined otherwise.

One of the relevant factors to be considered in evaluating a proposed guardian is the interest and commitment of the proposed guardian. Mr. Wanglie's commitment to his wife and to the vow he had made to her on their wedding day was so strong that he was willing to risk contempt of court in order to provide for her welfare. The court appointed Mr. Wanglie as guardian for his wife, and she died peacefully a few days later.

REFERENCES: *Cruzan v. Director*, 110 S. Ct. 2841 (1990); *In re Jobes*, 529 A.2d 434 (N.J. 1987), *In re Torres*, 357 N.W.2d 322 (1984); *In re Wanglie*, Hennepin Cnty. Dist. Crt. PX-91-283 (1991); *Missouri Department of Health v. Busalacchi* (1991) No. 73677, M. S. A. 525.531–525.554.

BARRY McKEE

INSTITUTE OF MEDICINE

The IOM is a private, not-for-profit center for health policy research established in 1970 under the charter of the National Academy of Sciences (NAS)*.

The IOM was formed to be "composed of individuals of distinction and achievement, committed to the advancement of the health sciences and education and to the improvement of health care." It has eight divisions, each of which is assisted by an advisory board: Health Sciences Policy, Health Care Services, Health Promotion and Disease Prevention, International Health, Biobehavioral Sciences and Mental Disorders, the Food and Nutrition Board, the Medical Follow-up Agency, and the Health Policy Fellowship Programs.

Among its publications, available through the National Academy Press, are *Ethics in Health Care* (1974); *The Elderly and Functional Dependency* (1977); *Nursing and Nursing Education: Public Policy and Private Action* (1983); *Preventing Low Birthweight* (1985); *For-Profit Enterprise in Health Care* (1986); *Medically Assisted Conception: An Agenda for Research* (1989); *The Responsible Conduct of Research in the Health Sciences* (1989); *The Artificial Heart: Prototypes, Policies, and Patients* (1991); *Biomedical Politics* (1991); *Extending Life, Enhancing Life: A National Research Agenda on Aging* (1991); *Research and Service Programs in the Public Health Service: Challenges in Organization* (1991); *Access to Health Care in America* (1993); *An Assessment of the National Institutes of Health Women's Health Initiative* (1993); *Adopting New Medical Technology* (1994).

In addition to compiling reports, the IOM also initiates colloquia, workshops, and lectures to address important issues in health reform. Future plans include, for example, a broad study of methods of bioethical problem solving by society, including government, community bodies, professional societies, and religious groups; research concerning the development and use of tests for genetic disorders; and a workshop exploring the informed consent process.

REFERENCES: Bulger, R. E. 1992. "The Institute of Medicine." *Kennedy Institute of Ethics Journal* 2:73–77; National Academy of Sciences. 1994. *1994 Report to Congress.* Washington, D.C.: National Academy Press.

DEBORAH R. MATHIEU

INSTITUTIONAL ETHICS COMMITTEE

An Institutional Ethics Committee (IEC), commonly hospital based and composed of a mixture of health care professionals and laypeople, is designed to ensure ethical integrity in patient care decisions and institutional policy and procedures. Historically, there have been six varieties of IECs. Each had distinctive patient care and ethical issues, specific mandates, and a different legal status. Each also contributed to some aspect of the common role and functioning of the Hospital Ethics Committee (HEC), which is the most prevalent of IECs.

The earliest version of the IEC was the Kidney Dialysis Admission and Policy Committee. It was occasioned by the invention of the arteriovenous ("Scribner") shunt and cannula (1961) at the Swedish Hospital of the University of Washington (Seattle). This technological innovation made it possible, for the first time, to provide hemodialysis for chronic, end-stage renal patients. Because the cost was great and there was more demand than supply, this IEC had the task of deciding which candidates for dialysis would receive it. Their decisions were based on other than medical grounds, since all the patients were medically eligible. This was a committee mainly of laypersons who applied social value criteria to the problem of allocating a scarce medical resource. The problem disappeared when all end-stage renal therapy was reimbursed under Medicare, starting in 1972. The Seattle Kidney Dialysis Admission and Policy Committee was the first committee to provide moral scrutiny of medical decision making by society.

The Medical-Moral Committee is mandated and encouraged by the U.S. and Canadian Catholic hierarchy for all Catholic hospitals. In its contemporary form, it originated in 1971 with the express purpose of communicating the ethical implications of developing technology "from the front line of experience to the rear line of policy making." Its concerns were religious, mainly doctrinal, values, and in particular, the protection of the sanctity of life. Although concerned with the scrutiny of the full range of medical decision making, there was special focus on reproduction issues and particularly termination of pregnancy decisions. These committees aimed at establishing consensus interpretation of the *Ethical and Religious Directives for Catholic Health Facilities* (1949; revised in 1954 and 1971). Originally conceived as the "moral conscience of the hospital," the Medical-Moral Committee functioned as a predecessor to the current Hospital Ethics Committee as they currently exist in many Catholic institutions.

The Institutional Review Board* (IRB) is required by federal law of every hospital that participates in Food and Drug Administration* (FDA) clinical trial protocols or federal patient care funding. Its establishment was a major recommendation of the National Commission for the Protection of Human Subjects of Biomedical and Behavioral Research* (1976) in order to protect the human subjects of advanced clinical biomedical research. The ethical concern of the IRB is to ensure the autonomy of the patient as a research subject by protecting his or her privacy through confidentiality and especially through rigorous and meticulous processes of informed consent.

The Prognosis Committee derived from the decision in the New Jersey case of *In re Quinlan** (1976) in which the parents of a young woman in a persistent vegetative state petitioned for the removal of respirator support. *Quinlan* was a landmark decision for support of the privacy of the individual over the state's duty to protect life and the role of the family in the substitution of judgment for this aspect of patient autonomy. That support is contingent on the medical determination that the treatment matches the prognosis. Chief Justice Richard Hughes suggested, in his ruling, that the medical determinations in future cases be assisted by an ad hoc "ethics committee."

Regulation of this committee's function was subsequently developed in New Jersey (1977) by a joint task force of the department of health, board of medical examiners, and attorney general's office. It stipulated that such a Prognosis Committee would be composed of two neurologists or neurosurgeons and a third nonphysician and would be convened to render a medical judgment to confirm (or not) the likelihood of a patient's return to "a cognitive and sapient state." Although its jurisdiction is exceedingly narrow, the Prognosis Committee model is frequently activated in order to ensure the integrity of patient care decisions involving cases of persistent vegetative state.

The Infant Care Review Committee (ICRC)* is similar in many ways to the Prognosis Committee in that its role is closely constrained in legal precedent and mandate to medical prognosis judgments. It has become an important agency in the implementation of the Federal Child Abuse Amendments.

The Bioethics Committee or Hospital Ethics Committee (HEC) is the most common and widespread of the IECs in the United States. It was initially a hospital response to the President's Commission for the Study of Ethical Problems in Medicine and Biomedical and Behavioral Research* (1982). The President's Commission recommended an "internal mechanism" for hospitals to deal with prospective ethical problems in patient care decision making. In addressing this broad concern, the HEC has emerged as an agency with three areas of activity: education, development of hospital ethics policy and procedures, and case consultation.

Education is universally the first function of these committees, starting with self-education of its members and the hospital staff and expanding out to the larger community, including public education. This function has been given additional impetus by various national and state policies (e.g., Organ Donation and Transplantation Act, Neurological Criteria for Death legislation, Patient Self-Determination Act, etc.), the implementation of which requires broad educational and communication efforts.

HECs also develop hospital policies and procedures to ensure patients' rights in the context of changes in law, regulation, accreditation, licensing, and professional practices with ethical significance. The development of a Do Not Resuscitate (DNR) policy, for example, was often the first order of business for HECs. Hospital-based policies/procedures on such topics as brain death,* organ donation, withholding and withdrawal of treatment, informed consent, and the like, continue to exercise HECs' policy and procedure activities.

Case consultation was the last function to develop and is still not universally practiced by HECs. At one end of the spectrum, hypothetical case presentations are used as part of the educational function. At the other end of the spectrum is the highly proactive role of a "consultation service" in which a team of HEC members are invited to consult, and provide advice or opinion, on an active patient care dilemma. Typically, HECs move across this spectrum over a period of time, experimenting first with retrospective review, then the application of policy to cases, later providing informal prospective review of a troublesome case, and perhaps finally developing a consultation service. This variation from one institution to another is a reflection of the culture of the institution, the leadership of the committee, and the enthusiasm of committee members. The Patient Self-Determination Act, and the mandates of the Joint Commission of the Accreditation of Healthcare Organizations (JCAHO) that support it, require that hospitals develop a process by which disputes in the implementation of advance directives may be resolved. This requirement has given impetus for some HECs to move further along the case consultation spectrum in order to provide this "dispute resolution" function.

No definitive national survey of HECs exists. Several state-based studies, however, provide guides to best estimates of some salient characteristics of the HECs. By extrapolation from such studies, we estimate that approximately 30 to 35 percent of U.S. hospitals support HECs. Extrapolation of this sort is exceedingly precarious, however, and differentiation of institutions by type, size, and location needs to be taken into account. Although the JCAHO has not yet required HECs as a standard, some states have regulations that require such committees or some of the functions they provide. The HECs in these states generally conform to the letter, but not all to the spirit, of the law.

Hospitals in densely populated areas are more likely to have committees than rural hospitals. Likewise, medium-large (200- to 500-bed) hospitals are more likely to support an HEC than either smaller or larger institutions. The existence of residency training programs in community hospitals is a good predictor of bioethics programs in general and of an HEC in particular. Service modalities were initially important differentiation, but the presence of intensive care units (ICUs) or combined ICU/CCU (critical care unit) is no longer a distinctive characteristic of larger hospitals.

Unlike the IRB, the Prognosis, and the Infant Care Review Committees, the HEC has no defined legal mandate or charges. Lacking such standards, individual HECs vary widely in their specific structures and functions. Typically interdisciplinary, HECs may range in size from 6 to 30 or more members, with an average of between 15 and 20 individuals actively involved. Most committees are composed of physicians (who commonly chair the HEC) and nurses, in equal numbers, and a member of the clergy, an administrator, a lawyer, and a social worker. Other members might include an academic or consulting bioethicist, a member of the governing board of the hospital, a patient advocate professional, and a representative of the lay community. HECs typically meet at least quarterly, with monthly meetings a common level of activity.

Current issues for an HEC include developing standards for its various activities either through JCAHO requirements or the various professional bioethics societies; determining the extent and nature of liability for its role in specific patient care decisions; extending HEC activities to other settings, most notably nursing homes; continually redefining the scope of its activities, with such matters as resources allocation determination; involvement in bioethical aspects of public policy (e.g., health care delivery reform); and developing a consultation service, taking notable attention.

REFERENCES: *Cambridge Quarterly of Health Care Ethics.* 1994. Edited by David Thomasma, Thomasine Kushner, and Steve Helig. New York: Cambridge University Press; Cranford, Ronald E., and A. Edward Doudera, eds. 1984. *Institutional Ethics Committees and Health Care Decision Making.* Ann Arbor: Health Administration Press; Fleetwood, Janet, and Stephanie S. Unger. 1994. "Institutional Ethics Committees and the Shield of Immunity." *Annals of Internal Medicine* 120:320–325; *Hospital Ethics Committee (HEC) Forum.* 1994. Edited by Stuart F. Spicker and Judith W. Ross. Hingham, MA: Kluwer Academic Publishers; La Puma, John, and David Schiedermayer. 1994. *Ethics Consultation: A Practical Guide.* Boston: Jones and Bartlett; President's

Commission. 1983. "Deciding to Forego Life-Sustaining Treatment: Ethical, Medical and Legal Issues in Treatment Decisions." In *Report on the Ethical Problems in Medicine and Biomedical and Behavioral Research.* Vol. 2. Washington, D.C.: U.S. Government Printing Office.

JOSEPH C. d'ORONZIO

INSTITUTIONAL REVIEW BOARDS

IRBs, also commonly known as Human Subjects Research Committees, are research review committees designed to protect the rights and well-being of human subjects of research. The Common Federal Rule for the Protection of Human Subjects, which governs all federally funded biomedical research in the United States involving human subjects, requires that an IRB review and approve each human subject research protocol before implementation and monitor the research on a continuing basis. Although an institution may refuse to allow an IRB-approved research project to be implemented, it may not permit federally funded research to proceed without explicit IRB approval. (The U.S. government also mandates that a research institution receiving federal grants and using animal subjects in biomedical research appoint a similar review committee, called an Institutional Animal Care and Use Committee, to protect the interests of the animals.) Federal regulations do not mandate IRB approval for nonfederally funded research, but research institutions tend to require it anyway for all human subjects research, regardless of support source. Thus, the authority by which an IRB evaluates research protocols derives from both federal regulation and institutional policy.

It is the responsibility of each institution sponsoring an IRB to develop and publish official principles and guidelines for protecting the rights and welfare of human subjects in research. This assurance, which bears the imprimatur of institutional authority, must contain a statement of the codes, declarations, and ethical principles underpinning the specific institutional policies. Within the institution, there must be an authorized official who has the legal and administrative authority to ensure effective oversight of research activities and investigator/institutional compliance with federal regulations and IRB decisions. The research institution must also provide its IRB with adequate staff and resources to conduct its review process and recordkeeping duties. "Independent" (i.e., noninstitutional) IRBs may be established to review projects from individual investigators or small groups when institutional support is not available or feasible.

It is customary for each IRB to have a written manual of procedures and guidelines to be followed by investigators and the IRB for conducting initial and continuing review and for reporting decisions and recommendations to the investigator. The IRB must also document its review and approval of all research with human subjects, its review and approval of all research changes, unanticipated problems involving subject risk, and its notification process for adverse event reporting.

The IRB chairperson is selected or elected and should have appropriate professional skills and sufficient institutional prestige to ensure IRB decisions are immune from pressure by investigators, institutional administration, or other professional/nonprofessional sources. Diversity and societal representation are the goal of federal policy for IRB committee composition. There must be at least five members with varying backgrounds in scientific activity, behavioral expertise, and so on, and at least one noninstitutional member. Every effort should be made to have an appropriate gender and ethnic balance in the committee.

Each approved research project must be reevaluated by the IRB at least annually, or at more frequent intervals appropriate to the degree of subject risk. This review focuses largely on any changes in the risk/benefit ratio, assuring adequate safety and data monitoring, and evaluating unanticipated adverse events. The IRB may require research modifications, or consent changes on the basis of these periodic reviews, and has the authority to suspend or terminate the project.

Protection of the research subjects' rights of privacy and confidentiality is an important responsibility of the IRB. Subjects have a right to know the extent to which the research may compromise their self-control and the extent to which information about them will be disclosed to others. Concerns often arise with the issue of the identifiability of the subject, either in the selection process or from the research records maintained. To protect the subject, the IRB requires the establishment of safeguards to protect the information from unauthorized disclosure (e.g., limited access to data, locked record storage, record destruction, removal of identifiers) to which the subject must consent. On occasion, this becomes so paramount that waiver of the consent form is granted when the form may be an identifiable link to the subject. The IRB may be called upon to make difficult decisions when the research involves covert observation of private or public activities. All such research in children and minors must be reviewed by the IRB committee. IRB review is also required when identifiers are recorded, and the observations would place the subjects at risk for criminal or civil liability, financial harm, employability, or reputation. Research investigators may obtain an advance grant of confidentiality in particularly sensitive research that even precludes subpoena. The IRB has the authority to waive the requirement for prior consent, however, if it feels the interests of the subject are adequately protected.

In theory, requiring prior and continuing review of research involving human and other animal subjects ensures that their interests are adequately protected. In practice, however, the committee structure is often problematic. Since most committee members belong to the research institution, for instance, there is often an institutional bias that constrains discussion and consideration of options. And while IRB decisions are supposed to be immune from pressure by others—investigators, for example, and institutional administrators—it is difficult to guarantee this in all cases. Finally, those committees who use majority rule may often override a more compassionate or more knowing minority opinion. Despite its flaws, however, the requirement for ongoing local committee review is a significant step toward protecting vulnerable research subjects.

REFERENCES: Anonymous. 1992. "Tales of Informed Consent: Four Years on an Institutional Review Board." *Health Matrix* 2:193; Greenwald, R. A., Ryan, M. K., and Mulvihill, J. E., eds. 1982. *Human Subjects Research: A Handbook for Institutional Review Boards.* New York: Plenum Press; Kim, D. T. 1994. "A Retrospective Analysis of Institutional Review Boards and Informed Consent Practices in EMS Research." *An-*

nals of Emergency Medicine 23:70; Porter, Joan P. 1991. "The Federal Policy for the Protection of Human Subjects." *IRB* 13:8–9; Veatch, R. M. 1987. *The Patient as Partner: A Theory of Human Experimentation Ethics.* Bloomington: Indiana University Press.

WILLIAM F. DENNY

INTRACERVICAL DEVICES (ICDS)

Demand for reversible fertility control has led to the development of a variety of ICDs. A prototype has been tested successfully in Britain. This ICD is a mushroom-shaped device that is inserted in the cervical canal. The main portion of the device is a hollow cylinder made of inert polycarbonate plastic containing a nontoxic silicone rubber valve that prevents the ascent of sperm while allowing exit of menstrual flux. The cap of the ICD prevents penetration of any sperm cells that may have gained access to the area between the cervical walls and the cylinder. The device is kept in place by two anchors of stainless steel on the outside of the cylinder; the ICD is inserted or removed with a specially designed inserter.

Another form of intracervical device releases a relatively constant level of levonorgestrel from a Silastic reservoir that is placed in the cervical canal. Horizontal arms located in the uterine opening hold it in place. Although it presently has an unacceptably high rate of expulsion, researchers are attempting to refine the design to reduce this rate.

Research continues on the Silastic vaginal ring. One method being tested releases a combination of levonorgestrel and estrogen to virtually eliminate ovulation. The ring is designed to stay in place for up to three weeks. The woman then removes it for one week and reinserts it herself. The same ring can be used for up to six months. A variation on this device now being investigated is a low-dose ring that releases levonorgestrel but not estrogen. Although it does not stop ovulation, this vaginal ring blocks conception by making the cervical mucus impermeable to sperm for the two months it is in place.

Other devices that are now being tested or used include the cervical cap, which was approved for general use by the U.S. Food and Drug Administration (FDA) in May 1988. This small, rubber, thimble-shaped barrier contraceptive fits tightly across the cervix, thus preventing sperm from entering the uterus. The cap has been shown to be 85 percent effective in preventing pregnancy, comparable to the diaphragm but significantly less effective than long-term subdermal implants. The cap is inserted by the woman for up to 60 hours at a time, but problems remain concerning cap fit and dislodgement.

REFERENCES: Darney, P. D. 1991. "Subdermal Progestin Implant Contraception." *Current Opinion on Obstetrics and Gynecology* 3(4): 470–476; Katz, Z., M. Lancet, and S. Shiber. 1986. "New Intracervical Contraceptive Device." *British Journal of Sexual Medicine* (May): 153–154; Klitch, Michael. 1988. "FDA Approval Ends Cervical Cap's Marathon." *Family Planning Perspectives* 20(3): 137–138; Liskin, Laurie, and R. Blackman. 1987. "Hormonal Contraception: New Long-Acting Methods." *Population Reports* (March–April): K57–K87; Rastula, K. 1988. "Clinical Performance of a Levonorgestrel-Releasing Intracervical Device During the First Year of Use." *Contraception* 36(6): 659–664.

See also **DEPO-PROVERA; SUBDERMAL HORMONAL IMPLANTS (SHI).**

ROBERT H. BLANK

IN VITRO FERTILIZATION (IVF)

IVF is the procedure by which eggs are removed from a woman's ovaries and fertilized outside her body. The resulting embryos are kept in a culture medium for approximately two days until they reach the four- to eight-cell stage, at which point they are transferred via catheter into the uterus of the woman. When successful, the embryos will implant within six to nine days, resulting in a pregnancy. Usually, the retrieval of the mature eggs via laparoscopic surgery is preceded by ovulation induction in which the woman takes a combination of hormones that stimulate her ovaries to "superovulate"—to produce an abnormal number of eggs to be fertilized, thus increasing the chances of conception and, ultimately, pregnancy. This procedure is indicated when the oviducts are blocked, preventing the egg from passing through the fallopian tubes to be fertilized.

One variation of IVF is gamete intrafallopian transfer (GIFT) in which sperm and eggs are transferred separately to the fallopian tubes. Because fertilization takes place in the fallopian tubes instead of a petri dish, GIFT is more acceptable than IVF to some religions. A second is zygote intrafallopian transfer (ZIFT) in which the embryo is placed in the fallopian tube about 18 hours after fertilization. All of these techniques (IVF, GIFT, ZIFT) can use donor ova and sperm where appropriate and increasingly make use of frozen embryos.

The short history of IVF demonstrates the demand for a diffusion of this technology. In 1978 in England, Louise Brown became the first baby conceived via IVF. In January 1980, after considerable political debate, Norfolk General Hospital in Virginia obtained governmental approval to make the technique available. On December 28, 1981, Elizabeth Carr became the first baby conceived with the help of IVF in the United States. By 1990, the number of clinics offering IVF expanded to over 200. The U.S. IVF Registry has documented 70,000 stimulation cycles, resulting in approximately 8,200 deliveries and 10,600 babies. In 1991 alone, approximately 4,000 IVF clinical pregnancies were reported by the approximately 200 clinic members of the Society for Assisted Reproductive Technology (SART) for a rate of about 19 percent per retrieval. Corresponding figures for GIFT were 1,500 and 34 percent.

The potential clientele for IVF is approximately 1 million persons with an estimated income of $2 billion annually. Most clinics continue to have waiting lists of couples who are willing to pay between $4,000 and $6,000 for each chance to become pregnant. In many cases the final cost of attempting pregnancy through IVF approaches $50,000, counting multiple cycles, incidental costs, and loss of employment for the duration of treatment, which might last for over six months. Despite this investment, up to 80 percent of the women who undergo IVF do not become pregnant.

As a result of the high costs, pressures are mounting for insurance companies to pay for all or part of the procedure. Advocacy groups have lobbied states for insurance coverage. At least seven states have responded by adopting statutes that mandate insurance coverage or the provision of policy options that reimburse all or some of the costs of IVF and related fertility treatment. Until now, Medicaid has been spared the costs of IVF, leading to questions of inequitable access.

In addition to its clinical application to circumvent infertility caused by blocked fallopian tubes, IVF expands considerably the possible combinations of germinal material and further complicates the concept of parenthood. There is no biological reason why the fertilized egg cannot be transferred to a woman other than the one who supplied the egg. IVF, then, enables collaborative conception and the use of surrogate mothers who carry another genetic mother's baby to term. Moreover, there is evidence that the embryo might be transferred to the abdominal cavity of a male, thus enabling male pregnancy.

The removal of conception from the secrecy of the womb to under the microscope of the laboratory also enables a wide range of preembryo research possibilities, as well as genetic screening, selection, and modification of embryos as these techniques develop. Techniques in which the embryo is physically divided to create twins will permit screening of one embryo—only if it "passes the test" will its twin be transferred to the womb for implantation and eventual birth. Cryopreservation of eggs and embryos, in addition to sperm, permits combination of germ materials from persons across generations. Embryo freezing, perhaps combined with twinning, will allow for twins to be born years or even generations apart.

Because the IVF process is designed to override the natural reproductive mechanisms, questions have been raised about its safety. To date, however, it appears that the overall rate of congenital abnormalities of IVF babies is not significantly higher than for those conceived naturally, although there are some suggestions that IVF babies exhibit a higher incidence of low birth weights (Bonnicksen, 1989, 85). Potential sources of damage, however, could be related to development of the ovum (especially if superovulation is employed), the selection of sperm (the female reproductive tract selects against some types of abnormal sperm), the fertilization itself, and the use of freezing techniques to preserve gametes or embryos (Schenker and Ezra, 1994).

REFERENCES: Bonnicksen, Andrea L. 1989. *In Vitro Fertilization: Building Policy for Laboratories to Legislatures.* New York: Columbia University Press; Ingram, John D. 1993. "Should In Vitro Fertilization Be Covered by Medical Expense Reimbursement Plans?" *American Journal of Family Law* 7: 103–108; "MRI, SART, and AFS." 1990. *Fertility and Sterility* 55(1): 14–23; Neumann, Peter J., Soheyla D. Gharib, and Milton C. Weinstein. 1994. "The Cost of a Successful Delivery with In Vitro Fertilization." *New Zealand Journal of Medicine* 331(4): 239–242; Neumann, Peter J., and Magnus Johannesson. 1994. "The Willingness to Pay for In Vitro Fertilization." *Medical Care* 32(7): 686–699; Schenker, Joseph G., and Yossef Ezra. 1994. "Complications of Assisted Reproductive Technologies." *Fertility and Sterility* 61(3): 411–422; Society for Assisted Reproductive Technology. 1993. "Assisted Reproductive Technology in the United States and Canada." *Fertility and Sterility* 59(5): 956–962.

See also **EGG DONATION; PREIMPLANTATION GENETIC DIAGNOSIS; PRENATAL GENETIC DIAGNOSIS.**

ROBERT H. BLANK

J

JOHNSON V. CALVERT

In 1989, Anna Johnson agreed to serve as a gestational surrogate for Mark and Crispina Calvert, a married couple. Crispina was unable to gestate the fetus due to a partial hysterectomy that left ovaries and the ability to ovulate but not to gestate. An agreement was signed in which Mark and Crispina agreed to pay Anna a fee for gestating a fetus fertilized ''in vitro'' utilizing sperm and ovum from Mark and Crispina. Part of the money was to be paid before the birth, and part, after. Mark and Crispina also agreed to take out a $200,000 life insurance policy on Anna. Anna agreed to relinquish parental rights.

The in vitro fertilization and implantation of the zygote were successful; however, the relationship between the gestational surrogate and the genetic parents of the child began to break down when Mark and Crispina learned that Anna had withheld medical information. Her reproductive history included several stillbirths and miscarriages, making her a less-than-ideal candidate as a gestational surrogate. Anna thought that Mark and Crispina had violated their agreement by not doing enough to obtain the required insurance. She also ''felt abandoned'' when premature birth was threatened. Anna threatened to refuse to give up the child if Mark and Crispina did not pay the remainder of the surrogacy fee prior to the birth of the child. Mark and Crispina sued to be declared the legal parents of the child. Anna filed an additional suit to be declared the legal mother. The suits were consolidated.

Blood tests were done following the birth of the child that excluded Anna as the biological mother. Crispina was thus recognized by the court as the ''natural mother'' of the child. The child was placed with Mark and Crispina until a judgment could be made by the court as to who was the ''legal mother'' of the child. Anna was permitted to visit with the baby. The subsequent ruling of the Superior Court of Orange County recognized Crispina and Mark as the ''genetic, biological, and natural'' parents of the child (*Anna J. v. Mark C.,* 1991, 373).

The contract was viewed as legal and enforceable; therefore, Anna had no parental rights. The court terminated her visitation rights. Anna responded by appealing the case.

The appellate court utilized the California Civil and Evidence Codes to guide its decision on the question of who is the legal mother of the child. Under the civil code, the legal parent is either the natural or adoptive parent. The California Statute (Civil Code Section 7015) allows for determination or exclusion of natural maternity in the same manner as paternity (Civil Code Section 7004) by meeting the conditions of the California Evidence Code. Under Evidence Code Section 621, there is a presumption of paternity if the husband of the mother of the child is living with her. However, paternity may be rebutted by blood tests as prescribed in the Evidence Code, beginning with Section 890. Thus, if blood tests determine that the husband of the mother of the child is not genetically related to the child, then he is not to be considered the natural father of the child. Similarly, if blood tests exclude the woman who gives birth to the child as the genetic mother, then she is not the genetic mother of the child.

The court addressed the issues of the relative importance of gestation and genetics. Anna argued that Civil Code Section 7003—which states, ''The parent and child relationship may be established as follows: '(1) Between a child and the natural mother it may be established by proof of her having given birth to the child, or under this part' ''—established her as the natural mother of the child (*Anna J. v. Mark C.,* 1991, 377). The court disagreed. They interpreted the statute to indicate that giving birth was one way, but only one way, in which motherhood might be established. The birth mother may be ruled out as the natural mother by blood tests.

Anna also argued that to deny her claim to parenthood would be to deny her due process liberty interest. In examining this argument, the court recognized the ''profound'' contributions that a woman makes to a child's development during gestation. However, it noted that the rights of a gestational surrogate have not been traditionally protected and that to enforce these rights would infringe on the liberty rights of the natural parents of the child, which have been traditionally protected. They noted that Anna could apply for visitation rights and that granting of these rights would be decided, based on the best interests of the child.

Neither was equal protection violated by this application of the state statutes, according to the court, since the status of natural mother and natural father was determined in the same manner. Therefore, there was no basis for an accusation of gender discrimination. As to making a decision on the status of two women, they gave greater weight to the importance of genetics over gestation. The issue of enforceability of surrogate motherhood contracts was not decided.

In 1992, the California Supreme Court granted a review. As a result of that review, the California Supreme Court concluded that Crispina and Mark Calvert are the natural parents of the child and that ''this result does not offend the state or federal constitution or public policy'' (*Johnson v. Calvert,* 1993, 778). The

California Supreme Court disagreed with the appellate court that genetics should be weighted heavier than gestation. In the opinion of this court, both women had provided "acceptable proof of maternity" under the California statutes (*Johnson v. Calvert*, 1993, 782). However, as the statutes did not give preference of one type of proof over another, the California Supreme Court examined the intentions of the parties to determine maternity. As it was clear from the surrogacy agreement that Crispina was the intended mother, the California Supreme Court recognized her intention as determining maternity.

Anna argued that surrogacy contracts violate social policy, including statutes prohibiting payment for consent to adopt a child (California Penal Code Section 273), public policy underlying adoption statutes that would prohibit prebirth waiver of parental rights, federal statutes prohibiting involuntary servitude, and public policy concerning exploitation and dehumanization of women and commodification of children. The California Supreme Court rejected these arguments and distinguished between surrogacy and adoption. They concluded that the element of coercion was absent in surrogacy agreements and that there was "no proof that surrogacy contracts exploit poorer women to any greater degree than economic necessity in general exploits them" or will foster the idea that children are mere commodities (*Johnson v. Calvert*, 1993, 785). The California Supreme Court also rejected arguments that the court decision naming Crispina as the natural mother of the child interfered with Anna's constitutional rights.

Johnson v. Calvert was cited in *In re Marriage of Moschetta* (30 Cal. Rptr 2d 893) (Cal. App. 4 Dist. 1994), involving a custody dispute over a child conceived in a traditional surrogacy arrangement. The appellate court noted the difference between the determination of the natural mother in a gestational surrogacy and a traditional surrogacy in which the surrogate is both the genetic and gestational mother of the child in declaring the surrogate to be the natural mother of the child. The court refused to enforce the surrogate motherhood contract, as enforcement would be incompatible with the rationale of *Johnson v. Calvert*.

REFERENCES: *Anna J. v. Mark C.,* 286 Cal. Rptr. 369 (Cal. App. 4 Dist. 1991); *In re Marriage of Moschetta,* 30 Cal. Rptr. 2d 893 (Cal. App. 4 Dist. 1994); *Johnson v. Calvert,* 851 P.2d 776 (Cal. 1993).

CHERYLON ROBINSON

L

"LIVING WILL" STATUTES

Living will statutes in general sanction the execution of declarations to with-hold and withdraw "life-sustaining" or "life-prolonging" treatment that apply when the declarant has a "terminal condition" and is no longer able to make medical treatment decisions. The first statute that authorized living will decla-rations was enacted in California in 1976. By 1994, 47 states, the District of Columbia, and Puerto Rico enacted statutes that authorize such declarations in one form or another. Only Michigan, New York, and Massachusetts have no such statute.

Living will statutes all include provisions that bestow civil and criminal im-munity on physicians who abide by declarations; requirements that the decla-ration voluntarily be signed and witnessed by competent adults (with restrictions on the identity of those who witness); revocation procedures; penalties for fal-sifying, forging, canceling, or destroying a declaration without the declarant's consent and for concealing a revocation; provisions stating that the implemen-tation of a declaration does not constitute suicide for any purpose and that declarations do not affect the sale, issuance, or terms of life insurance; and provisions that govern the transfer of declarants when health care providers are unwilling to comply with declarations. Regardless of the specifics in a decla-ration, the statutes all authorize the use of pain relief and comfort care measures.

Most statutes include suggested living will forms and provisions that specif-ically decline to authorize euthanasia, mercy killing, or intentional acts or omissions to end life other than to permit the natural process of dying. Under some statutes, a declaration is inoperative while a woman is pregnant. Some statutes provide that food and fluids must always be provided, while some more recent statutory formulations provide that artificially provided food and fluids may be declined when one has a terminal condition or is in a "persistent veg-etative state"*—frequently by way of a feature in the statutory form that permits the declarant to request or decline artificially provided food and fluids in such circumstances. Many statutes have been revised to bring them in closer conformity with the Uniform Rights of the Terminally Ill Act, issued by the Uniform Commissioners on State Law in 1985.

The purpose of the living will is to ensure that the terminally or severely ill patient's right to refuse life-supportive treatment will be honored when the patient is no longer able to make treatment decisions. Since living wills may be directed toward prospective, perhaps remote contingencies, they do not necessarily represent an expression of "informed" consent to forgoing treatment, which involves disclosure of specific risks and alternatives of a treatment in the context of specific circumstances. Because of the general terms used in living will forms, open to various interpretations by both the declarant and health care providers, and because of the often potentially variable interpretations of critical statutory definitions, a living will in practice may represent only a general, somewhat symbolic memorial of the patient's wish to decline extraordinary treatment as the patient is dying. Indeed, because most of the living will statutes provide subjective, good-faith immunity to physicians in implementing living wills, it would be practically difficult to hold physicians liable for failure to abide by the terms of a declaration. Moreover, a living will becomes operative only when the declarant becomes incapable of making treatment decisions, and the physician makes this determination as well. Thus, whether the declaration should be honored or not also falls to the physician in this regard.

These potential inadequacies of living will declarations may be somewhat remedied by inclusion of specific directions regarding specific forms of treatment in specific circumstances within the document and by providing copies of the document to third parties who might advocate for compliance. Inclusion of directions that fall outside the scope of the authorizing statute (for example, directions on forms of treatment that are not "life-sustaining" or for conditions that are not "terminal"), however, would not have the force or protection of statutory law—although they might otherwise be deemed sufficient evidence of patient intent to refuse or accept treatment by the judiciary. Similarly, living will declarations in those states without authorizing statutes would likely be generally enforceable under common law or constitutional law, although the usual statutory substantive and procedural safeguards and immunities would not apply.

Living will statutes and their statutory forms are strongly ratcheted in favor of assuring the declarant's right to refuse, rather than to accept, medical treatment or care. Hence, it becomes especially important that the declarant include specific directions on any treatment or care the declarant may wish to *receive* (for example, food and fluids by tube, resuscitation, antibiotics) and what circumstances in which it should be provided.

Because of the limited circumstances in which living will statutes govern treatment decisions, the general nature of the terms of declarations, and problems in assuring compliance, appointment of a health care decision-making agent (by which the declarant appoints another to make health care decisions for the declarant when the declarant is no longer able to do so by way of a durable power of attorney for health care or a similar instrument) is usually preferable in those states that authorize the appointment of such an agent. Nevertheless, the living will may be the only option for those who have no trusted third party who is available or willing to act as a health care decision maker.

REFERENCES: Marzen, Thomas J. 1986. "The 'Uniform Rights of the Terminally Ill Act': A Critical Analysis." *Issues in Law & Medicine* 1: 441–475; Meisel, Alan. 1989 & 1994 Supp. *The Right to Die.* §§ 10.1–10.27. New York: John Wiley & Sons; *Right to Die Law Digest.*

THOMAS J. MARZEN

M

MATERNAL SERUM ALPHA-FETOPROTEIN TESTING

Approximately 6,000 infants are born annually in the United States with neural tube defects, the majority equally divided between anencephaly and spina bifida. Although there is a 2 to 3 percent risk that the defect will recur after one affected pregnancy, over 90 percent of neural tube defects occur without prior indication that prenatal testing is warranted. In 1973, however, an association between elevated levels of maternal serum alpha-fetoprotein (AFP) and open neural tube defects was reported.

The level of AFP is determined from either amniotic fluid or maternal serum collected between the fourteenth and twentieth week of pregnancy. At present, approximately 90 percent of neural tube defects can be diagnosed through use of these tests. Because dynamic changes in AFP levels occur normally during this period of gestation, more critical control data and more advanced techniques for quantification are required. Also, since there is some overlap in the distribution of AFP levels in amniotic fluid and maternal serum both in pregnancies with neural tube defects and in normal pregnancies, there is still a false-positive rate in approximately 1 in 10,000 cases.

Although measurement of AFP in amniotic fluid samples taken from women at known risk for fetal neural tube defects is recommended, mass serum AFP screening from unselected pregnant women is regarded as premature. Approval by the Food and Drug Administration (FDA) of diagnostic kits to test for neural tube defects spurred controversy by consumer groups and scientists. Primary objections focused on the high rate of false positives, the gross nature of the test, and the possibility that women would abort fetuses solely on the basis of this preliminary screening device, when the actual probability of having an affected child is very low. Furthermore, because of heightened levels of maternal serum AFP in the pregnancies of black women not affected by open spina bifida as compared to white women, an adjustment must be made when used on black women. In 1986, California passed legislation requiring physicians to inform pregnant patients of the availability of AFP tests.

REFERENCES: Bombard, A. T., S. Nakagawa, C. D. Runowicz, et al. 1994. "Early Detection of Abdominal Pregnancy by Maternal Serum AFP + Screening." *Prenatal Diagnosis* 14(12): 1155–1157; Brazerol, W. F., S. Grover, and A. E. Donnenfeld. 1994. "Unexplained Elevated Maternal Serum Alpha-Fetoprotein Levels and Perinatal Outcome in an Urban Clinic Population." *American Journal of Obstetrics and Gynecology* 171(4): 1030–1035; Haddow, James E., Glenn E. Palomaki, and George J. Knight. 1992. "Prenatal Screening for Down's Syndrome with Use of Maternal Serum Markers." *New England Journal of Medicine* 327(9): 588–592; Johnson, A. M., G. E. Palomaki, and J. E. Haddow. 1990. "Maternal Serum- α -Fetoprotein Levels in Pregnancies Among Black and White Women with Open Spina Bifida: A United States Collaborative Study." *American Journal of Obstetrics and Gynecology* 162(3): 328–331; Reichler, A., R. F. Hume, Jr., A. Drugan, et al. 1994. "Risk of Anomalies as a Function of Level of Elevated Maternal Serum Alpha-Fetoprotein." *American Journal of Obstetrics and Gynecology* 171(4): 1052–1055; Steinbrook, Robert. 1986. "In California, Voluntary Mass Prenatal Screening." *Hastings Center Report* 16(5): 5–7.

See also **PRENATAL DIAGNOSIS.**

ROBERT H. BLANK

MATERNAL SUBSTANCE ABUSE DURING PREGNANCY

There has been much discussion in the 1990s regarding maternal use of chemical substances during pregnancy. While there is an ongoing debate in the United States whether abuse of chemical substances is an illness or a matter of choice, one alternative to dealing with such abuse has been to prosecute women. Two cases have reached state supreme courts.

Perhaps the most noteworthy case is that of Jennifer Johnson. Her first child, a son, tested positive for cocaine at birth in 1987. Two years later, Johnson advised hospital personnel that she was addicted to cocaine when she admitted herself to the hospital for delivery of her second child, a daughter. This child also tested positive for cocaine shortly after delivery. Neither child was addicted, suffered withdrawal symptoms, or was disabled. Johnson was then charged with child abuse and also with illegally delivering a controlled substance to her children during the birth process. In July 1989, the trial court convicted her on the controlled substance charge, and she was sentenced to 15 years' probation, community service, random drug testing, participation in educational and vocational training, and participation in a prenatal care program, should she become pregnant again. She was acquitted on the child abuse charge.

Johnson's conviction was upheld by Florida's Fifth District Court of Appeals (1991) but reversed by the Florida Supreme Court on the grounds that the intent of the state legislature was to treat drug-dependent mothers and newborns as a public health problem, not a criminal problem, and there was insufficient evidence to prove that the delivery of the cocaine occurred during the birth process (as opposed to prior to the birth process).

In 1988, Tammy Gray was indicted by a grand jury for child endangerment because she used cocaine during the last trimester of pregnancy. The trial court dismissed the indictment, finding that the statute applied to born children, not fetuses. The Ohio Supreme Court upheld the trial court's dismissal in *State v. Gray* (1992) because the statute did not apply to use of drugs by pregnant women.

Other noteworthy cases that have not reached state supreme courts include the 1986 case of Pamela Rae Stewart who was advised by her physician that she had placenta previa (a condition where the placenta blocks the birth canal) and therefore should not have intercourse and should seek prompt medical attention if she began to bleed vaginally. She was also advised not to use drugs during the pregnancy. Her son was born brain damaged and tested positive for amphetamines; he subsequently died. Stewart was charged under a California criminal statute that required parents to provide medical care, food, shelter, and clothing for their children, both born and unborn. An investigation revealed that Stewart had taken amphetamines, had smoked marijuana, had intercourse, and had failed to seek prompt medical attention when she began to bleed. In 1987, the trial court dismissed the charges against Stewart, finding that the California legislature had not intended for the statute to be used to prosecute women for not obtaining prenatal care and for not following physicians' recommendations.

In 1977, a California court of appeals ruled in *Reyes v. Superior Court* that a pregnant woman who was advised by a public health nurse not to use heroin could not be tried under the child abuse statute because the statute did not refer to the fetus. In 1988, Brenda Vaughn was incarcerated in the District of Columbia because she tested positive for cocaine during her sixth month of pregnancy. In 1989, Melanie Green was charged in Illinois with involuntary manslaughter and delivery of a controlled substance after her infant daughter died. Both mother and daughter tested positive for cocaine. Charges were dropped after a grand jury refused to issue an indictment. In 1990, Diane Pfannenstiel was charged with child abuse in Wyoming because she was intoxicated while pregnant. She was arrested at a hospital where she had been taken after an incident of family violence. Charges were dropped because the prosecution failed to provide that an injury had occurred because the child was yet unborn.

REFERENCES: Blank, Robert H., and Janna C. Merrick. 1995. *Human Reproduction, Emerging Technologies, and Conflicting Rights.* Washington, D.C.: Congressional Quarterly Press; *California v. Stewart,* No. M5081997, *slip op.* (San Diego, Cal. Mun. Ct. Feb. 26, 1987); "Criminal Law and Procedure: Pregnant Defendant." 1989. 17 *Daily Washington Law Reporter* 441; *Johnson v. Florida,* 578 So.2d 419 (Fla. App. 1991); *Johnson v. State,* 602 So.2d 1288 (Fla. 1992); *Reyes v. Superior Court,* 75 Ca. App. 3d 214, 141 Cal. Rptr. 912 (1977); *State v. Gray,* 584, 710 (Ohio 1992); *Wyoming v. Pfannenstiel,* Crim. Complaint No. 1–90–8CR (Albany County, Wyo. Jan. 5, 1990).

JANNA C. MERRICK

MEDICARE/MEDICAID

Medicare and Medicaid were both created as amendments to the Social Security Act of 1965. The programs are closely linked politically and can most succinctly be described by initially focusing on the legislative history of Medicare, the federal program for senior citizens over age 65.

Unlike Europe, health and welfare programs in American politics have always been looked on with suspicion. Even the Roosevelt administration treated the issue gingerly. In 1935 the Social Security bill mentioned that health insurance should be "studied," and efforts to legislate in the area were opposed by the Ways and Means Committee and by organized medicine. By 1939 the Wagner bill included comprehensive medical insurance, but the provision was deleted at committee level. Health insurance was introduced between 1939 and 1949, but committees refused to hold hearings during that period. President Harry Truman's proposals for health insurance, covering medical, dental, hospital, and nursing care for all contributors to the plan and their dependents, and providing block grants to the states, were equally opposed by organized medicine and many others associated with the conservative coalition between 1948 and 50. Although the Truman Plan included choice of physician, fees set by physicians, and fee for service, the Democratic Party lost control of the Senate in 1950, and its House majority was also reduced. An American Medical Association (AMA) campaign in 1950 that assessed each member $25 also helped to defeat the Truman Plan.

Remarkably, the ideological issues and economic groups in the 60-year debate over universal health care have not changed greatly. Opponents in the 1950s argued that federal insurance (1) represented creeping socialism, (2) would increase utilization beyond the capacity of the hospitals, and (3) lacked a means test for Americans who could afford private insurance and therefore represented a "giveaway" program. Professional and trade associations such as the AMA and the Life Insurance Association of America were deeply concerned about government agencies controlling prices and reducing markets.

I. S. Falk and Wilbur Cohen, the two principal drafters of the Truman Plan, recognized the ideological unacceptability of Truman's proposal and crafted an alternative that would become the model and strategy for all health insurance models, leading to the passage of Medicare in 1966. In 1951, Oscar Ewing, then head of the Federal Security Agency, introduced a new plan based on this strategy that proposed to insure the 7 million aged Social Security beneficiaries for 60 days of hospital care a year (Marmor, 1973). Although this early version of Medicare never survived the legislative gauntlet—it was opposed by President Dwight D. Eisenhower as "socialized medicine" and by the Ways and Means Committee that had to mark up the bill—the overall strategy influenced all subsequent legislation leading up to the passage of Medicare in 1966.

The strategy for Medicare's successful passage was to finance Medicare out of Social Security taxes and also avoid a large price tag and a welfare label by focusing only on seniors. If a means test were employed, Medicare would be viewed as welfare, and it would not have enough support from conservatives. Those without private insurance and especially those on welfare were considered by conservatives as "nondeserving," but everyone thought of senior citizens as those who had worked hard and deserved the fruits of their Social Security payments. Moreover, younger members of families financially supporting elderly parents would also support such a policy. Medicare was promoted as a program for "deserving" seniors, yet a foot in the door for a general national health insurance program.

From 1952 to 1958, the Ways and Means Committee refused hearings on a Medicare bill, with one exception, and that was never reported out of committee. In 1960, John Kennedy campaigned for an insurance program for the elderly. His campaign resulted in the first cracks in the opposition of the Ways and Means Committee to a reported bill. The Kerr-Mills bill of 1960 was offered as a substitute for the Forand bill that proved unacceptable to the conservative coalition in Congress. Kerr-Mills was authored by Senator Robert Kerr of Oklahoma and Representative Wilbur Mills of Arkansas and chair of the Ways and Means Committee. In 1961, after initial opposition, the AMA signed on to Kerr-Mills, the first bill the medical association had ever sponsored. Clearly, the election of a young president pledged to support compulsory health care insurance for Social Security recipients had altered the political landscape.

Kerr-Mills actually provided broad coverage, 50 to 80 percent matching federal funds, with higher percentages going to poor states. Beneficiaries were limited to those in financial need, and standards of need and benefits were generally left to the states. But Kerr-Mills raised problems for the Kennedy White House. To begin with, Kerr-Mills required a state match, and only 32 of the 50 states had programs in effect by 1963, with 90 percent of federal funding going to only 5 states with 32 percent of the population (Marmor, 1973, 36–37). Moreover, the legislation depended upon a means test, which weakened the development of a constituency. Many liberal democratic leaders believed that the program would not be supported, and opted for an alternative.

The alternative was supported by John Kennedy on February 9, 1961, and introduced by Senator Clinton Anderson of New Mexico and Representative Cecil King of California, both high-ranking members of the Senate Finance Committee and House Ways and Means Committees, respectively. Unlike the 1960 statute, King-Anderson was financed by Social Security taxes rather than general revenues, did not rely on the states for funding or determining benefits, and did not include a means test. All individuals over 65 were eligible for hospitalization and limited nursing home costs but not surgery. The president followed the strategy outlined by Cohen and Falk previously. Freedom of choice of physician and hospital would be guaranteed, and prepaid insurance rather than "socialist" government administration would characterize the program.

Kennedy still had to contend with opposition from Ways and Means with 16 votes—including 5 Democrats—opposed to King-Anderson and only 9 in favor (Marmor, 1973, 41). Wilbur Mill's committee had broad support from the conservative coalition in the House (southern Democrats and partisan Republicans) and had just authored a rival statute, Kerr-Mills. Mills also had strong support from interest groups, specifically the AMA, who, through speeches, pamphlets, and high school debate materials, reached a wide spectrum of opinion. Yet the key barrier for passage was the ideological disposition of Ways and Means members. Between 1961 and the elections of November 1964, three pro-Medicare congressmen replaced three retiring opponents. Finally, the Democratic liberal landslide in the 1964 election changed the makeup of the Ways and Means Committee and of the Rules Committee, which made health care legislation possible.

The Johnson administration Medicare proposal in 1964 still included coverage for hospitalization and nursing home care for those over 65 without a means test. This was met with Republican, insurance, and medical trade association counterproposals supporting extensions of Kerr-Mills that would cover physician care, surgical and drug costs, diagnostic services, laboratory fees, and other costs only for those elderly in financial need. The most serious alternative to the Johnson administration's Medicare proposal was the senior Republican member of Ways and Means, John Byrnes. Byrnes preferred a voluntary insurance program that would be scaled to the elderly's Social Security case benefits, while the government's share would be financed by general tax revenues.

Previously opposed to a federal health program for the elderly, Wilbur Mills merged the content of AMA, Republican, and Johnson administration proposals in a manner that greatly expanded the scope of care for seniors while adding services for the nonelderly poor. Physician services, now known as Part B of Medicare, were financed out of general revenues and partly out of voluntary insurance by recipients. The AMA plan to extend Medicare through state programs for only the needy was transformed into what we now call Medicaid, a program administered by the states and partially funded by the federal government for low-income people. Hospitals and physicians were permitted to charge their "usual and customary fees," a provision of the Byrne bill. The assumption was that insurance companies would put some limitation on prices since they were to act as intermediaries for the medical insurance. Once the fiscally conservative Mill had expanded the coverage of the bill, the more liberal Senate and House general membership found it easy to go along.

By 1964, however, the forces in support of Medicare and Medicaid were on the verge of passing legislation based on government-financed care for the elderly regardless of ability to pay. Opponents continued to insist on the sanctity of the patient-doctor relationship, which required autonomy for two individuals to freely contract; charity for those who could not afford to contract; and when charity was not forthcoming, some kind of a means test for eligibility to government assistance that would be administered by the states. Supporters were opposed to a means test and opposed to state administration of the program. However, passage was possible only as long as the legislation was not perceived as "socialized medicine." Nor could legislation be perceived as threatening free-market investment in health care or as interfering with professional discretion to set fees, diagnose and treat patients, or alter consumer choice of health care providers.

Chairman Mills was acutely aware of the above. He knew that support for government-financed Medicare was strong as long as financing did not interfere with traditional "freedom of choice," local autonomy, and physician/hospital-controlled pricing structure. Consequently, a compromise financing scheme, a sweetener for the physician and hospital lobby, was worked out that avoided a floor fight on the House. Financing would be open-ended; that is, hospitals would be able to charge a per diem fee based on their operational costs, plus a percentage for-profit for Medicare patients. Physician prices would continue to be set by the doctors and based on "usual and customary fees." Government would finance Medicare but not set prices. Moreover, doctors could charge patients directly if they wished, rather than depend on insurance companies as intermediaries for Medicare. That left open an opportunity for physicians to charge more than insurance companies would pay, but it avoided a fight over fee schedules that would have doomed the bill.

Reimbursing hospitals according to their operating costs (per diem) plus profit and physicians according to whatever they thought "reasonable" meant that the federal government would not establish fixed budgets. Budgets raised fears that government would control prices or choice of provider or employ some variant of a means test to determine eligibility. Supporters of Medicare, and of other federally financed medical program initiatives that quickly followed such as Medicaid, were reluctant to tamper with the physician's professional discretion to treat and charge as he saw fit, for fear of losing Medicare and Medicaid support. Medicare simply piggybacked privately operated medicine on top of open-ended government funding for health care. With the advent of Medicare and Medicaid, Congress combined open-ended financing, Medicare-Medicaid entitlements, tax-free third-party payments, physician and consumer autonomy, and fee-for-service medicine.

No health care system can continue to provide open-ended financing for all perceived health needs without experiencing rapidly increasing expenditures. Such financing left no incentive to the hospital to reduce operating costs. Rather than establishing limits and priorities on government-sponsored health care resources, Medicare accepted hospital operational costs plus profit formulas and physician-determined reasonable and customary fees. Excluding research, construction, and public health costs, health care expenditures in the United States rose from 5.3 percent of gross domestic profit (GDP) in 1960 to 13.9 percent in 1994 (Levit et al., 1994, 15). When inflation is held constant, the estimated sources for real growth in the cost of medical care between 1950 and 1985 are led by technology (Freeland and Schendler, 1983, 1–58). Other estimates are considerably higher, but technology was a major cost factor.

Of course, much of this increase was a function of an aging population and secular inflationary trends in the 1970s. But the particularities of the compromise created a system that encouraged construction of hospitals, development of specialization, overutilization by consumers who demanded specialization and hospitals, and above all, the purchase of technology (whose expense would be paid by open-ended financing) to attract both consumers and specialists to the medical center.

Medicaid, the state-administered program to assist the indigent with health care, has been closely tied to the ideological politics of Medicare. The federal government provided financial incentives for state participation and established mandates and criteria for state-administered programs for the poor. Both state and federal governments shared in funding, while the states established, with approval from the federal government, eligibility, coverage, and outreach programs.

By 1991, Medicaid was the fastest-growing cost in state governments. States devoted 6 percent of their budgets for Medicaid in the early 1980s and 12 percent of their budgets by 1989 (*Health Week,* 1989, 4). Health care represented only 12 percent of state and local budgets in 1970 (Letsch, 1993, 100). The current cost for health care in the states is second only to education and consumes between 15 and 18 percent of state and local budgets. Most of the growth was from Medicaid.

Paradoxically, as of 1993 more than a third of all those below the poverty line in the United States remain without access to health care, and almost all of those between the poverty level and 130 percent of the poverty level, referred to as the *working poor,* do not qualify for Medicaid, are not covered by medical insurance, and cannot privately pay for medical assistance. What explains the paradox? There are several reasons. First, Medicaid, which totaled $118 billion in 1993 (Levit et al., 1994, 26), is distributed to those groups who are demographically in important political categories, rather than to individuals who have demonstrable medical needs. For example, 14 percent of those under the poverty line had employer-provided insurance, while 40 percent had no insurance at all, public or private. Thirty-nine percent of all those under the poverty line were covered by Medicaid in 1992—65 percent in the 1970s. One reason is that between 1975 and 1985 there was a 30 percent decrease in Medicaid for single parents and children and a 10 percent increase in supplemental security income (SSI) for the aged, blind, and disabled. In 1972, Aid to Families with Dependent Children (AFDC) received 18.1 percent, SSI, 52.8 percent. In 1988, AFDC received 12 percent, SSI, 73.4 percent. Eligibility based on poverty has sharply declined for those over six years of age and especially for those in the ranks of the working poor. One of the consequences is that pressures increase on the working poor to leave employment, reduce their income, and allow ill family members to become eligible for medical assistance.

Second, federal mandates require states to treat pregnant women and the disabled, provide dental exams, and support orthodontics and organ transplants. Recent federal mandates built into Omnibus Budget Reconciliation Acts (OBRAs) required the states, without additional federal appropriations, to provide that the unemployed (excepting those dismissed) could purchase their former health coverage for 102 percent of its costs for 18 months and, in some instances, for 36 months (OBRA, 1985); expand nursing home facilities, prenatal care, and care for welfare beneficiaries for one year after they start working (OBRA, 1987); and provide income tax credits for low-income working families to purchase health care, $13,000 approximately for a family of four (OBRA, 1990). Future federal mandates will expand Medicaid coverage for all children under age 6 in families with incomes under the 133 percent of poverty line and for all poor children under 18 by 2000. Current mandates expand coverage for children of the unemployed and pregnant women even when not eligible in terms of income. Following the 1994 congressional elections, however, interest in removing federally unfunded mandates was very strong in Congress, leaving the future structure of Medicaid in doubt.

REFERENCES: Freeland, M. S., and Schendler, C. E. 1983. ''National Health Expenditure Growth in the 1980s: An Aging Population, New Technologies, and Increasing Competition.'' *Health Care Financing Review* 4: 1–58; *Health Week,* April 3, 1989, 4; Letsch, Suzanne M. 1993. ''National Health Care Spending in 1991.'' *Health Affairs* 12: 100; Levit, Katharine R., Cowan, Cathy A., Lazenby, Helen C., McDonnell, Patricia A., Sensenig, Arthur L., Stiller, Jean M., and Won, Darleen K. 1994. ''Health Spending Analysis.'' *Health Affairs* 13: 26; Marmor, Theodore R. 1973. *The Politics of Medicare.* Chicago: Aldine Publishing Company; Omnibus Budget Reconciliation Act of 1985 100 Stat. 201, 29 USC §§ 1161–3; Omnibus Budget Reconciliation Act of 1987 101 Stat. 1330–141; Omnibus Budget Reconciliation Act of 1990 104 Stat. 1388-164-9; Somers, Herman, and Somers, Anne. 1967. *Medicare and the Hospitals: Issues and Prospects.* Washington, D.C.: Brookings Institute.

ROBERT P. RHODES

MOORE V. REGENTS OF THE UNIVERSITY OF CALIFORNIA

In a case of first impression, the California Supreme Court held in *Moore v. Regents of the University of California* (1) that a patient does not own tissues removed from his body or have rights to profits from any product that researchers derive from those tissues but that (2) a physician has a fiduciary duty to disclose any personal interest that he may have in a patient's genetic material.

John Moore had sued his physician, Dr. David Golde of the University of California at Los Angeles (UCLA), both for breach of fiduciary duty and for conversion. As Golde's patient, Moore had been treated for hairy-cell leukemia and, in that context, had undergone surgery for the removal of his affected spleen. Without informing his patient, Golde used Moore's spleen cells and other later-removed tissues to develop a cell line upon which Golde and the Regents of the University of California later received a U.S. patent directed, in part, to biopharmaceutical substances, such as the lymphokine granulocyte-macrophage colony stimulating factor (GM-CSF), obtainable from the cell line.

Apparently concerned over a potentially devastating effect on scientific research, a majority of the California Supreme Court rejected the contention that Golde's unauthorized use of Moore's cells constituted wrongful conversion of a patient's personal property right in bodily materials, including genetic material. Rather than basing its decision on the law of conversion, the court invoked specialized statutes that govern the disposition of human tissue. The *Moore* decision suggests, however, that any property right in genetic material must arise by operation of law, with respect to the creativity and ingenuity of the physician/ researcher, in the form of a patent right. In light of *Moore,* investigators also are obliged to draft with particular care any agreement that entails a patient's consent to a research use of his tissues.

REFERENCES: Elman, Gerry J. 1990. "Physician's Self-disclosure Emerges as a Key Issue from the Moore Case." *Genetic Engineering News* 9: 3; Hartman, Rhonda G. 1993. "Beyond *Moore:* Issues of Law and Policy Impacting Human Cell and Genetic Research in the Age of Biotechnology." *Journal of Legal Medicine* 14: 463; *Moore v. Regents of the University of California,* 793 P.2d 479 (Cal. 1990), 271 Cal. Rptr. 146 (1990), 15 U.S.P.Q.2d 1753 (Cal. 1990), *cert. denied,* 111 S. Ct. 1388 (1991); Office of Technology Assessment. 1991. *New Developments in Biotechnology: Ownership of Human Tissues and Cells.* Special Report 31–46 (OTA-BA 337 1991); "The Ownership of Cells." July 23, 1990. *U.S. News and World Report;* Shaffer, Gary L. 1990. "*Moore* Defines the Issues But Only Legislation Will Settle the Controversy." *Biotechnology Law Report* 9: 261.

STEPHEN A. BENT

N

NATIONAL ACADEMY OF SCIENCES (NAS)

A private, not-for-profit organization established by congressional charter in 1863 to advise the government on scientific matters, it instead functions more as an honorific rather than an advisory body, although it continues to sponsor symposia and publishes a research journal, *Proceedings of the National Academy of Sciences.*

The NAS is part of a complex of private not-for-profit research organizations located in Washington, D.C. The National Academy of Engineering (NAE) was founded in 1964 under NAS's charter. It sponsors studies, encourages education and research, promotes international cooperation, and recognizes the superior achievements of engineers. The Institute of Medicine* (IOM), established under NAS's charter in 1970, examines policy matters pertaining to the health of the public. The National Research Council (NRC) was created as part of the NAS in 1916 to offer technical advice during World War I and operates now as the principal operating agency of the NAS and the NAE, carrying out most of the studies done in their names (the IOM carries out its own studies). The NRC has no research laboratories and does not usually conduct its own research; instead, it generally evaluates and compiles research done by others. In a few cases, though, and increasingly so in recent years, the NRC has been funding research in a variety of areas (e.g., transportation and medical care). Approximately 85 percent of the NRC's work is funded by the U.S. government in the form of sole-source awards. The NRC is administered jointly by the NAS, the NAE, and the IOM, and its work is overseen by a Governing Board and an Executive Committee.

The NAS, NAE, and IOM jointly publish a quarterly research journal, *Issues in Science and Technology,* and they sponsor two other research organizations: the Committee on Science, Engineering and Public Policy, which carries out broad, cross-disciplinary studies related to the strength of U.S. science and technology, and the Government-University-Industry Research Roundtable, which provides a forum where scientists, engineers, administrators, and policymakers can explore research issues.

The range of research conducted by these research organizations is impressive. In 1992, for instance, the NAS, NAE, IOM, and NRC completed over 200 studies on such diverse subjects as controlling infectious diseases, improving mathematics education, increasing automotive fuel efficiency, reexamining the federal role in technology development, using DNA technology in forensic science, including women and children in health care reform, and dealing with misconduct in scientific research. All publications appear through the National Academy Press.

REFERENCES: Cochrane, R. C. 1978. *The National Academy of Sciences.* Washington, D.C.: National Academy Press; National Academy of Sciences. 1994. *1994 Report to Congress.* Washington, D.C.: National Academy Press.

DEBORAH R. MATHIEU

NATIONAL ADVISORY BOARD ON ETHICS IN REPRODUCTION (NABER)

NABER is an independent, nonpartisan body founded in 1992 by the American College of Obstetricians and Gynecologists and the American Fertility Society to provide a forum for consideration of the ethical aspects of research and medicine in the fields of human reproduction, fetal research, fetal tissue use, and contraception. The board is composed of 14 professionals with nationally recognized expertise in medicine, reproductive sciences, bioethics, theology, and law. Funding comes from foundations. A Consultants' Working Group of 18 individuals has been formed to help the board define and develop the central issues related to the topics under investigation by participating in workshops and developing background papers. In addition, individual consultants in areas under study are invited to participate in NABER meetings and workshops.

Major activities of NABER include:

1. Disseminate reports identifying and addressing major ethical issues related to research and practice in human reproduction and fetal research.

2. Evaluate existing ethical guidelines concerning research and practice in human reproduction and fetal research from America and abroad in light of these issues.

3. Develop a set of ethical guidelines with explanatory commentary that may be used to assist in resolving these issues.

4. Hold conferences to encourage public discussion and provide education concerning these issues.

5. Review in an advisory capacity proposed research policies and practice questions related to human reproduction and fetal research that raise new ethical issues.

REFERENCES: Hilton, Bruce. 1993. "Board to Consider Reproduction Ethics." *Washington Times* (July 6), A3; Hilts, Philip J. 1991. "Groups Set Up Panel on Use of Fetal Tissue." *New York Times* (January 8); Jonsen, Albert R., and Cynthia B. Cohen. 1993. "An Improved Tissue Bank." *The Washington Post* (February 4), A20.

ROBERT H. BLANK

NATIONAL CANCER INSTITUTE

NCI is the U.S. government's primary agency in cancer research and one of the National Institutes of Health (NIH).* NCI conducts and supports programs relating to the cause, diagnosis, treatment, and prevention of all cancers and the continuing care of cancer patients and the families of cancer patients. These programs include basic and applied research, patient screening programs, health professional training, and information dissemination (among the NCI's publications is the biweekly *Journal of the National Cancer Institute*).

NCI was established in 1937 by the National Cancer Institute Act (P.L. 244) to conduct research relating to cancer. In 1944, the Public Health Service Act (P.L. 78–410) incorporated NCI into the NIH. In 1971, the National Cancer Act (P.L. 92–218) created the National Cancer Program (to oversee and coordinate cancer research) and the National Cancer Center Advisory Board (responsible for advising the NCI's director regarding the activities of the National Cancer Program as well as approving cancer research grants); it also authorized the establishment of 15 extramural cancer centers as well as an international cancer data research bank. NCI's mandate was expanded in 1974 by the National Cancer Act Amendments (P.L. 95–352) to include greater emphasis on the role of nutrition, and the mandate was expanded again by the 1978 amendments to the National Cancer Act (P.L. 95–622) to emphasize cancer caused by occupational and environmental factors and to include more education and training programs in cancer treatment and prevention.

In 1980, the institute was reorganized to reflect its emphasis on "applied prevention." The research and research-related activities of the institute are now conducted by five divisions: the Division of Cancer Biology and Diagnosis, the Division of Cancer Prevention and Control, the Division of Cancer Etiology, the Division of Cancer Treatment, and the Division of Extramural Activities. In addition, the Director's Office includes the Biometry Branch (which tracks the extent and impact of cancer control and develops research and evaluation methodology and related computer systems) and the Smoking, Tobacco and Cancer Branch. NCI is the largest of the National Institutes of Health, with the most full-time intramural researchers, the greatest access to NIH clinical beds, and the biggest budget.

The institute has made significant contributions to the understanding, prevention, and treatment of cancer. For example, the first malignancy was cured with chemotherapy at the institute in 1957; one of the institute's scientists discovered the first human ribonucleic acid (RNA) virus in 1979; in 1983, the institute launched the Community Clinical Oncology Program to bring the advantages of clinical research to cancer patients in their own communities; in 1984, institute scientists identified HTLV-III (now called human immunodeficiency virus [HIV]) as the etiologic agent for acquired immunodeficiency syndrome (AIDS), enabling the development of an effective blood screening test (approved by the Food and Drug Administration* in 1985); in 1986, the institute adopted a more sensitive drug screen, replacing the traditional test system of mouse leukemia with a panel of 100 tumor cell lines from human cancer cells; the institute is currently undertaking the largest intervention research program in tobacco use prevention and cessation in the world; the Cancer Information Service, which is located in 20 cities around the United States, relays the latest cancer information to patients, the public, and health care professionals.

REFERENCES: Office of the Director, National Institutes of Health. 1994. *NIH Almanac 1994*. Bethesda, MD: NIH Publication; Rettig, R. A. 1977. *Cancer Crusade: The Story of the National Cancer Act of 1971*. Princeton, NJ: Princeton University Press.

DEBORAH R. MATHIEU

NATIONAL COMMISSION FOR THE PROTECTION OF HUMAN SUBJECTS OF BIOMEDICAL AND BEHAVIORAL RESEARCH

Known as the National Commission, the 11-member multidisciplinary body was established in 1974 by the U.S. Congress to conduct "a comprehensive investigation and study [of] the basic ethical principles which should underlie the conduct of biomedical and behavioral research involving human subjects." The National Commission was also to develop guidelines to ensure that federally funded research using human subjects is conducted in accordance with such principles; identify the requirements for informed consent for participation in research by children, prisoners, and the mentally infirm; investigate and make recommendations regarding research on living fetuses; investigate and make recommendations regarding "psychosurgery"; and study the "implications of advances in biomedical and behavioral research and technology" (P.L. 93–348).

Congress granted the National Commission considerable authority. For example, the secretary of the Department of Health, Education, and Welfare (DHEW) was required to publish the recommendations of the National Commission in the *Federal Register* within 60 days of receiving them to allow for public comment. More strikingly, the secretary was required to accept these recommendations and act upon them within six months or publish reasons for not accepting the recommendations in the *Federal Register*.

The National Commission was born as a result of public and, ultimately, federal attention to the ethical issues involved in research involving human subjects. In 1966, for instance, the *New England Journal of Medicine* published Henry Beecher's description of 22 unethical experiments that had appeared in important peer-reviewed journals. This was a source of considerable concern, as all of the experiments were conducted after the Nuremberg Code (1949) and the Declaration of Helsinki (1964) were adopted. In 1972, the public learned about the federally funded and highly unethical research involving hundreds of human subjects in Tuskegee, Alabama. In addition, public ire was raised by reports about alleged research on decapitated heads of dead fetuses, stimulated by a National Institutes of Health (NIH) announcement that this type of research was ethically acceptable. These three events, among others, raised the specter of federally funded research gone awry, without oversight or accountability. Public awareness led eventually to governmental action. From 1971 to 1974, the Subcommittee on Health of the Senate Committee on Labor and Public Welfare conducted a series of hearings on ethically suspect research, and as a result, the U.S. Congress passed the National Research Act, establishing the National Commission (P.L. 93–348).

The National Commission, which functioned from 1974 until 1978, was the first national body to operate under the newly enacted Federal Advisory Committee Act (P.L. 92–463), and so it established a precedent for public involvement in bioethics policy. All meetings, hearings, and discussions were conducted in open session, transcribed, and documented. The reports and appendixes were published and made available through the U.S. Government Printing Office in Washington. All recommendations for establishing federal regulations governing human subjects research were published in the *Federal Register* with requests for comment.

The National Commission produced ten reports. Three of these reports— *Research on the Fetus* (1975), *Research Involving Prisoners* (1976), and *Research Involving Children* (1977)—led directly to federal regulations to protect these groups of human subjects, considered to be especially vulnerable to research. A fourth report, *The Belmont Report* (1978), described the ethical principles and guidelines for research involving human subjects. The cumulative result of the National Commission's recommendations was an extensive revision to existing federal regulations governing human subjects research. These revisions were proposed in the *Federal Register* on August 14, 1979, and, after extensive public comment was received, codified in regulations (45 CFR 46) and published on January 26 and 27, 1981. The regulations set out for the first time the standards by which research involving human subjects funded by the U.S. Public Health Service could proceed. The report and appendixes on *Institutional Review Boards* (1978) have been of considerable scholarly value, providing the first comprehensive assessment of the role, structure, and function of the committees used to evaluate the ethical acceptability of human research. Many of the recommendations found in this latter report were incorporated into the U.S. regulations and adopted in guidelines by countries throughout the world. Several of the National Commission's other reports were either ignored or of less direct use for establishing regulations. For example, the reports on *Psychosurgery* (1977) and *Research on Those Institutionalized as Mentally Infirm* (1978) never resulted in regulations, despite the National Commission's recommendations.

The National Commission has had a significant impact on bioethics in general and human research in particular, in both obvious and subtle ways. The most obvious impact was the effect of the National Commission's recommendations in the drafting of federal regulations. These regulations defined in unambiguous ways terms such as *research, minimal risk,* and *informed consent,* which became important foci for both philosophical scholarship and institutional guidelines. The second general impact of the National Commission's work has been the influence of the philosophical framework it articulated in *The Belmont Report.* The commission satisfied its mandate to identify "the basic ethical principles which would underlie the conduct of biomedical and behavioral research" by articulating three ethical principles it took to be fundamental to the conduct of research: respect for persons, beneficence, and justice. These abstract principles were then applied to or used to justify three specific requirements for assessing the ethical appropriateness of research involving human subjects: informed consent, risk-benefit assessment, and subject selection. Never before had philosophic reasoning and language been used so directly in the establishment of research policy in the United States.

A relatively underappreciated but important effect of the National Commission was the success that it had in avoiding political interference, even though it was administratively responsible to the federal agency for whom its recommendations were being written. As the first major bioethics advisory body created in the United States, this group set a precedent for future government panels and commissions. Indeed, one important legacy of the National Commission was its recommendation that the DHEW establish the Ethics Advisory Board (EAB) to review research involving the human fetus, pregnant women, and in vitro fertilization (IVF). The EAB was intended to serve as a standing board to review specific research protocols for the DHEW secretary but was eventually disbanded, in part because the executive branch reassigned its budget to the President's Commission for the Study of Ethical Problems in Medicine and Biomedical and Behavioral Research in 1978.

The National Commission brought together a diverse group of individuals to debate controversial and highly charged topics and, in a relatively short period of time, was able to achieve consensus on matters of urgency in a pragmatic way. However, given that the regulations resulting from the National Commission's recommendations were superseded in 1991 by the Common Federal Rule for the Protection of Human Subjects, the commission's final legacy may be that bioethical input in public policymaking is both possible and productive.

REFERENCES: Beecher, Henry K. 1966. "Ethics and Clinical Research." *New England Journal of Medicine* 274:1354–1360; Faden, Ruth R., and Beauchamp, Tom L. 1986. *A History and Theory of Informed Consent.* New York: Oxford University Press; Frankel, Mark S. 1975. "The Development of Policy Guidelines Governing Human Experimentation in the United States." *Ethics in Science & Medicine* 2:43–59; Greenwald, Robert A., et al. 1982. *Human Subjects Research: A Handbook for Institutional Review Boards.* New York: Plenum Press; Hanna, K. E., et al. 1993. "Finding a Forum for Bioethics in

U.S. Public Policy." *Politics and the Life Sciences* 12:205–219; Veatch, Robert M. 1987. *The Patient as Partner: A Theory of Human Experimentation Ethics.* Bloomington: Indiana University Press; Yesley, Michael S. 1978. "The Use of an Advisory Commission." *Southern California Law Review* 51:1451–1469.

ERIC M. MESLIN and CHARLES R. McCARTHY

NATIONAL EYE INSTITUTE

The NEI investigates the cause, prevention, diagnosis, and treatment of disorders of the eye and visual system. Established as one of the National Institutes of Health (NIH)* in 1968 (P.L. 90–489), the institute conducts and supports basic and applied research and educational programs and supports the construction or renovation of vision research facilities throughout the United States.

Evolving over time, the institute has added a laboratory of sensorimotor research (1978), a laboratory of molecular and developmental biology (1981), a laboratory of ophthalmic pathology (1984), a laboratory of mechanisms of ocular diseases (1987), a laboratory of retinal cell and molecular biology (1987), a laboratory of immunology (1987), and a laboratory of ocular therapeutics (1991).

Studies supported by the institute have contributed significantly to the improved vision of millions of people by, for instance, demonstrating that treatment with a laser dramatically reduces the risk of visual impairment from the ocular complications of a variety of diseases; improving corneal transplantation techniques; developing a simple, rapid, and extremely sensitive method for diagnosing herpesvirus in superficial corneal lesions; and advancing techniques for correcting eye movement disorders.

REFERENCE: Office of the Director, National Institutes of Health. 1994. *NIH Almanac 1994.* Bethesda, MD: NIH Publication.

DEBORAH R. MATHIEU

NATIONAL HEART, LUNG, AND BLOOD INSTITUTE

One of the larger institutes among the National Institutes of Health (NIH),* the NHLBI advances the national attack on diseases of the heart, lung, blood vessels, and blood and conducts research and training programs on the use of blood and blood products.

In 1948, the National Heart Act established the National Heart Institute as part of the NIH to investigate diseases of the heart and circulatory system (P.L. 80–655). In 1969, the National Heart Institute was renamed the National Heart and Lung Institute to reflect the expansion of its functions. In 1972, the institute became more deeply involved with diseases of the blood. First, the National Sickle Cell Anemia Control Act (P.L. 92–294) established a national program for the diagnosis, control, and treatment of sickle-cell anemia, a program that was coordinated by the institute. And later that year, the National Heart, Blood Vessel, Lung and Blood Act of 1972 enlarged the mandate of the institute to investigate all heart, blood vessel, lung, and blood diseases (P.L. 92–423). Reflecting its new responsibilities, the institute was redesignated the National Heart, Lung, and Blood Institute in 1976, and its authority was expanded even further to include research in the use of blood and blood products and in the management of blood resources (P.L. 94–278).

Institute researchers have contributed significantly to biomedical policy. In 1979, for instance, the institute published results of a major clinical trial, begun in 1971, that provided solid evidence that tens of thousands of lives are being saved through treatment of mild hypertension and recommended that all people with mild hypertension undergo treatment. In 1984, institute studies showed that reducing total blood cholesterol reduces the risk of coronary heart disease in men. This study, in addition to a large body of evidence from laboratory, epidemiological, and clinical studies, provided the impetus for NIH to inaugurate the National Cholesterol Education Program in 1985. The institute administers four other education programs as well, on high blood pressure, blood resources, asthma, and smoking.

REFERENCE: Office of the Director, National Institutes of Health. 1994. *NIH Almanac 1994.* Bethesda, MD: NIH Publication.

DEBORAH R. MATHIEU

NATIONAL INSTITUTE OF ALLERGY AND INFECTIOUS DISEASES

One of the larger institutes within the National Institutes of Health (NIH),* the NIAID is divided into five divisions, reflecting its intersecting spheres of responsibility: the Division of Microbiology and Infectious Diseases; the Division of Allergy, Immunology, and Transplantation; the Division of Acquired Immunodeficiency Syndrome (AIDS); the Division of Intramural Research; and the Division of Extramural Activities.

The National Institute of Allergy and Infectious Diseases began in 1948 as the National Microbiological Institute, which was created by combining four existing entities: the Rocky Mountain Laboratory, the Biologics Control Laboratory, the Division of Infectious Diseases, and the Division of Tropical Diseases. In 1955, the National Microbiological Institute was reorganized, with part of it becoming the National Institute of Allergy and Infectious Diseases.

Over the years, the institute has expanded its areas of concern, adding a laboratory of parasitic diseases (1959), a laboratory of viral diseases (1967), allergic disease centers (1971), centers for the study of sexually transmitted diseases (1974), centers for the study of influenza (1974), a laboratory of immunogenetics (1977), a maximum containment facility for recombinant DNA research (1978), centers for the study of immunologic diseases (1978), a laboratory of immunoregulation (1980), a laboratory of molecular microbiology (1981), a laboratory of immunopathology (1985), a laboratory of cellular and molecular immunology (1987), a laboratory of intracellular parasites (1990), and a laboratory of host diseases (1991). In addition, the Office of Tropical Medicine and International Research was established in 1984 to coordinate the institute's international research activities. The Acquired Immunodeficiency Syndrome (AIDS) Program was established in 1986 as well, to coordinate the institute's extramural AIDS research efforts; one of its first major thrusts was to fund 14 centers to evaluate experimental drugs in the treatment of AIDS. The Office of Recombinant DNA Activities was part of the institute from 1979 until it was transferred to the NIH Director's Office in 1988.

The institute has contributed to biomedical policy by, for example, demonstrating the efficacy of influenza vaccines and a variety of bacterial vaccines, developing a new technique to detect the hepatitis C virus, improving the treatment of asthma, and leading the fight to understand and control sexually transmitted diseases (including AIDS).

REFERENCE: Office of the Director, National Institutes of Health. 1994. *NIH Almanac 1994*. Bethesda, MD: NIH Publication.

DEBORAH R. MATHIEU

NATIONAL INSTITUTE OF ARTHRITIS AND MUSCULOSKELETAL AND SKIN DISEASES

One of the smaller of the National Institutes of Health (NIH),* the NIAMSD conducts and supports basic and clinical research on arthritis and other rheumatic diseases (e.g., Lyme disease), diseases of the musculoskeletal system (e.g., osteoporosis), and diseases of the skin (e.g., allergic contact dermatitis). The institute also conducts and supports research on the normal structure and function of joints, muscles, bones, and skin, as well as training programs for health professionals.

Major arthritis research programs were established at the NIH in 1950 as a component of the National Institute of Arthritis and Metabolic Diseases (P.L. 81–692). The name of the institute was changed in 1972 to the National Institute of Arthritis, Metabolic and Digestive Diseases (P.L. 92–305), and again in 1980 to the National Institute of Arthritis, Diabetes, and Digestive and Kidney Diseases (P.L. 96–538). In 1985, the institute was split into two separate institutes: the National Institute of Arthritis and Musculoskeletal and Skin Diseases, and the National Institute of Diabetes and Digestive and Kidney Diseases (P.L. 99–158).

Among the institute's recent contributions to biomedical policy have been the development of a test for detecting the presence of Lyme disease bacteria, the determination of the complete structure of a key protein critical in triggering allergic reactions, the discovery of the gene that causes osteoarthritis, and the demonstration that regular exercise and adequate calcium intake throughout life may significantly delay the onset of osteoporotic fractures in women.

REFERENCE: Office of the Director, National Institutes of Health. 1994. *NIH Almanac 1994*. Bethesda, MD: NIH Publication.

DEBORAH R. MATHIEU

NATIONAL INSTITUTE OF CHILD HEALTH AND HUMAN DEVELOPMENT

One of the National Institutes of Health (NIH),* the NICHHD supports and conducts research on the reproductive, developmental, and behavioral processes that determine the health of children, adults, families, and populations; it also supports medical rehabilitation research to restore or enhance function in individuals affected by diseases, injury, or birth defects; and it supports research training and public information efforts.

Legislation establishing the National Institute of Child Health and Human Development as part of the NIH was passed in 1962 (P.L. 87–838), and in 1963, the institute was created when two centers—the Center for Research in Child Health (established in 1961) and the Center for Research in Aging (established in 1956)—were transferred from NIH's Division of General Medical Sciences to the new institute. The institute has undergone a series of reorganizations (in 1965, for instance, it was expanded by the transfer of the National Heart Institute's Gerontology Branch and the National Cancer Institute's Endocrinology Branch, and in 1968, the four-story Gerontology Research Center building in Baltimore, Maryland, was opened; in 1975, however, the entire gerontology research program was transferred to the newly established National Institute on Aging).

The institute now has five major research components. Three of them are extramural programs. The Center for Population Research, which began in 1968, offers research and training grants in family planning and population issues. The Center for Research for Mothers and Children, which began in 1975, is responsible for increasing knowledge about pregnancy, infancy, childhood, adolescence, and adulthood. The National Center for Medical Rehabilitation Research, which began in 1990, conducts and supports programs regarding the rehabilitation of individuals with physical disabilities or disorders resulting from congenital defects, injuries, or diseases. The institute's two other major components are intramural programs: the Division of Intramural Research and the Division of Epidemiology, Statistics, and Preventive Research.

Notable achievements in the institute's history include its contributions to the lowering of the nation's infant mortality rate, its elucidation of the female reproductive cycle, and its progress toward understanding how a one-cell fertilized egg becomes a complex organism. Institute grantees were the first to demonstrate the successful use of recombinant DNA technology to create transgenic animals and to create an animal model for a genetic disease using "gene knock-out" technology. Institute studies have also documented the effectiveness of neonatal screening and dietary restriction in preventing mental retardation due to phenylketonuria (PKU), and an institute scientist made possible the simultaneous screening of newborns for PKU and congenital hypothyroidism. These two advances have prevented thousands of new cases of mental retardation each year. Intramural scientists developed a vaccine for *Hemophilus influenzae* effective in infants; meningitis due to *Hemophilus influenzae* was the leading cause of acquired mental retardation in the United States, with 6,000 new cases annually. Widespread use of this vaccine has the potential to eliminate this cause of mental retardation. In addition, institute studies have demonstrated the safety and accuracy of amniocentesis* and chorionic villus sampling (CVS)* in the prenatal diagnosis of congenital disorders.

REFERENCE: Office of the Director, National Institutes of Health. 1994. *NIH Almanac 1994.* Bethesda, MD: NIH Publication.

DEBORAH R. MATHIEU

NATIONAL INSTITUTE OF DENTAL RESEARCH

One of the National Institutes of Health (NIH),* the NIDR is the primary sponsor of dental research and related training in the United States. Its mandate is to support and conduct research and training on the cause, prevention, diagnosis, and treatment of oral, dental, and craniofacial disorders and related systemic conditions. Its programs include clinical and laboratory research aimed at the eradication of the two major oral diseases—tooth decay and periodontal diseases—as well as research on a broad variety of conditions affecting soft and mineralized tissues of the mouth.

In 1931, the Public Health Service created a Dental Hygiene Unit at NIH, which in 1948 became the National Institute of Dental Research (P.L. 80–755). In its early years, the institute was instrumental in establishing water fluoridation as a safe, effective, and economical procedure for the control of dental caries. As a result, about 8,000 American communities—representing over one half of the U.S. population—have adopted municipal water fluoridation programs, and many thousands of children participate in school-based fluoride programs. The institute has continued its leadership role in oral health science—for example, initiating school demonstration projects through the National Caries Program (in 1975), creating the first multidisciplinary pain clinic in the United States (in 1983), completing the first and most comprehensive nationwide survey on the dental health of American adults (in 1986), and supporting 22 extramural research centers.

REFERENCE: Office of the Director, National Institutes of Health. 1994. *NIH Almanac 1994.* Bethesda, MD: NIH Publication.

DEBORAH R. MATHIEU

NATIONAL INSTITUTE OF DIABETES AND DIGESTIVE AND KIDNEY DISEASES

The NIDDKD conducts and supports basic and clinical research and research training in diabetes, endocrinology; and metabolic diseases (such as cystic fibrosis), digestive diseases and nutrition, and kidney, urologic, and blood diseases. One of the National Institutes of Health (NIH),* the institute conducts research at laboratories in Bethesda, Maryland, and in Phoenix, Arizona, and funds researchers at more than 400 other medical institutions.

The institute was established in 1950 as the National Institute of Arthritis and

Metabolic Diseases (P.L. 81–692) to conduct and support research in arthritis, rheumatism, and metabolic diseases. In 1972, the institute was renamed the National Institute of Arthritis, Metabolic and Digestive Diseases (P.L. 92–305) and, in 1980, the National Institute of Arthritis, Diabetes, and Digestive and Kidney Diseases (P.L. 96–538) to emphasize research in diabetes and digestive and kidney diseases. In 1985, P.L. 99–158 changed the name of the institute to the National Institute of Diabetes and Digestive and Kidney Diseases and established the National Institute of Arthritis and Musculoskeletal and Skin Diseases* as a separate NIH institute.

Recent contributions to biomedical research by the institute include the discovery of the cystic fibrosis gene; completion of the Diabetes Control and Complications Trial, showing that intensive treatment of insulin-dependent diabetes slows the onset and progression of long-term diabetes complications; advances in parathyroid hormone research, leading to combination therapy with other hormones in preserving cancellous bone in osteoporosis patients; and development of a new technique that doubles the period of time a donor liver can remain viable for transplantation. In addition, the institute has sponsored consensus development conferences on the morbidity and mortality of dialysis, physical activity and obesity, and impotence. Current research priorities include obesity and nutritional disorders, kidney disease of diabetes, acquired immunodeficiency syndrome, and gene therapy of human disease.

REFERENCE: Office of the Director, National Institutes of Health. 1994. *NIH Almanac 1994.* Bethesda, MD: NIH Publication.

DEBORAH R. MATHIEU

NATIONAL INSTITUTE OF ENVIRONMENTAL HEALTH SCIENCES

The NIEHS works to develop the research base, advanced scientific methodology, and trained scientists necessary to understand and ultimately prevent adverse effects of environmental agents. It also works to investigate the chemical, physical, and biological effects of environmental hazards.

The institute began as a division of the National Institutes of Health (NIH)* in 1966 and was elevated to institute status in 1969; it did not receive legislative authorization, however, until 1985 (P.L. 99–158). Unlike the other components of the NIH, which are in Maryland, the National Institute of Environmental Health Sciences is located in Research Triangle Park, North Carolina. And unlike most of the other components of NIH, the institute focuses on chemical and physical agents in the environment instead of on specific body organs or diseases.

The institute is composed of four divisions—intramural research, extramural research and training, toxicology research and testing, and biometry and risk assessment—all of which have made important contributions to biomedical policy. For instance, institute studies showing that there is no threshold value at which the common manufactured contaminant dioxin is safe have led the Environmental Protection Agency and the Food and Drug Administration* to review their regulations governing acceptable exposure levels. Institute studies documenting neurobehavioral problems in children whose blood has been contaminated by lead have led to new safety standards and to a national campaign to identify children with blood lead levels above the level of concern and to environmental and therapeutic programs to prevent childhood lead poisoning. The institute also plays a significant role in the nation's management of hazardous wastes. The Superfund Amendments and Reauthorization Act of 1986 requires the institute to support basic research regarding the health effects of releasing hazardous substances and wastes into the environment and to train people working with hazardous wastes to meet health and safety standards when responding to emergencies as well as when transporting or managing hazardous substances.

REFERENCE: Office of the Director, National Institutes of Health. 1994. *NIH Almanac 1994*. Bethesda, MD: NIH Publication.

DEBORAH R. MATHIEU

NATIONAL INSTITUTE OF GENERAL MEDICAL SCIENCES

One of the National Institutes of Health (NIH),* the NIGMS supports research and research training in the basic biomedical sciences that form the foundation needed to make advances in the understanding of disease. It emphasizes areas such as the structure and function of cell components, basic genetic processes, and mechanisms of drug action. It also supports the development of new techniques and tools to facilitate further studies (e.g., the institute supports the Human Genetic Mutant Cell Repository, which establishes and stores cultured cell lines representing metabolic and chromosomal disorders as an aid to the study of the role of mutations and other genetic errors in disease).

The institute has five main program areas. Four of them—Cellular and Molecular Basis of Disease, Genetics, Pharmacology and Biorelated Chemistry, and Biophysics and Physiological Sciences—fund grants for research projects and research training. The fifth, Minority Opportunities in Research, aims to increase the number and capabilities of minority individuals engaged in biomedical research by funding research and research training grants at colleges and universities with substantial minority enrollments. The goals of the institute's programs are to supply new knowledge, theories, and concepts for the disease-targeted studies supported by the other institutes within the NIH and to provide well-trained scientists. The institute is a major source of NIH research training support, funding nearly half of the predoctoral trainees and about 30 percent of all the trainees who receive assistance through the NIH.

The institute began as a division within the NIH in 1958 and was elevated to institute status in 1962 (P.L. 87–838). It is the only one of the National Institutes of Health with no laboratories on the NIH campus (although it does sponsor a small program in which research fellows work in the laboratories of other NIH institutes in areas related to the pharmacological sciences). All of the other activities the institute supports take place at diverse research institutions throughout the country.

REFERENCE: Office of the Director, National Institutes of Health. 1994. *NIH Almanac 1994.* Bethesda, MD: NIH Publication.

DEBORAH R. MATHIEU

NATIONAL INSTITUTE OF MENTAL HEALTH

One of the National Institutes of Health (NIH),* it is the largest research institute in the world, with a primary focus on mental disorders. Its mission is to sponsor research, training, and the dissemination of information on the cause, diagnosis, treatment, and prevention of mental disorders.

In 1946, President Harry Truman signed the National Mental Health Act, which called for the creation of the National Institute of Mental Health (P.L. 79–487), but Congress failed to allocate funds to it until 1948. When the institute was established as part of the NIH the following year, its precursor, the Public Health Service's* Division of Mental Hygiene, was incorporated into it. Like the other NIH institutes, the National Institute of Mental Health (NIMH) focused on basic and applied biomedical research, but unlike them, it also supported behavioral and social science research as well as direct services (e.g., grants to states for the establishment of clinics and treatment centers). In 1966, NIMH was expanded by the addition of two new centers—the National Center for Prevention and Control of Alcoholism and the Center for Studies of Narcotic Addiction and Drug Abuse; the NIMH was taken out of the NIH and elevated to bureau status within the Public Health Service the following year; in 1968, it was moved into a new federal agency, the Health Services and Mental Health Administration; in 1973, it was moved back to the NIH; in 1974, the institute was moved to the newly created Public Health Service agency, the Alcohol, Drug Abuse, and Mental Health Administration* (P.L. 93–282); and upon the demise of that agency in 1992, the institute was transferred back to NIH (P.L. 102–321).

The institute has had profound effects on policies governing mental health care in the United States. For instance, the institute's Joint Commission on Mental Illness and Health, which was created in 1955 (P.L. 84–182), conducted a historic study on the human and economic problems of mental health, which was reported in *Action for Mental Health* (1961). President John F. Kennedy used this report as a basis for his special message to Congress on mental health issues, and in response, Congress voted to allocate funds to provide grants for the nationwide construction of community health centers (P.L. 88–164) and for staffing the centers (P.L. 89–105). In 1970, the Food and Drug Administration* used studies supported by the institute to approve lithium for use as an antimanic drug, which resulted in a sharp drop in the number of suicides and institutionalizations.

Currently, the institute supports intramural and extramural research and training on all areas of the brain, mental illness, and mental health. Among its various programs are the Division of Clinical and Treatment Research, which studies mental disorders (e.g., schizophrenia, mood disorders, Alzheimer's disease) and their etiology, diagnosis, psychopathology, and treatment; the Division of Neuroscience and Behavioral Science, which supports basic biomedical and behavioral research (e.g., studies of learning processes and neuronal mechanisms); the Division of Epidemiology and Services Research, which tracks the frequency and types of mental disorders, the availability of treatment programs, the causes of interpersonal violence, and so on; the Office on AIDS, which supports intramural and extramural research at the biological, psychological, and behavioral levels; and the Office of Rural Mental Health Research, which concentrates its research on the special problems of those living in rural areas. The institute also places a strong emphasis on information dissemination, producing a wide variety of journal articles, publications, and audiovisual materials. In addition, the institute has launched a long-term, nationwide public education campaign on depression (the Depression, Awareness, Recognition and Treatment [D/ART] program), to provide information on the symptoms, causes, and treatments of various depressive disorders. And the Office of Prevention sponsors conferences and workshops that bring together experts and policymakers to improve prevention programs.

REFERENCES: Brand, J. L. 1965. "The National Mental Health Act of 1946: A Retrospect." *Bulletin of the History of Medicine* 39:231–244; Connery, R. H., et al. 1968. *The Politics of Mental Health*. New York: Columbia University Press; Joint Commission on Mental Health. 1961. *Action for Mental Health*. New York: Basic Books; Kolb, L. C. 1994. "Research and Its Support Under the National Mental Health Act 1949." *American Journal of Psychiatry* 151:210–215; Pincus, H. A., and Fine, T. 1992. "The 'Anatomy' of Research Funding of Mental Illness and Addictive Disorders." *Archives of General Psychiatry* 49:573–579.

DEBORAH R. MATHIEU

NATIONAL INSTITUTE OF NEUROLOGICAL DISORDERS AND STROKE

One of the National Institutes of Health (NIH),* the NINDS conducts and supports research and research training programs relating to the cause, prevention, diagnosis, and treatment of stroke and neurological disorders (such as Huntington's disease, Alzheimer's disease, Parkinson's disease, cerebral palsy, multiple sclerosis, and epilepsy).

The institute has undergone several changes of function since it was established in 1950 as the National Institute of Neurological Diseases and Blindness (P.L. 81–692). In 1968, the blindness program was separated from the institute to become the nucleus of the National Eye Institute* (P.L. 90–489), and the National Institute of Neurological Diseases and Blindness was renamed the National Institute of Neurological Diseases (P.L. 90–489); its name was changed a few months later to the National Institute of Neurological Diseases and Stroke (P.L. 90–639). In 1975, communication disorders (hearing loss, language difficulties, speech deficiencies, and so on) were added to the institute's mission, and the name was changed again, to the National Institute of Neurological and Communicative Disorders and Stroke. It received its present name in 1988, when part of the institute was transferred to the new National Institute on Deafness and Other Communication Disorders* (P.L. 100–553). The institute is now organized into six divisions, reflecting its current areas of research interest: (1) convulsive, developmental, and neuromuscular disorders (e.g., cerebral palsy and epilepsy), (2) demyelinating, atrophic, and dementing disorders (e.g., Alzheimer's disease and Parkinson's disease), (3) stroke and trauma, (4) fundamental neurosciences, (5) extramural activities, and (6) intramural research.

Although the institute has been embroiled in considerable controversy over its use of primates as research subjects, it has also enjoyed some real successes. Institute researchers have developed motor prostheses to restore hand and arm movement in paralyzed individuals, for instance, as well as cochlear implants for the deaf. They have been involved in the development of important new diagnostic tools: computed tomography (CT), positron emission tomography (PET), magnetic resonance imaging (MRI), and ultrasound imaging. In addition, the institute has supported scientific advances in understanding and treating a variety of diseases: discovering the gene for Huntington's disease, Duchenne muscular dystrophy, the familial form of ALS (amyotrophic lateral sclerosis, or Lou Gehrig's disease), and neurofibromatosis type 1, among others; developing an enzyme replacement therapy for the most common genetic metabolic disease, Gaucher's disease; and demonstrating that aspirin is effective in reducing the risk of stroke in some patients, as is surgical removal of fatty deposits from the carotid artery.

REFERENCE: Office of the Director, National Institutes of Health. 1994. *NIH Almanac 1994*. Bethesda, MD: NIH Publication.

DEBORAH R. MATHIEU

NATIONAL INSTITUTE OF NURSING RESEARCH

The NINR strives to improve nursing care by expanding the scientific foundation for nursing practice. As one of the National Institutes of Health (NIH),* it supports research and research training in a variety of areas: promoting health and preventing disease, understanding and mitigating the effects of acute and chronic illnesses and disabilities, improving patient care, and comprehending the physiological and behavioral processes that relate to sickness and health.

The Health Research Extension Act of 1985 (P.L. 99–158) authorized the establishment of the National Center for Nursing Research within the NIH; in 1993, the center was elevated to institute status (P.L. 103–43). The institute has identified four principal concerns among its many research areas—low birth weight, the human immunodeficiency virus (HIV), long-term care for older adults, and symptom management—and it promises to make valuable contributions to each of them. Institute researchers are developing social support interventions for pregnant, low-income black women, for instance; they are identifying culturally sensitive behavioral interventions that reduce HIV transmission in inner-city black women of childbearing age; they are funding research on the special caregiving problems associated with Alzheimer's patients; and they are working to improve the ability of nurses to assess and manage acute pain, especially in infants and children.

REFERENCE: Office of the Director, National Institutes of Health. 1994. *NIH Almanac 1994.* Bethesda, MD: NIH Publication.

DEBORAH R. MATHIEU

NATIONAL INSTITUTE ON AGING

One of the National Institutes of Health (NIH),* the NIA is responsible for biomedical, social, and behavioral research and training related to the aging process and diseases and other special problems and needs of the aged. In particular, the institute's programs aim to discover the basic processes of aging; understand normal changes associated with aging; identify age-related changes brought about by disease; determine ways of coping with disease and disability in old age; and promote disease prevention and maintenance of effective functioning.

In 1971, the White House Conference on Aging recommended the creation of a National Institute on Aging as a component of the National Institutes of Health, but Congress did not establish the institute until 1974 (P.L. 93–296), and the institute did not really begin to take shape until 1975, when two NIH components—the Adult Development and Aging Branch and the Gerontology Research Center—were separated from the National Institute of Child Health and Human Development* to form the nucleus of the new National Institute on Aging.

The institute's extramural programs provide grants to nonfederal institutions to develop research, train researchers, and provide research resources. The Biomedical Research and Clinical Medicine Program supports research in a variety of areas: The Molecular and Cell Biology Branch plans, implements, and supports fundamental molecular, cellular, and genetic research on the mechanisms of aging (e.g., age-associated patterns of cell growth and age-related changes in the immune system); the Geriatrics Branch supports the development of clinical research on the special medical needs and problems of the growing aging population in the United States (e.g., alterations in blood pressure regulation with age and age-related changes in bones and muscles). The Neuroscience and Neuropsychology of Aging Program works to further the understanding of the neural and behavioral processes associated with the aging brain; one of the program's highest priorities is research on dementias of old age, especially Alzheimer's disease. The Behavioral and Social Research Program focuses on understanding how psychological and social aging interact with biological aging processes, how older people relate to social institutions (such as the family), and the consequences of population aging.

The bulk of the institute's intramural research program is conducted at the Gerontology Research Center in Baltimore, Maryland, while a small proportion is undertaken at the NIH campus in Bethesda, Maryland. One of the best known of the intramural research studies is the Baltimore Longitudinal Study of Aging, a unique source of data on normal human aging. The study population is a group of volunteers from 20 to 95 years of age—over 500 men and 500 women—who are evaluated via a battery of clinical, biochemical, and psychological tests every 2 years over the course of their lifetimes. In contrast, the Epidemiology, Demography, and Biometry Program has initiated a multicenter prospective study of 14,000 older Americans to plan and conduct disease-oriented epidemiologic studies. Among the other intramural programs are the Laboratory of Behavioral Sciences (focusing on the interaction between behavioral aging and physiological processes), the Laboratory of Personality and Cognition (focusing on individual differences in psychosocial and intellectual functioning with aging), the Laboratory of Cellular and Molecular Biology (emphasizing genetic information transfer and environmental effects related to the aging process), and the Laboratory of Biological Chemistry (focusing on the biochemical, biophysical, and molecular mechanisms by which physiological functions change with age).

REFERENCE: Office of the Director, National Institutes of Health. 1994. *NIH Almanac 1994.* Bethesda, MD: NIH Publication.

DEBORAH R. MATHIEU

NATIONAL INSTITUTE ON ALCOHOL ABUSE AND ALCOHOLISM

One of the National Institutes of Health (NIH),* the NIAAA conducts and supports research on all aspects of alcohol dependence, alcohol abuse, and alcohol-related problems.

In 1970, the institute was established within NIH as part of a comprehensive federal attack on alcohol abuse (P.L. 91–616); in 1974, it was given the status of an institute within the newly created federal agency, the Alcohol, Drug Abuse, and Mental Health Administration* (ADAMHA) (P.L. 93–282). It remained part of ADAMHA until 1992, when it was transferred to the NIH (P.L. 102–321).

The institute's mission has changed over time. It began as a comprehensive program on alcoholism and alcohol abuse, responsible for supporting and conducting research as well as developing treatment and prevention programs. But in 1981 Congress transferred responsibility and funding for treatment services to the states (P.L. 97–35), and in 1986, Congress transferred the nonresearch prevention programs to the new Office for Substance Abuse Prevention in ADAMHA, leaving the institute to concentrate on its research efforts (P.L. 99–570). Despite losing these programs, the institute's budget grew steadily, from about $9 million in 1971 to over $180 million in FY 1994. The institute is now responsible for conducting and supporting biomedical and behavioral research on the causes and effects of alcoholism as well as on prevention and treatment strategies; conducting policy and epidemiological studies; serving as a national information resource; training researchers; coordinating federal research activities on alcohol abuse and alcoholism; and facilitating international cooperation and collaboration. Among its major research programs are studies of the mechanisms of alcohol intoxication and alcohol-induced brain damage; the effects on the fetus of alcohol use during pregnancy; neurotransmitter and hormonal signaling mechanisms in the brain; genetic predisposition to alcoholism; the effects on consumption of price and availability of alcoholic beverages and of alcohol warning labels; and alcohol problems among special populations (such as women, ethnic minorities, and the elderly).

REFERENCES: Clark, W. D., and Hilton, M. E., eds. 1991. *Alcohol in America: Drinking Practices and Problems.* Albany: State University of New York Press; Levine, H. G. 1984. ''The Alcohol Problem in America: From Temperance to Alcoholism.'' *British Journal of Addiction* 79:109–119.

DEBORAH R. MATHIEU

NATIONAL INSTITUTE ON DEAFNESS AND OTHER COMMUNICATION DISORDERS

The institute conducts and supports research and research training on the normal and disordered processes of hearing, balance, smell, taste, voice, speech, and language. The institute also conducts and supports research and training related to disease prevention and health promotion, as well as the development of devices that can substitute for lost and impaired sensory and communication functions. Established as one of the National Institutes of Health (NIH)* in 1988 (P.L. 100–553), the institute conducts and supports research in its own laboratories in Rockville, Maryland, and through programs of extramural research grants.

Among the research programs the institute has emphasized are noise exposure (the most common preventable cause of hearing loss), head and neck surgery, computerized devices to detect balance disorders, communication problems of acquired immunodeficiency syndrome (AIDS) patients, the incidence and prevalence of communication disorders across the life span, the mechanics of ordinary speech, and understanding how certain diseases may affect women, men, and members of minority populations differently. In 1991, the institute established the National Information Clearinghouse as a national resource center to broaden the dissemination of information about disorders of human communication. The clearinghouse provides information services and access to materials from the institute and other organizations with an interest in deafness and other communication disorders.

REFERENCE: Office of the Director, National Institutes of Health. 1994. *NIH Almanac 1994.* Bethesda, MD: NIH Publication.

DEBORAH R. MATHIEU

NATIONAL INSTITUTE ON DRUG ABUSE

The NIDA is the U.S. government's primary research agency on drug abuse and addiction and one of the National Institutes of Health (NIH).*

Federal involvement in drug abuse research and treatment began in the 1930s when the Public Health Service* established a Narcotics Division (renamed the Division of Mental Hygiene), opened two treatment centers, and created a research facility (later to become the institute's Addiction Research Center). In 1966, Congress demonstrated its increased concern by providing support for the rehabilitation and treatment of opiate abusers (P.L. 89–793) and expanded the program in 1970 to include all drug abusers (P.L. 91–513). In 1972, Congress created the National Institute on Drug Abuse as a division within the National Institute of Mental Health* (P.L. 91–513), and in 1974, the NIDA became a component of the new federal agency, the Alcohol, Drug Abuse, and Mental Health Administration* (ADAMHA) (P.L. 93–282). When Congress reorganized ADAMHA in 1992, the NIDA was transferred to the NIH (P.L. 102–321).

The mission of the NIDA is to support both extramural and intramural research (at its clinical center in Baltimore, Maryland) on the biological, social, behavioral, and neuroscientific bases of drug abuse, as well as its causes, prevention, and treatment. In addition, the NIDA supports research training as well as public education and research dissemination (through, for instance, its research monograph series and its bimonthly newsletter). Among its many programs are studies to assess the effectiveness of drug rehabilitation and identify factors associated with success; the Drug Abuse Information and Treatment Referral Hotline (a toll-free information telephone line); the Office of Workplace Initiatives, which was created in 1986 to implement the president's call for a drug-free workplace; the National AIDS Demonstration Research Project, which was implemented in 1987 to study and change the high-risk behaviors of injection drug users; a special division for developing new medications to aid in drug rehabilitation efforts; data collection efforts (such as the Drug Abuse Warning Network, which collects information on hospital emergency room deaths related to drug abuse); research into the neurobiological, behavioral, and social mechanisms underlying drug abuse as well as the specific biomedical and behavioral effects of drug abuse; investigation of the relationship of drug use to other problem behaviors; and epidemiologic studies (such as the National Household Survey on Drug Abuse, which has been conducted periodically since 1972, and the National High School Senior Survey, conducted annually since 1975).

REFERENCES: Musto, D. F. 1991. "Opium, Cocaine and Marijuana in American History." *Scientific American* (July): 40–47; National Institute on Drug Abuse. 1991. *Drug Abuse and Drug Abuse Research.* Rockville, MD: DHHS Publication No. (ADM) 91–1704.

DEBORAH R. MATHIEU

NATIONAL INSTITUTES OF HEALTH (NIH)

NIH is the U.S. government's principal biomedical research agency. The NIH has three main functions: (1) acquire knowledge to help prevent, detect, diagnose, and treat all human diseases and disabilities and improve human health; (2) train health professionals; and (3) disseminate biomedical information. The NIH fulfills these functions in a variety of ways. It supports biomedical research in universities, hospitals, and research institutions throughout the United States and abroad. It conducts biomedical research in its own laboratories and clinics. It supports the training of researchers as well as the development and maintenance of research resources. It identifies research advances that have significant potential for clinical application and facilitates the transfer of such advances to the health care system. It promotes effective ways to communicate biomedical information to scientists, health practitioners, and the public. In these capacities, the NIH typically accounts for between 20 and 30 percent of all U.S. dollars spent annually on biomedical research and development. With a budget of over $10 billion, the NIH is the largest single supporter of biomedical research in the United States and the largest biomedical research center in the world.

The NIH began in 1887 as a one-room bacteriological laboratory with a budget of $300. The Ransdell Act (P.L. 71–251) redesignated the laboratory as the National Institute of Health in 1930 and authorized funds for constructing buildings and providing research fellowships. In 1944, the Public Health Service Act (P.L. 78–410) gave NIH, now a bureau within the Public Health Service* (PHS), the legislative authority for a broad research program and incorporated the National Cancer Institute* into it. The name of the organization was changed to the National Institutes of Health in 1948, when four more institutes were established and construction of the Clinical Center was begun (P.L. 80–165, P.L. 80–655, P.L. 80–755). Currently, among NIH's major components are 17 institutes, 3 centers, a research hospital, and a library (the National Library of Medicine).

The NIH is under the aegis of the Public Health Service within the U.S. Department of Health and Human Services (DHHS). Its director, who reports to the DHHS assistant secretary for health, is assisted by three deputy directors and ten associate directors. In addition to leading the NIH, the Office of the Director oversees new and/or specialized programs, such as acquired immunodeficiency syndrome (AIDS) research and research on diseases of particular relevance and concern to women. Of special interest is the Office for Protection from Research Risks* (OPRR), established in 1974. On behalf of the NIH, the PHS, and the entire DHHS, the OPRR spearheads efforts to protect human and other animal subjects of biomedical research.

Also in the Director's Office is the Office of Recombinant DNA Activities (ORDA), which was established in 1974 as a result of nationwide concerns over the safety of research involving the manipulation of genetic material. First located in the National Institute of General Medical Sciences,* ORDA was transferred to the National Institute of Allergy and Infectious Diseases* in 1979 and transferred again in 1988 to the Office of the Director of NIH. Overseen by the Recombinant DNA Advisory Committee, ORDA is responsible for ensuring compliance with NIH guidelines for research involving recombinant DNA. In 1990, the Advisory Committee approved the first experiments involving transfer of human genes for therapeutic purposes.

The 17 research institutes composing the NIH are the National Institute on Aging,* National Institute on Alcohol Abuse and Alcoholism,* National Institute of Allergy and Infectious Diseases,* National Institute of Arthritis and Musculoskeletal and Skin Diseases,* National Cancer Institute,* National Institute of Child Health and Human Development,* National Institute on Deafness and Other Communication Disorders,* National Institute of Dental Research,* National Institute of Diabetes and Digestive and Kidney Diseases,* National Institute on Drug Abuse,* National Institute of Environmental Health Sciences,* National Eye Institute,* National Institute of General Medical Sciences,* National Heart, Lung, and Blood Institute,* National Institute of Mental Health,* National Institute of Neurological Disorders and Stroke,* and National Institute of Nursing Research.* With the exception of the National Institute of Environmental Health Sciences, which is in Research Triangle Park, North Carolina, all of the institutes are located in Maryland.

Each NIH institute has its own director, budget (separately negotiated with Congress), and three-member Advisory Council appointed by the president (to set institutional policy and award grants). The institutes vary greatly in budget size, number of personnel, space allocation for intramural laboratories and clinical facilities, and extent of their extramural programs. Typically—but not always—an institute includes both an intramural and an extramural program component, each with its own director. The extramural programs are responsible for roughly 80 percent of NIH resources in the form of research grants or contracts to medical schools, universities, and other nonfederal institutions. Extramural awards are based on a two-tiered peer review assessment: one for technical merit and one for program relevance. The intramural programs account for considerably fewer dollars (less than 20 percent) but require more than half of all NIH personnel to maintain the laboratory and clinical research programs conducted at the clinical centers. Intramural researchers need not undergo the peer review process imposed on extramural researchers but instead are overseen by Boards of Scientific Counselors.

The Warren Grant Magnuson Clinical Center, which was authorized by Congress in 1944 (P.L. 78–410), has been the research hospital for the NIH since it was completed in 1953. The 14-story, 500-bed facility was designed to place patient care facilities close to research laboratories. Each of the NIH's resident institutes is allotted a group of beds in the clinical center, an allocation that varies according to the institutes' needs and commitments (in one recent year, for instance, the National Cancer Institute had 24 percent of the beds; the National Institute of Allergy and Infectious Diseases had 10 percent; the National Institute of Child Health and Human Development had 9 percent; and the National Eye Institute had 2 percent). Physicians from the various institutes provide medical care for patients from all over the world who are referred by their physicians because they have the precise kind or stage of illness under investigation at the NIH. "Healthy" volunteers are also invited to the center to participate in studies of "normal" body functions.

Originally called simply the Clinical Center, it was renamed in 1981 to honor Warren Grant Magnuson, the former chairman of the Senate Committee on

Appropriations. The center has continually evolved to include state-of-the-art technology and techniques, and new buildings have been added, such as a 13-story Ambulatory Care Research Facility—which was opened in 1981 to provide space for the center's outpatient program as well as additional laboratory space—a radiation oncology building, and a facility for the department of transfusion medicine.

The National Center for Research Resources (NCRR) is responsible for supporting the research infrastructure necessary for NIH's biomedical and behavioral research. It was established in 1990 through a merger of two divisions within the NIH: the Division of Research Resources (which provided extramural resources to NIH-supported institutions) and the Division of Research Services (which provided resources to NIH's intramural research programs). Among NCRR's major extramural programs are the general clinical research centers program, which supports therapeutic experiments on human patients; seven primate research centers, located in universities, which conduct biomedical experiments on primates; the Chimpanzee Breeding and Research Program and the Specific-Pathogen-Free Rhesus Monkey Breeding and Research Program; a laboratory animal sciences program, which oversees the creation and use of mammals on which to conduct experiments; the Biological Models and Materials Research Program, which develops and supports nonmammal research models such as cell systems and lower organisms; a program to establish a variety of biomedical research technology resource centers, such as computer centers and engineering centers; the biomedical research support program, which provides relatively small grants to qualified research institutions for a variety of purposes such as pilot programs, equipment and facilities, unanticipated or urgent research needs; and the Research Centers in Minority Institutions program. Among its major intramural programs are the Biomedical Engineering and Instrumentation Program, the Veterinary Resources Program, and the Medical Arts and Photography Branch.

The John E. Fogarty International Center for Advanced Study in the Health Sciences is the component of the National Institutes of Health responsible for fostering worldwide scientific cooperation. It became operational in 1968 when the Office of International Research within the National Institutes of Health was abolished, and several of its functions were transferred to the Fogarty Center, named for late Representative John E. Fogarty (RI). In 1985, it was formally established in law (P.L. 99–158). The center funds basic research and training programs, providing opportunities for foreign scientists to pursue their research interests on the NIH campus and in other laboratories throughout the United States, as well as providing the means for U.S. researchers to work in foreign laboratories. It also administers bilateral and multilateral agreements and supports conferences and special studies. In addition, the center supports the Gorgas Memorial Institute of Tropical and Preventive Medicine, Inc., in Washington, D.C., and its operating arm, the Gorgas Memorial Laboratory, in Panama City, Panama. The director of the Fogarty Center is also the NIH associate director for International Research, advising the NIH director on the development of international policies and procedures related to biomedical science.

The National Center for Human Genome Research coordinates the participation of the various components of the NIH in the Human Genome Project,* a worldwide research effort to map and sequence the human genome and improve genetic research technology. In the United States, the project is jointly managed by the Department of Energy's Office of Health and Environmental Research and the NIH. Established in 1990, the center plans genome project research goals, supports related research and research training programs, coordinates with other U.S. and foreign agencies engaged in genome research, advises the NIH director, and disseminates information. The center is divided into three branches. The Research Centers Branch directs an extramural program for the establishment and support of multidisciplinary human genome research centers. The Office of Scientific Review plans and conducts peer review activities (e.g., establishes review criteria and organizes review groups). The Research Grants Branch provides a variety of extramural research grants, fellowships, and training grants and oversees the Bioethics Research Program, which focuses on the social and ethical implications of genome research and which, through the Ethical, Legal, and Social Implications Programs,* funds bioethics research related to the Human Genome Project.

With over 3.5 million items, the National Library of Medicine is the world's largest research library in a single scientific field. It was established in 1836 as the Library of the Army Surgeon General's Office; in 1956, the library was redesignated the National Library of Medicine and placed within the Public Health Service (P.L. 84–941); it became a component of the NIH in 1968. In addition to acquiring and preserving the world's biomedical literature, the library extends access to biomedical information and literature in a variety of ways: It disseminates over 75 publications (including, since 1879, *Index Medicus,* a comprehensive monthly listing of articles appearing in the world's leading medical journals); it also provides automated information retrieval services (the Medical Literature Analysis and Retrieval System [MEDLARS]) and databases (e.g., MEDLINE, CANCERLINE, TOXLINE). The collection is housed in two buildings on the NIH campus: the main building and the Lister Hill National Center for Biomedical Communications, which holds the library's research and development component as well as its grants, toxicology, and audiovisual programs.

REFERENCES: Aherns, Edward H., Jr. 1992. *The Crisis in Clinical Research.* New York: Oxford University Press; Anonymous. 1992. "Consensus Conference on Research Funding." *FASETS Journal* 6:813–20; Healy, Bernadine. 1994. "NIH and the Bodies Politic." *New England Journal of Medicine* 330:1493–98; Moore, G. W. 1980. *The N.I.H., How It Works.* Bethesda, MD: National Health Directory.

DEBORAH R. MATHIEU

NATIONAL LEGAL CENTER FOR THE MEDICALLY DEPENDENT AND DISABLED, INC.

The National Legal Center for the Medically Dependent and Disabled, Inc., was organized in 1984 and is a not-for-profit public interest law office and national support center funded through the Legal Services Corporation. Attorneys of the National Legal Center provide legal expertise on issues concerning the civil rights of persons with disabilities, particularly the right to receive life-sustaining treatment and other health services, such as personal attendant care and rehabilitation.

The National Legal Center's chief function is to provide its legal expertise to lawyers serving indigent clients. The National Legal Center also acts as a clearinghouse of information regarding disability rights, medical decision making, advance directives, and advocacy/prevention programs concerned with medical neglect and abuse. The center's information and litigation services extend to Americans with Disabilities Act* (ADA)–based cases and non-ADA cases involving unlawful medical discrimination; this area includes matters where access to medical treatment and related services is denied or limited on the basis of disability, age, and quality-of-life assessments.

People with disabilities, especially the indigent, often encounter discrimination in the delivery of medical and personal assistance services. Older persons and persons with medical needs are often placed in confining institutional settings without adequate rehabilitation services. They are often denied access to less restrictive, more appropriate home environments that would meet or better address the individual's abilities, emotional needs, and overall best interests. In other instances, some older adults and persons with disabilities are cognitively impaired, unconscious, or otherwise legally incompetent when critical, life-saving medical decisions must be made. Many are in nursing homes and hospitals and receive public assistance. Therefore, these persons often require representation by pro bono and public interest attorneys or by court-appointed guardians.

Persons subject to guardianship proceedings are particularly vulnerable to infringements and deprivations of their basic rights. Availability of expert legal assistance, such as that offered by the National Legal Center, is often crucial in such cases. For example, numerous courts have addressed, and continue to address, controversies concerning the medical treatment of persons with disabilities in general and people with complex medical needs in particular. In some instances, a relative or guardian, doctor, or hospital refuses to provide beneficial and essential medical treatment for a person in need of care. These cases involve newborns, young children, adults, and older persons. They are typically referred to as "medical discrimination cases" because the decision maker attempts to forgo or halt the patient's receipt of essential medical treatment on the basis of "quality-of-life" judgments or on the basis of other prejudicial and pejorative assessments of persons who live with disabilities or grave illnesses.

Recent court cases and federal laws, such as Section 504 of the Rehabilitation Act of 1973 and the Americans with Disabilities Act, prohibit disability-based discrimination. However, current notions and attempts to ration health care and limit health insurance coverage compete with the goals set forth in the ADA and related civil rights laws. In particular, rationing proposals often focus on providing care for short-term illnesses. Therefore, in providing priority or exclusive access to persons who have only few, and relatively uncomplicated, medical needs, such proposals tend to discriminate against persons with disabilities or chronic and severe illnesses.

The National Legal Center was created to address these various issues and to ensure the protection of persons with disabilities in the context of medical treatment and related services. The National Legal Center provides the public with general information and assists attorneys in every stage of the litigation process by offering the following services.

- *Technical assistance.* The National Legal Center provides legal research, preparation of appellate briefs, and consultation on litigation strategy.
- *Direct assistance.* Staff attorneys serve as counsel in selected cases.
- *Informational assistance.* The National Legal Center publishes a peer reviewed quarterly journal, *Issues in Law & Medicine,* conducts conferences, and compiles litigation and reference manuals, each providing timely materials on recent federal and state court rulings, statutes, and regulations. Upon request, staff attorneys present in-service workshops, conference papers, and other educational outreach programs to inform and train attorney and nonattorney organizations alike—for example, elder law attorneys, social workers, medical case managers, nursing home residents, care providers, ombudspersons, and protection and advocacy systems.

Two major activities of the National Legal Center are (1) an annual national training conference on legal and medical issues related to the rights of persons with disabilities to receive beneficial medical care and related assistance services and (2) the quarterly publication *Issues in Law & Medicine,* which provides updates on current court cases and legislation and publishes scholarly articles on important legal and medical issues in this area. *Issues* was first published in 1985.

The National Legal Center offers its legal expertise and informational and referral services with five goals in mind:

- To protect the rights of indigent persons who have disabilities or serious medical needs to secure essential medical treatment, regardless of age, health, function, or condition of dependency or disability;
- To protect the rights of persons with disabilities to secure personal assistance services and access to care and treatments;
- To increase the understanding of the Legal Services community, as well as pro bono and public interest attorneys, regarding the legal and medical concerns of persons with disabilities or complex medical needs;
- To gather and disseminate information on legal and medical developments that affect persons with disabilities and their rights to access care, treatment, rehabilitation, and personal assistance services;
- To coordinate efforts of Legal Services and pro bono attorneys by eliminating duplication of research and services.

The National Legal Center serves the public interest as a clearinghouse on information, research, and litigation to protect people with complex medical needs and persons with disabilities through the provision of legal services.

REFERENCES: "An Introduction to the National Legal Center for the Medically Dependent & Disabled, Inc." 1985. *Issues in Law & Medicine* 1:1; National Legal Center Staff. 1994–95. "Quarterly Report[s] of the National Legal Center for the Medically Dependent and Disabled, Inc." *Issues in Law & Medicine* 9–10:v.

JAMES BOPP, JR.

NATIONAL ORGAN TRANSPLANT ACT OF 1984

NOTA (P.L. 98–507) established the Task Force on Organ Transplantation and prohibited the sale or purchase of human organs for use in transplantation. NOTA also required the secretary of the Department of Health and Human Services (DHHS) to develop and maintain a scientific registry of organ transplant recipients and to convene a conference on the feasibility of establishing a national registry of voluntary bone marrow donors. In addition, NOTA empowered the secretary to make grants to qualified nonprofit organ procurement organizations and to create and operate a national Organ Procurement and Transplantation Network (OPTN), which would establish a national list of individuals who need organs and a national system to match organs and individuals included in the list, especially those whose immune systems make it difficult for them to receive organs.

In the years preceding the act's submission to Congress, the success rate of organ transplants had improved; fewer organs were being rejected and patients were living longer. This improvement was linked to the development of the immunosuppressant drug cyclosporin, which could subdue the body's immune system so that it does not reject transplanted organs. Cyclosporin had significantly increased the one-year organ survival rate for human kidney, heart, and liver transplants; and this increased the demand for human organs. An organized organ procurement system, however, was absent, and NOTA was passed in an effort to decrease the gap between supply and demand.

NOTA established the Task Force on Organ Transplantation to conduct a comprehensive examination of the medical, legal, economic, ethical, and social issues presented by human organ procurement and transplantation, to assess immunosuppressive medications, and to prepare a detailed report of its findings. The Task Force issued its final report, *Organ Transplantation: Issues and Recommendations,* in April 1986.

The Task Force recommended that all states enact "routine inquiry" legislation in order to increase organ donation. Hospitals would be required to establish a system to ensure that the families of all suitable organ donors are informed of opportunities for donating organs and tissues. A system of routine inquiry differs from a system of "required request" insofar as the former does not require that an unwilling health care professional make a request nor that families be asked to donate. The Task Force also recommended that the OPTN be promptly established to facilitate organ sharing by procurement organizations. This network would improve donor and recipient matching, decrease organ wastage, and increase the access of disadvantaged groups to organs. In addition, the Task Force urged public and private health insurers to make funds available to their clients for organ transplant procedures. The Task Force argued that a combined effort by public insurers, private insurers, and the federal government (for those with no other source of funds) would make equitable access to transplantation more possible. The Task Force also recognized the importance of enhanced and continued research into transplant procedures and recommended that the federal government increase the funding for such research. Finally, the Task Force provided a specific legislative proposal for the establishment of the National Organ Transplantation Advisory Board. This organization would be charged with ensuring that the recommendations of the Task Force on Organ Transplantation be implemented.

Subsequent legislation has addressed NOTA and the recommendations of the Task Force. The Omnibus Budget Reconciliation Act of 1986 required that all hospitals, as a condition of participating in Medicaid and Medicare, adopt routine inquiry protocols to identify and assist potential organ donors. This act also precluded Medicaid and Medicare payments for those organ procurement agencies that do not meet the standards specified in NOTA.

The Health Omnibus Programs Extension of 1988 (P.L. 100–607) revised and extended the programs of assistance to organ procurement organizations, authorizing the appropriation of $5 million for each fiscal year from 1988 through 1990. It also extended the duties of the OPTN. It required the OPTN to establish membership criteria and medical criteria for allocating organs and to adopt standards for preventing the acquisition of those organs infected by the human immunodeficiency virus (HIV). It also required the secretary of DHHS to establish a registry of voluntary bone marrow donors by October 1, 1988, and to report on the clinical and scientific status of organ transplantation by October first of each year. Finally, the act appropriated an Immunosuppressive Drug Therapy Block Grant of $5 million for each of the fiscal years 1988 through 1990 for allotments to states.

REFERENCES: Eyskens, E. 1994. "Ethics in Actual Surgery: Ethics and Organ Transplantation." *Acta Chirirgica Belgica* 94: 185–188; McDonald, John C. 1988. "The National Organ Procurement and Transplantation Network." *Journal of the American Medical Association* 259: 726–727; Salvatierra, Oscar, Jr. 1988. "Optimal Use of Organs for Transplantation." *New England Journal of Medicine* 318: 1329–1331; Task Force on Organ Transplantation. 1986. *Organ Transplantation: Issues and Recommendations.* Washington, D.C.: U.S. Department of Health and Human Services.

TIM DUVALL

NATIONAL RIGHT TO LIFE COMMITTEE, INC.

The purpose of the National Right to Life Committee, (NRLC) Inc., is to promote protection of innocent human life, including unborn children from the moment of conception, infants subject to infanticide, and persons of all ages subject to euthanasia and assisted suicide. NRLC is opposed to the rationing of health care or other actions that would put innocent human life at risk unnecessarily. It engages in various lawful political, legislative, legal, and educational activities to protect and promote the concept of the sanctity of innocent human life.

NRLC is incorporated as a not-for-profit corporation in the District of Columbia. The executive and publishing headquarters of NRLC are in Washington, D.C. NRLC also has a Western Office in Sacramento. The National Right to Life Committee is composed of a board of directors representing 51 state affiliate organizations and about 3,000 local chapters. The membership of NRLC and its affiliated organizations represents a cross-section of American racial, ethnic, religious, and socioeconomic groups.

The National Right to Life Committee was organized in June 1973 by local and state pro-life leaders because states were beginning to enact permissive abortion laws in the wake of the decision of the U.S. Supreme Court in *Roe v. Wade,* 410 U.S. 113 (1973), and *Doe v. Bolton,* 410 U.S. 179 (1973), which declared abortion a constitutional right. It was felt by these leaders that a national organization was needed to resist the passage of weakened abortion laws.

The members of the National Right to Life Committee have been the primary promoters of laws restricting abortion to only those instances in which the mother's life is in danger. Since the decisions of the U.S. Supreme Court in *Roe v. Wade* and *Doe v. Bolton,* the members of the National Right to Life Committee have supported legislation to protect unborn human life within the limits set by those decisions and have sought, through lawful means, those changes in the law that would allow full legal protection for the unborn.

The educational arm of NRLC is called the National Right to Life Educational Trust Fund. NRLC has a federal political action committee and various state political action committees, which are involved in promoting pro-life candidates. NRLC also publishes a pro-life newspaper, *NRL News,* which enjoys wide distribution.

REFERENCE: *NRL News.*

RICHARD E. COLESON

NATIONAL SCIENCE FOUNDATION (NSF)

An independent agency of the federal government, the NSF serves to preserve the well-being of all scientific fields and to promote progress in science and engineering by sponsoring scientific research and education projects. In general, the NSF meets its mission by funding basic science research grants to academic, industrial, and nonprofit institutions. At present, the NSF receives greater than 30,000 requests for grants and funds more than half of them, accounting for approximately 25 percent of the federal support to academic institutions for basic research.

Grants may be used for a variety of purposes including the development of science curricula, of fellowships and traineeships in science and engineering, and of data processing and dissemination methods. Funds to colleges and universities are targeted to improve the scientific quality of the institution by obtaining research equipment and facilities and by upgrading their research and scientific educational activities.

The NSF maintains four national research centers that are open to all qualified scientists: the National Radio Astronomy Observatory in Green Bank, West Virginia; Kitt Peak National Observatory near Tucson, Arizona; Cerro Tololo Inter-American Observatory in Chile; and the National Center for Atmospheric Research in Boulder, Colorado. In addition, the NSF initiates and supports specific international scientific projects, such as the U.S.-Antarctic Research Program, the Ocean Sediment Coring Program, the International Biology Program, the Global Atmospheric Research Program, and other cooperative scientific programs.

The NSF was established by the National Science Foundation Act of 1950 (P.L. 81–507) in recognition of scientific contributions during World War II. The National Science Board is the NSF's policymaking body. Each of the 24 members of the board is a prominent person in his or her field of science. The director of the NSF sits on the board as an ex officio member. All individuals sitting on the board are appointed by the president with Senate approval.

REFERENCES: Kleinman, D. L. 1994. "Layers of Interests, Layers of Influence Business and the Genesis of the National Science Foundation." *Science, Technology and Human Values* 19: 259; Massey, W. E. 1992. "The Future of the National Science Foundation." *Notices of the American Mathematical Society* 39: 1021; Mazuzan, G. T. 1992. " 'Good Science Gets Funded': The Historical Evolution of Grant Making at the National Science Foundation." *Knowledge* 14:63.

ANA MARIA LOPEZ

NEURAL GRAFTING

Neurological disorders are a significant cause of illness, disability, and death in the United States. They can result from either injury or disease. Injury to the central nervous system (CNS) can result from physical damage to the brain or spinal cord or disruption in the normal flow of blood to the brain. Similarly, the CNS is susceptible to a number of diseases. Neurodegenerative disorders are marked by the loss of specific nerve cell populations in the brain or spinal cord. In most cases, the disease is progressive and the cell loss is gradual. Examples of neurodegenerative disorders include Parkinson's disease, Huntington's disease, and Alzheimer's. Demyelinating disorders are marked by the loss of myelin, the fatty material that surrounds many axons in the brain or spinal cord. When a cell loses this myelin sheath, its ability to send messages is impaired. The most common demyelinating disorder is multiple sclerosis. The final form of neurological disorder is epilepsy or the disruption of the normal electrical activity in the brain either in a specific confined area or in the entire brain.

Neural grafting represents a controversial but promising intervention for treating neurological disorders. One approach would focus on the provision of a continuous supply of chemical substances that have been depleted by injury or disease in affected regions of the brain or spinal cord. A second function would be to introduce new substances or cells that promote neuron survival, stimulate neuron regrowth, or both. The third function would be to replace nerve cells in the brain or spinal cord that are lost to injury or disease.

In order to accomplish these varied functions, appropriate materials for transplantation must be selected. Many scientists consider the most effective material for neural grafts to be human fetal CNS tissue (Freed et al., 1992). Fetal tissue is especially well suited for grafting because it replicates rapidly and differentiates into functioning mature cells. Unlike mature CNS tissue, fetal tissue has been found to readily develop and integrate into the host organism. Nutritional support provided by blood vessels from the host is readily accepted and likely promoted by fetal tissue. In animal experiments, fetal CNS tissue has displayed a considerable capacity for survival within the CNS of the graft recipient. Moreover, of all the graft materials available, fetal tissue is most capable of reconstituting nerve cell structure and function. Furthermore, fetal CNS tissue is amenable to cell culture and storage via cryopreservation and enjoys immunological advantages over other sources of material.

The use of fetal CNS tissue for neural grafting is highly controversial because a dependence on spontaneously aborted fetuses or ectopic pregnancies is impractical due to the limited numbers available, the inability to control the timing, and the rapid deterioration of fetal tissue after the death of the fetus. The major supply of fetal tissue, therefore, is likely to come from induced abortions on unwanted pregnancies. This has raised vehement objections from antiabortion groups as well as questions regarding consent protocol, impact on timing and method of abortion, ownership, and payment.

On March 22, 1988, in response to a growing political controversy surrounding the publicity over the Mexican and Swedish attempts at grafting fetal CNS tissue into Parkinson's patients, Robert Windom, assistant secretary for the Department of Health and Human Services (DHHS), imposed a moratorium on federal support for fetal tissue transplantation applications, pending a report from a special panel he directed the National Institutes of Health (NIH)* to convene in order to answer ethical and legal questions posed by a proposal for transplanting fetal brain tissue into patients with Parkinson's disease.

In September 1988, the Human Fetal Tissue Transplantation Research Panel recommended that funding be restored. By a 17–4 vote, the panel concluded that such research is "acceptable public policy." In order to protect the interests of the various parties, the panel recommended guidelines to prohibit financial inducements to women; prohibit the sale of fetal tissue; prevent directed donations of fetal tissue to relatives; separate the decision to abort and the decision to donate; and require consent of the woman and nonobjection of the father.

Although the pro-life lobby accused the panel of being stacked in favor of the research community, there was considerable consensus across the various interests represented on the panel concerning the appropriateness of fetal tissue transplantation research. The panel was chaired by retired federal Judge Arlin Adams, who is a known opponent of abortion but open to discussion of the use of fetal tissue. Membership on the panel, whose nomination required White House approval, included persons committed to a pro-life, antiabortion philosophy that includes opposition to the use of any tissue obtained from what they view as an immoral act.

In December 1988, the NIH Director's Advisory Committee unanimously approved the special panel's report without change and recommended that the moratorium be lifted (NIH, 1988). The committee concluded that existing procedures governing human research and organ donation are sufficient to regulate fetal tissue transplantation. In January 1989, James Wyngaarden, the director of NIH, concurred with the position of the Advisory Committee and transmitted the final report to the assistant secretary for health. The report languished in the department without action until November 1989, when Secretary Louis Sullivan, under pressure from Senator Gordon Humphrey (R—NH), Congressman William Dannemeyer (R—CA), and other pro-life congressmen, announced, in direct conflict with the recommendations, an indefinite extension of the moratorium. The secretary concluded:

I am persuaded that one must accept the likelihood that permitting the human fetal research at issue will increase the incidence of abortion across the country. Providing the additional rationalization of directly advancing the cause of human therapeutics cannot help but tilt some already vulnerable women toward a decision to have an abortion. (Sullivan, 1989)

This extension of the ban on fetal research funding was challenged by Congressman Ted Weiss (D—NY) on technical grounds. He warned that making the moratorium permanent could be construed legally as a rule and should thus be made subject to the formal rule-making process rather than a simple announcement by the administration.

In April 1990, the House Committee on Energy and Commerce Subcommittee on Health and the Environment held hearings on human fetal tissue transplantation research. The House passed H.R. 2507 in July 1991, which would have limited the authority of executive branch officials to ban federal funds for areas of research without support of an ethics advisory board. In May 1992, the House voted to approve the language of the conference committee, which included privacy and consent provisions added by the Senate, and sent the bill on to the president for a certain veto. In anticipation of a likely override of his veto, George Bush issued an executive order directing the National Institutes of Health to establish a fetal tissue bank from spontaneously aborted fetuses and ectopic pregnancies, even though there was little evidence that such a bank could provide sufficient amounts of high-quality tissue for transplantation.

The political controversy continued in June 1992, when a compromise bill was introduced in both houses. This bill in effect gave the administration one year to demonstrate that the tissue bank would work. If researchers were then unable to obtain suitable tissue from the bank within two weeks of a request, they could obtain tissue from other sources including elective abortions. In October 1992, a Senate filibuster by opponents of fetal research cut off attempts at passage, leading Majority Leader Mitchell to vow that the bill would be the first order of business when the Senate reconvened in January 1993. On his second day in office, President Bill Clinton issued an executive order removing the ban on the use of fetal tissue for transplantation, thus opening the door for intensified research on neural grafting.

REFERENCES: Branch, D. Ware, Lee Ducat, Alan Fantel, et al. 1995. "Suitability of Fetal Tissues from Spontaneous Abortions and from Ectopic Pregnancies for Transplantation." *Journal of the American Medical Association* 273(1): 66–68; Freed, Curt P., Robert E. Breeze, Neil L. Rosenberg, et al. 1992. "Survival of Implanted Fetal Dopamine Cells and Neurologic Improvement 12 to 46 Months After Transplantation for Parkinson's Disease." *New England Journal of Medicine* 327(22): 1549–1555; National Institutes of Health. 1988. *Human Fetal Tissue Transplantation Research.* Report of the Advisory Committee to the Director. Bethesda, MD: National Institutes of Health (December 14); Office of Technology Assessment. 1990. *Neural Grafting: Repairing the Brain and Spinal Cord.* Washington, D.C.: U.S. Government Printing Office; Sanberg, P. R., T. K. Koutouzis, T. B. Freeman, et al. 1993. "Behaviorial Effects of Fetal Neural Transplants: Relevance to Huntington's Disease." *Brain Research Bulletin* 32(5): 493–496; Sullivan, Louis W. Statement. Sec. H. H. S. Nov. 2, 1989; Turner, D. A., and W. Kearney. 1993. "Scientific and Ethical Concerns in Neural Fetal Tissue Transplantation." *Neurosurgery* 33(6): 1031–1037; Vawter, Dorothy E. 1993. "Fetal Tissue Transplantation Policy in the United States." *Politics and the Life Sciences* 12(1): 79–85.

ROBERT H. BLANK

NUREMBERG CODE

The Nuremberg Code is a code of ethics setting out basic guidelines governing experimentation with human subjects. At the conclusion of World War II, the Allied governments brought legal action against physicians and certain other professional and government officials of Nazi Germany for their performance of medical experiments on unwilling human subjects. An outcome of those legal processes was the Nuremberg Code for the conduct of medical experiments using humans. The code requires the following: The human subject must give his/her voluntary consent to participate in the experiment; the experiment should be based on initial animal studies; the experiment should avoid all physical and mental suffering; the experiment should not anticipate the death of the subject; the degree of risk should be in proportion to the humanitarian importance of the problem to be solved; planning and facilities should be designed to facilitate the safe conduct of the experiment; the experiment should be conducted by qualified persons; the study subject should be free to leave the experiment at any time; the scientist in charge should be prepared to terminate the experiment any time the experiment is judged to be a hazard to the subject.

Fundamental to ethical considerations for medical experiments involving humans is the test of social good—that experiments yield results for the good of society—and the requirement that the subject give his/her consent to participate. In the United States, these principles have been codified in the Common Rule for the Protection of Human Subjects (*Federal Register,* June 18, 1991).

REFERENCES: Annas, G. J., and Grodin, M. A. 1992. *The Nazi Doctors and the Nuremberg Code.* New York: Oxford University Press; Ivy, A. C. 1947. "Nazi War Crimes of a Medical Nature." *Federal Bulletin* 33: 133–146; Jonas, H. 1969. "Philosophical Reflections on Experimenting with Human Subjects." *Daedalus* 98: 219–247.

GERALD GOODMAN

O

OFFICE FOR PROTECTION FROM RESEARCH RISKS

The OPRR exercises authority on behalf of the secretary of the U.S. Department of Health and Human Services (DHHS) for the protection of human subjects and for the care and use of laboratory animals involved in research. Although OPRR is located within the National Institutes of Health (NIH)* for organizational purposes, its responsibility for the protection of human subjects extends to all research conducted or supported by any component of the DHHS. Similarly, OPRR's responsibility for the care and use of laboratory animals extends to all vertebrate animals involved in research conducted or supported by any component of the Public Health Service* (PHS).

The first major responsibility of the OPRR is to provide protections for human subjects involved in biomedical and behavioral research conducted or supported by the DHHS. The Public Health Service Act as amended by the Health Research Extension Act of 1985 directs the secretary, DHHS, to protect, by regulation, the rights and the welfare of human research subjects (P.L. 99–158, Sec. 491). That responsibility has been delegated by the secretary, DHHS, to OPRR, which develops, promulgates, and exercises oversight over the implementation of the DHHS Regulations for the Protection of Human Subjects (Regulations) (45 CFR 46).

The second major responsibility of the OPRR is to provide for the humane care and use of laboratory animals. The Public Health Service Act as amended by the Health Research Extension Act of 1985 directs the secretary, DHHS, acting through the director, NIH, to develop guidelines for the proper care of laboratory animals used in biomedical and behavioral research and for the proper treatment of animals while being used in such research (P.L. 99–158, Sec. 495). Responsibility for humane care and use of research animals has also been delegated to OPRR. In the case of laboratory animals, the only components within DHHS that conduct or support research involving animals are found within the

PHS (the health agencies within DHHS). As a consequence, in compliance with the provisions of the law cited above, OPRR has issued the *Public Health Service Policy on Humane Care and Use of Laboratory Animals* with the concurrence of the director, NIH, the assistant secretary for health, and the secretary, DHHS.

OPRR is an organizational hybrid unlike most other government components. For programmatic purposes, the OPRR answers directly to the secretary, DHHS, from whom it derives its authority and responsibility. For organizational and administrative purposes, OPRR is located within the Office of the Director, NIH. The director, OPRR, answers to the director, NIH, through the deputy director for Extramural Affairs.

For purposes of budget allocation, personnel, salaries, benefits, space, clearances, and travel, OPRR is a part of NIH. Nevertheless, under its Regulatory and Policy authority, OPRR can (and does) set standards, conduct investigations, and impose restrictions and penalties on NIH and other agencies within the DHHS, as well as on awardee institutions.

Created in 1972 by Dr. Robert Q. Marston, director, NIH, from the Institutional Relations Branch of the NIH's Division of Research Grants, OPRR has expanded both in terms of size and responsibility as a result of the legislation cited above and the delegation of authorities from the secretary, DHHS.

The human subjects regulations require each institution that conducts research involving human subjects supported in whole or in part by any component of the DHHS to provide an acceptable Assurance of Compliance (Assurance) to OPRR. An Assurance is a document signed by a senior official of the institution that sets forth in writing the commitment of the institution to protect the rights and welfare of human research subjects.

The first part of the Assurance identifies the code or principles that will guide the institution in making decisions about the rights and welfare of human research subjects. Most institutions in the United States have elected to follow the principles of (1) respect for persons; (2) beneficence; and (3) justice as set forth in the Belmont Report issued by the National Commission for the Protection of Human Subjects. Most foreign institutions prefer to identify the Declaration of Helsinki as their guiding code.

The second section of the Assurance provides a detailed description of the administrative structures in place in the institution to protect the rights and welfare of human subjects. Each institution is directed to create and describe a structure that is consistent with the needs, organization, history, and tradition of the institution. Among the items that must be included in the Assurance are the following: (1) identification of the qualifications of the chairperson and members of the Institutional Review Board* (IRB); (2) a commitment to IRB review of all research proposals covered by the Regulations prior to submission for funding; (3) provisions for certifying that each research project meets, at a minimum, the requirements of the Regulations; (4) a statement that informed consent from each research subject will be obtained and documented; (5) a determination that risks to subjects will be reasonable in the light of expected benefits to the subjects or to society; (6) a statement that selection of subjects will be equitable; (7) provision for additional protections for vulnerable subjects (e.g., the mentally disabled, prisoners, children, pregnant women, and fetuses); (8) assignment of meeting space; filing systems, and adequate staff for the IRB; and (9) methods that will be used to inform research investigators of their responsibilities for the rights and welfare of human research subjects.

More than 95 percent of the major research institutions in the United States have included in their Assurances a statement that they will provide the same protections to all subjects of research, irrespective of the source of funding. As a consequence, although the Regulations apply, literally speaking, only to research that is supported by DHHS funds, in practice most human subjects research in the United States is carried out in compliance with the Regulations. OPRR enforces the Regulations in situations where the research is not funded by HHS but where the Regulations are extended to unfunded research through the mechanism of the Assurance.

Since 1983 the OPRR, in accordance with the legislation cited above, has conducted more than 100 regional educational programs for research administrators, investigators, IRB members, and staff of institutions to clarify and guide institutions in meeting their responsibilities under the Regulations. OPRR operates on the assumption that most persons who conduct biomedical and behavioral research involving human subjects are dedicated to the well-being of their fellow human beings. Therefore, for the Regulations to achieve their purpose, it is necessary that these highly motivated individuals be educated concerning their responsibilities. It is for this reason that the primary enforcement mechanism of the Regulations is education. Through a variety of methods of communication, OPRR maintains close touch with the research community and attempts to keep that community well informed concerning the best ethical information available relative to a wide variety of research efforts.

The pattern of implementation of the Public Health Service Policy on Humane Care and Use of Laboratory Animals parallels that of the protections for human research subjects. Animal Welfare Assurances (Assurances) are negotiated with each institution that receives an award from any component of the PHS for research involving vertebrate animals.

In the first part of the Assurance, each institution is required to declare its willingness to follow the National Research Council's *Guide for the Care and Use of Laboratory Animals* and the provisions of the Animal Welfare Act (P.L. 89–544, P.L. 91–579, P.L. 94–279).

The second part of the Assurance sets forth administrative procedures that the institution will employ to implement the Policy. As is the case with human subjects, Animal Welfare Assurance Documents are tailored to the needs of each institution. Also similar to the protections for human subjects, the institution is required to establish a qualified Institutional Animal Care and Use Committee to review and to certify that each protocol that is conducted involving animal research subjects will be carried out in accord with the Policy.

OPRR conducts regional animal welfare educational efforts with respect to the implementation of the Policy in a manner similar to the efforts utilized for education concerning human subjects protections. The content of the education programs is very different. Because animals do not consent to participate in research, research investigators need not be concerned about informed consent. On the other hand, since facilities, sanitation, housing, and care are so critical to a sound animal research program, these issues receive special attention in the education program.

Regrettably, a few research investigators do not meet their responsibilities under the Policy or the Regulations. Others comply with the Policy or Regulations but are accused of not doing so. When an allegation of noncompliance occurs, OPRR deals with it in the following manner. Typically, OPRR requires the institution to make a thorough investigation of the allegation and to take appropriate steps. If the institution finds the investigator in noncompliance, it is both expected to provide administrative safeguards to prevent a repetition of the noncompliance and to exercise appropriate disciplinary action toward persons involved in the noncompliance.

If OPRR is not satisfied that the institution has made a thorough, good-faith effort to evaluate allegations of noncompliance, or if OPRR believes that the institution has not taken adequate preventive or disciplinary measures, OPRR may conduct its own investigation, impose appropriate preventive measures, and exercise disciplinary action.

Sanctions imposed by OPRR can extend to both research support and research personnel. With respect to research support, if the Policy or Regulations are not followed, OPRR can suspend or terminate payment of a single research award or terminate payment of all of the awards made to a component of the institution. If the regulatory breach is severe, OPRR may terminate all awards to an institution. Similarly, OPRR can take steps to debar individuals who fail to comply with the regulations from eligibility to compete for research support—for a limited period or for life. Such sanctions can have the practical effect of making a researcher unemployable.

Because decision making in investigations is based on a standard of ''preponderance of evidence'' rather than a standard of ''beyond a reasonable doubt,'' decisions whether noncompliance has occurred are usually reached in a relatively short space of time. Persons or institutions who have been disciplined under OPRR decisions have a right to appeal. Nevertheless, no OPRR decision has ever been overturned on appeal.

In carrying out its responsibilities, OPRR coordinates its efforts to protect human research subjects with the Food and Drug Administration,* which has responsibility for protecting human subjects involved in the testing of drugs, biologics, medical devices, and other test articles. OPRR also coordinates its efforts with the U.S. Department of Agriculture (USDA) in matters pertaining to the care and use of laboratory animals. Because OPRR can reach administrative decisions more quickly than USDA can obtain required court judgments under the Animal Welfare Act, OPRR often investigates violations of the Animal Welfare Act when USDA and PHS Policy jurisdictions overlap. Finally, the director, OPRR, serves as chairperson of the Interagency Human Subjects Coordinating Committee. That committee is responsible for standardizing the interpretation of the Common Federal Rule for the Protection of Human Subjects.

CHARLES R. McCARTHY and ERIC M. MESLIN

OFFICE OF SCIENCE AND TECHNOLOGY POLICY, WHITE HOUSE

In 1976, Congress enacted the National Science and Technology Policy, Organization, and Priorities Act, which outlined the role of the Office of Science and Technology Policy (OSTP, P.L. 94–282). The OSTP is mandated to advise the executive branch on the impact of science and technology on domestic and international affairs; evaluate the efficacy and quality of the federal effort in science and technology policies; develop and implement science and technology policies; promote and create strong partnerships among all levels of government and the scientific community; and work with the private sector to ensure federal investments in science and technology contribute to economic prosperity, environmental quality, and national security.

The director of the OSTP is responsible for the overall direction of the federal research and development activities and for developing a federal strategy for science and technology development that is consistent with national goals. Programs emerge from the efforts of interagency public sector teams in cooperation with the private sector.

The OSTP is divided into four divisions. The Technology Division develops and implements federal technology policies consistent with other federal policies. The Science Division leads the effort to maintain U.S. leadership in physical, life, and social sciences and supports the role of science in solving important problems in health, economy, education, and national security. Although the division supports basic science research, it also focuses on research that transcends traditional scientific boundaries.

The Environmental Division develops environmental policies that are consistent with federal energy and economic policies. This may be accomplished by the development and promotion of environmental education programs in global climate change, pollution assessment, and deforestation. The National Security and International Affairs Division provides links between scientific and technological development and national security. In addition, this division coordinates international policies on science and technology, negotiates international science and technology agreements, and directs the U.S. participation in the Organization for Economic Cooperation megascience forum.

ANA MARIA LOPEZ

OFFICE OF TECHNOLOGY ASSESSMENT

Established in 1972, the Office of Technology Assessment (OTA) of the U.S. Congress is a research organization charged with producing objective technological information from a broad spectrum of sources that members of Congress may utilize in making public policy decisions (P.L. 92–484). Congress created the OTA as an independent source of scientific and technical advice, and since its inception the OTA has maintained a reputation for clearly and accurately characterizing the scientific information involved in a wide range of policy debates.

REFERENCES: Office of Technology Assessment. 1987. *Life-Sustaining Technologies and the Elderly.* Washington, D.C.: Government Printing Office; Office of Technology Assessment. 1989. *New Developments in Biotechnology: Patenting Life.* Washington, D.C.: Government Printing Office; Office of Technology Assessment. 1992. *Cystic Fibrosis and DNA Tests: Implications of Carrier Screening.* Washington, D.C.: Government Printing Office; Office of Technology Assessment. 1993. *Biomedical Ethics in U.S. Public Policy.* Washington, D.C.: Government Printing Office; Office of Technology Assessment. 1994. *Guidelines for Special Care Units.* Washington, D.C.: Government Printing Office; Walters, Rhodri. 1992. "The Office of Technology Assessment of the United States Congress: A Model for the Future?" *Government and Opposition* 27: 89–108.

DEBORAH R. MATHIEU

ORGAN PROCUREMENT

The cornerstone of the American system of organ procurement is voluntariness. Because the transplant program met with a great deal of public apprehension at its inception, those asked to donate were seen to be in need of strict protection so that donations were not made under conditions of coercion or ignorance. These concerns resulted from the perception of transplantation as a highly experimental procedure. In addition, many worried that organ donation involved the mutilation of the body and violated the tenets of many religions. Voluntariness, by definition, means that donors (whether they are donating their own or a deceased's organs) must agree to do so free of coercion and in conformance with the doctrine of informed consent. The donor should understand what he is agreeing to donate, how the donation procedure works, and the consequences of donation (including possible benefits and risks). The system of voluntary donation can only work if altruism plays a significant role in the decision to donate organs. Supporters of a voluntary system of organ donation argue that the desire to help others is the overriding factor in the decision to donate. Moreover, a policy based on altruism and voluntariness is consistent with the American value of respecting individual autonomy and conveys respect for the dignity of the body after death.

Reflecting these values is the Uniform Anatomical Gift Act,* which Congress passed in 1968. The purpose of the act, which has been adopted by all 50 states and the District of Columbia, is to enable individuals to make anatomical bequests for a variety of purposes, especially to medical schools and for organ, tissue, and cornea transplantation. The process is simple: One need only sign a donor card or check a box on an application for a driver's license. It has not, however, been particularly successful. Very few people have signed up to be donors, and physicians rarely remove the organs without the permission of the deceased's family, even if the deceased had signed a donor card.

One result is that there remains a serious shortage of transplantable organs, tissues, and corneas. Initially, it was believed that this shortage was due to health care providers' refusal to ask the families of potential donors about donation. This belief resulted in the passage of a series of state and federal laws in an attempt to increase the supply of transplantable organs, tissues, and corneas. These laws have commonly been called *required request* or *routine inquiry laws* and are designed to encourage health care professionals to speak with families about organ or tissue donation. Two types of laws were passed: (1) "weak" laws—routine inquiry laws—which simply require that hospitals develop policies to ensure that families are made aware of the option to donate, and (2) "strong" laws—required request laws—which require that the health care professionals document that a request to donate was made as well as the outcome of the request. Forty-nine states and the District of Columbia have passed these laws; 26 are strong laws and 23 are weak laws. The Joint Commission on Health Care Accreditation of Hospital Organizations also requires hospitals to develop required request policies, including the establishment of written protocols. And in 1986, Congress enacted legislation requiring hospitals to establish written routine inquiry protocols or risk losing their Medicare funding (P.L. 99–509). It was hoped that this legislation would greatly ameliorate the shortage of transplantable organs and tissues, but this has not happened. Studies in a number of states have demonstrated that while there was a small immediate increase in procurement of organs, tissues, and corneas after passage of required request laws, these increases were modest and leveled off after the first two years of the laws' enactment to about 4,500 donors per year.

Routine referral has been proposed either as an alternative or as an adjunct to required request and routine inquiry policies. This policy would require hospitals either to routinely inform the local OPO (organ procurement organization) of admissions that are likely to lead to potential organ donors or to consult with the OPO about all hospital deaths. This policy could be construed in one of two ways. The policy could mandate that hospital personnel make referrals to OPOs in addition to performing their usual request functions with families. More likely, the policy is meant to shift responsibility for talking to families from hospital health care providers to OPO staff. This is based on the premise that the reason that families do not agree to donate is that the health care providers do a poor job of requesting donation. OPO staff, it is assumed, would do a better job and thus increase the consent rate. There are no data, however, to support this view.

Some have suggested that we institute public policies that force individuals to publicly decide either to agree to donate or to refuse and then strictly enforce the patient's (rather than the family's) wishes. Individuals could be required to decide when obtaining their driver's license, or all patients could be asked upon admission to the hospital. This type of policy—called *mandated choice*—is built on the following assumptions: (1) individuals are in favor of donation and if forced would agree to donate; (2) when families are asked about donation, they are under great stress and thus are less likely to donate than the individual would have been if forced to decide at an earlier time. Unfortunately, these assumptions are completely untested, and there are equally good theoretical reasons to doubt that such a policy would help. First, it is unclear that families are less willing to donate a loved one's organs than the individuals themselves; the available survey data would suggest the opposite. Second, given that one of the most common reasons that individuals do not fill out donor cards is the fear that doctors undertreat individuals with donor cards, mandated choice may lead to less, rather than more, prior consent to donation. Finally, it is unclear how these proposals will make OPOs more likely to take patient's organs when the families object since hospitals are extremely reluctant to do this for fear of becoming involved in a lawsuit.

Some proposals for increasing the number of donors appeal to the principles of self-interest and represent a significant divergence from the ideal of altruism. One suggestion is to encourage individuals to sign donor cards by promising payment to a beneficiary (designated beforehand by the deceased) if organs are procured. More complicated schemes set up a futures market for organs, offering such incentives as a reduction in health insurance premiums to those signing donor cards or a promise to put those agreeing to donate at some future date at the top of the transplantation waiting list if they should be in need of a transplant. A third proposal is to pay the donor family for the organs. At the time of death, the family would be asked to donate an eligible family member's organs in exchange for a financial reward. African-American families are a particular target of these programs, as they are underrepresented among organ donors. Advocates of this type of system have suggested everything from tax credits to a small amount of money to pay for burial expenses to payments as high as $30,000 per organ.

These proposals have come under both theoretical and empirical attack. Critics claim that allowing financial compensation reduces respect for the human body, raises issues of fairness, and devalues altruism. Even if these objections can be answered, there are empirical data suggesting that financial incentives will not increase, and may even decrease, donation. Prottas (1983) found that 78 percent of surveyed individuals rejected financial incentives for consent and that donor families were the most vehemently against these proposals.

A fourth method is to pay living donors for their organs. Such donations occur regularly in India and Egypt, where it is legal, and in Uruguay, where a black market in kidneys has been reported, but the practice is outlawed in the United States (P.L. 98–507). Obvious arguments against such a system are the tremendous potential for abuse, especially the exploitation of rich potential recipients buying the organs of desperately poor donors.

Presumed consent is a system in which no express consent for cadaver organ donation is sought from descendants or their families, and organs are removed for transplantation unless the donor or the family objects. This policy is in place in 15 foreign countries, including Austria, Belgium, and France, and recently has been suggested in the United States.

The following objections have been raised against presumed consent: First, for a presumed consent policy to be ethically acceptable, there would have to be a clear-cut societal consensus that people desire to donate. There is no evidence such a consensus exists in America. Second, presumed consent assumes that the general public is well educated about the policy and that a readily accessible system of opting out is in place. Third, greater information regarding how presumed consent works in other countries is needed. In many European countries the health care providers strenuously objected to presumed consent policies. Whether or not the policies are actually followed is unknown. This is important information, as the empirical success of presumed consent is controversial. The increase in kidney procurement in France was modest, and Austria's large increase in organ procurement occurred prior to the passage of its presumed consent law (postpassage figures have been almost flat). Fourth, in America, critics fear that presumed consent may negatively affect the public's desire to donate and undermine confidence in the procurement system. Interestingly, at least ten states allow organ procurement in medical examiner cases in which the family cannot be found and no prior objection to donation is known, and more states have presumed consent laws for corneal donation in coroner's cases. Further data regarding the ways in which these policies have been implemented and the public's response, however, are needed.

One problem with all of the above proposals is that they assume the pool of possible organ donors is roughly 20,000 to 30,000 per year. This number is based on two studies conducted in the mid-1970s. A study by the Centers for Disease Control and Prevention* in 1975 estimated that there were 55 to 116 kidney donors per million annually in the United States, while a concurrent study conducted by the Northwest Kidney Center in Seattle estimated 90 to 110 kidney donors per million annually. Two recent studies have downsized these estimates. It is now estimated that the total U.S. annual donor pool is between 6,900 to 14,000 potential donors per year. Given the number of persons on the transplantation waiting lists and the growing demand for transplants, it is likely that regardless of how successful a policy might be in increasing the rate of procurement, a shortage would soon ensue. Thus, new methods of increasing the donor pool have gained attention.

Prior to 1972, living donors were the most common source of donor kidneys for patients with end-stage renal disease. However, as dialysis became more widely available, and with the acceptance of brain death criteria, the use of living donors diminished. Currently, only one third of all transplanted kidneys in the United States still come from living donors. Many transplant programs have become reluctant to encourage living donation because improved immunosuppression techniques have greatly decreased rates of rejection with cadaver grafts. This has led some to question the risk/benefit ratio of potential harm to the donor versus benefit for the recipient. The urgency for finding a living kidney donor has also diminished since dialysis became universally available in 1972. The recent advent of split-liver and single-lung transplants, however, has led to an increased interest in living related donors. Ethical questions regarding the ability of parents to consent for their critically ill children and more data regarding the risks/benefits of these procedures will need to be resolved if these procedures are to become commonplace.

Nonrelated living donors are not an accepted practice in the United States. The general rules that currently govern the selection of living donors are: the donor must be a recipient's close blood relative; the donor may donate only a paired organ; the donor must be in excellent health. In the last few years, this consensus has come under attack; parents have donated parts of their liver, and authors have called for an expansion of nonrelated living donors. However, unrelated donation is unlikely to make much of an impact on the organ shortage, given the transplant community's distrust and suspicion regarding the donors' motivations and mental health. It should be noted, however, that there is little empirical evidence for these opinions and that some believe that nonrelated donors are subject to less coercion and evidence greater altruism than related donors.

Although procuring organs from anencephalic infants dates back to the early 1960s, the idea received national attention in the mid-1980s when transplant surgeons in Loma Linda began to seriously examine the ethical and practical feasibility of procuring organs from anencephalic infants. Since over 2,000 anencephalic infants are born annually in the United States (although most are stillborn), it was hoped that utilization of their organs would significantly decrease the organ shortage in infants. Three strategies have been suggested. The first strategy, redefining anencephalic infants as dead, was widely criticized as either requiring a radical change in our meaning of death (from whole brain to cortical death) or not understanding the difference between dying and death. The second strategy, permitting procurement from anencephalics as a special exception to the rule against procuring organs prior to death, did not fare much better. The proposal was seen as a utilitarian ploy to kill one living person to benefit another, a practice that traditionally has not met with societal approval. Moreover, critics pointed out that if society is willing to allow living people to choose to give up their organs rather than dying from their disease, it should start with competent adults rather than infants. Finally, given that most anencephalic infants die within a few days of birth, some have suggested supporting the infants and waiting for them to be declared dead by neurological criteria. In 1987, Loma Linda developed a model protocol for obtaining organs from anencephalic infants. The Loma Linda protocol stipulated: maintenance of the infant on a ventilator, medication to prevent distress, consistent comfort care, monitoring of brain stem activity, and organ removal following establishment of brain death. The protocol, however, was unsuccessful in procuring solid organs from anencephalic infants, and a moratorium on the program was called in 1988, pending further consideration of the complex ethical, biomedical, and psychological questions raised.

Many trauma patients are perfect potential donors: young, otherwise healthy individuals who suffer a single catastrophic event. Because these patients die of cardiopulmonary failure, however, there is a prolonged interval between the declaration of death and the process of removing and cooling the organ. During this time, the organs must endure warm ischemia, typically leading to such damage that the organs are not transplantable. (Individuals who are declared dead using neurological criteria do not have this problem, as their heart is kept beating until the time of procurement.) To salvage these organs in situ, organ preservation immediately following uncontrolled cardiopulmonary arrest is being used on an experimental basis. After failing resuscitation, a patient is declared dead, and catheters are inserted in the femoral artery and peritoneal cavity. A cold perfusant is then introduced that preserves the organs for up to five hours. These individuals are referred to as non–heart beating cadaver donors. The most significant problem is that the infusion must be accomplished quickly after the declaration of death to avoid warm ischemia. Unfortunately, obtaining family consent within this time frame is difficult, and thus one institution has proceeded with cold perfusion prior to obtaining family consent. This process has generated considerable controversy, as discussants debate whether the process is a minimal intervention designed to allow families the opportunity to donate or if it is unduly disrespectful to perform invasive procedures on a dead body without the deceased's or his family's consent. An alternative measure for procuring organs from non–heart beating organ donors allows the family and patients the option to donate organs after having decided to forgo life-sustaining treatment.

The use of non–heart beating organ donors raises numerous ethical questions, such as whether patients are actually dead when their organs are procured; whether the protocol interferes with the provision of optimal care to the dying patient or crosses the line from allowing death to take place to intentionally hastening death to procure organs; and whether there are potential conflicts of interest that may arise between the health care team and the dying patient when innovative protocols to procure organs are developed at major transplant centers. While there is a great deal of interest in this technique (and in fact a number of organ procurement organizations have developed protocols), a great public debate and consensus is needed prior to a widespread attempt to procure organs from non–heart beating cadaver donors.

Finally, some have suggested that the solution to the shortage of transplantable human organs is to use animal organs. Advances in genetics and immunosuppression raise the hope that xenograft transplantation will be possible in the near future. Recent attempts involving a baboon liver transplant at the University of Pittsburgh and a pig liver at the University of California at Los Angeles have fueled these hopes. In addition to the technological hurdles that remain before xenograft transplantation is a reality are a number of thorny ethical, psychosocial, and public policy problems that are likely to confront any effort to promote the use of animals for transplantation. Many feel that it is immoral to raise primates for the sole purpose of killing them for human benefit. Others are concerned that this attempt, like many of the others mentioned above, is evidence of our irrational reluctance to confront our mortality. In these critics' eyes, our attention and resources should be shifted from high-tech interventions that benefit a few at a great cost to interventions that could improve the lives of a greater number of individuals.

REFERENCES: American Medical Association. 1994. "Strategies for Cadaveric Organ Procurement." *Journal of the American Medical Association* 272: 809–12; Barnett, A. H., and Kaserman, D. L. 1993. "The Shortage of Organs for Transplantation." *Issues in Law and Medicine* 9: 117–37; Caplan, A. L., et al. 1993. "Financial Compensation for Cadaver Organ Donation." *Transplantation Proceedings* 25: 2740–42; Diaz, J. H. 1993. "The Anencephalic Organ Donor." *Critical Care Medicine* 21: 1781–86; Dunning, J. J., et al. 1994. "The Rationale for Xenotransplantation as a Solution to the Donor Organ Shortage." *Pathologie Biologie* 42: 231–35; Evans, R. W., et al. 1992. "The Potential Supply of Organ Donors." *Journal of the American Medical Association* 267: 239–46; Prottas, J. L. 1983. "Encouraging Altruism: Public Attitudes and the Marketing of Organ Donation." *Milbank Memorial Fund Quarterly* 6: 278–305; Spital, A. L. 1992. "Unrelated Living Donors: Should They Be Used?" *Transplantation Proceedings* 24: 2215–17; Virig, B. A., and Caplan, A. L. 1993. "Required Request: What Difference Has It Made?" *Transplantation Proceedings* 24: 2155–58; Younger, S. J., and Arnold, R. M. 1993. "Ethical, Psychosocial, and Public Policy Implications of Procuring Organs from Non-Heart-Beating Cadaver Donors." *Journal of the American Medical Association* 289: 2669–74.

LAURA A. SIMINOFF, ROBERT M. ARNOLD, and MOLLY SEAR

ORGAN TRANSPLANTATION

Organ transplantation is the surgical replacement of a nonfunctioning organ with a functioning one. Human organ transplantation has been in existence since the 1950s. The first attempts to transplant organs involved kidneys from living donors using close relatives, as no reliable methods existed to suppress rejection and no techniques existed that would allow preservation of organs outside the body for any appreciable time. These technical difficulties in procurement, as well as problems with surgical techniques and rejection of the donor organ by the transplant recipient, limited the feasibility of transplantation in the early years. Transplantation also raised many previously unresolved legal, ethical, and religious questions regarding what constituted mutilation of the body, the definition of death, and who "owned" the deceased's organs and who could donate them.

During the past 40 years, great progress has been made in overcoming the scientific barriers to transplantation. Of critical importance has been the development of immunosuppressant drugs, enabling wider use of cadaver organs. Transplants are now commonly performed with kidneys, livers, hearts, and lungs and are being extended to other digestive system organs. Success rates for renal transplantation are above 90 percent at one year and 70 percent for livers at three years. The average recipient lives for eight years with the transplanted organ, and available data suggest that transplantation improves the quality of life of the majority of kidney and liver transplant recipients. The result of these successes is that transplantation has become the treatment of choice for many previously terminal conditions and is currently being offered to an increasing number of patients.

The last 40 years also have seen the apparent resolution of many of the societal questions raised by organ procurement and transplantation. The move toward a legal definition of brain death* and the development of preservation solutions have meant that unlike in the 1950s most donor organs are from cadaver sources. Moreover, a consensus developed that voluntary choice and altruism should constitute the legal and ethical foundations of organ procurement in the United States. These values are the foundation of the Uniform Anatomical Gift Act,* the federal legislation governing organ donation.

Insufficient numbers of people agree to donate, however, and there remains a serious shortage of transplantable organs and tissues. Between 1988 and 1991, the number of candidates on the waiting list in the United States grew 55 percent, and every month 20,000 new patients are added. As of September 1993, there were 24,382 persons waiting for a kidney, 2,873 waiting for a heart, and 2,775 listed as waiting for a liver transplant. The shortage of organs for newborns and children is even more severe. In 1990, nearly 400 children born with congenital heart defects died before a donor heart was found for them. It has been estimated that about one third of all transplant patients will die before a transplantable organ can be found. In addition, between 2,500 and 4,000 patients are waiting for corneal transplants during any given month, while tens of thousands await other types of transplants (e.g., bone, skin, heart valves, and other tissues). There is every indication that the existing shortages will become more acute. Improvements in the performance of transplants and their subsequent medical management have expanded the number of diseases for which transplantation is viewed as an appropriate therapy. The standards for candidacy have also grown less stringent, increasing the gap between supply and demand. Organ scarcity has become the primary factor limiting the future growth of organ transplantation.

Proposals to increase the number of procured organs are being considered. Three general strategies have been suggested: (1) improving the current system while maintaining the emphasis on voluntary choice and altruism, (2) giving up voluntary choice and altruism and developing a new system based on self-interest or the societal good, and (3) developing new sources of transplantable organs. Most of these proposals raise thorny ethical questions, and even if these questions could be resolved, the lack of empirical data regarding many of the key assumptions underlying these programs makes it difficult, if not impossible, to determine if implementing any of the proposals to increase the number of transplantable organs would actually do so.

REFERENCES: Anonymous. 1990. "Uniform Anatomical Gift Act." *Uniform Law Annotated* 8A (Supp. 2):2–29; Caplan, A., et al. 1991. "Increasing Organ and Tissue Donation." In *Proceedings of the Surgeon General's Workshop on Increasing Organ Donation.* Washington, D.C.: Health and Human Services; Chaffin, J. S., et al. 1992. "Donor Organ Availability." *Journal of the Oklahoma State Medical Association* 85: 111–14; Eyskens, E. 1994. "Ethics in Actual Surgery: Ethics and Organ Transplantation." *Acta Chirirgica Belgica* 94: 185–88; Fox, R. C., and Swazey, J. P. 1992. *Spare Parts.* New York: Oxford University Press; Land, W., and Dossetor, J. B., eds. 1991. *Organ Replacement Therapy: Ethics, Justice, Commerce.* New York: Springer-Verlag; Mathieu, Deborah, ed. 1988. *Organ Substitution Technology: Ethical, Legal and Public Policy Issues.* Boulder: Westview Press; Molzahn, A. E. 1991. "Quality of Life After Organ Transplantation." *Journal of Advanced Nursing* 16: 1042–47.

LAURA A. SIMINOFF, ROBERT M. ARNOLD, and MOLLY SEAR

ORPHAN DRUG ACT

The U.S. Congress in 1983 enacted the Orphan Drug Act, Public Law 97–414, to stimulate the development of drugs for the treatment of rare diseases. The act empowers the U.S. Food and Drug Administration* (FDA) to designate a product as an "orphan drug" by virtue of its efficacy against a "rare disease or condition," defined as one affecting fewer than 200,000 individuals in the United States or, if there are more victims, one for which the sponsor cannot realistically anticipate U.S. sales sufficient to recover its costs. The Orphan Drug Act provides incentives for the development of orphan drugs by providing a seven-year period of market exclusivity, after FDA approval, to the first developer of the drug. That the act has spurred innovation, including the certification for marketing by 1989 of nine new orphan biopharmaceuticals, is evidenced by a 1990 dispute between Genentech and Eli Lilly (*Eli Lilly v. Genentech**) over an orphan drug designation pertaining to recombinant human growth hormone. There have been concerns expressed, however, that companies may abuse the act by seeking orphan drug status for drugs that are quite valuable commercially, for example, because a given drug may bring a high price or may be used in treatment of other conditions. In an attempt to address these concerns, Congress amended the act in 1988 to allow a second company that believes that the drug may be profitable, or that developed the drug independently, to share the seven-year period of market exclusivity with the first company. Legislation providing further amendments, directed to perceived "windfall profits" reaped from "unprofitable" orphan drugs, was introduced in Congress on March 24, 1994 (S. 1981 and H.R. 4160). The new legislation will change the period of market exclusivity for newly designated orphan drugs to four years, rather than seven, but will be granted three subsequent years if they continue to show limited commercial potential.

REFERENCES: "Do We Pay Too Much for Prescriptions?" 1993. *Consumer Reports* 58: 668–674; *Genentech, Inc. v. R. Bowen,* 676 F. Supp. 301 (D.D.C. 1987); "Legislation: Orphan Drug Act Amendments Are Introduced in Senate and House." 1994. *BNA's Patent, Trademark & Copyright Journal News & Comment* 47: 482; *Orphan Drug Amendments of 1988,* Public Law 100–290 (H.R. No 100–473); Thompson, Dick. 1992. "Your Money or Their Lives." *Time* 140: 66.

STEPHEN A. BENT

P

PATENTS AND BIOTECHNOLOGY

Patents are a type of property created and recognized under the laws of almost every nation. Patents are intended to promote the progress of science by creating a trade-off; in exchange for publicly disclosing the details of an invention, the inventor may exclude others from making, using, or selling that invention for a period of time. Public disclosure enables other people to build upon an inventor's achievements, while the patent gives the patent owner the opportunity to financially gain through licensing the invention to others.

The fate of the American biotechnology industry is linked to the American patent system. Patents protect the time and money invested in the discovery of new and useful inventions. Furthermore, companies owning patents to critical technologies are in a position to receive lucrative royalties from anyone that practices the patented technology. Biotechnology companies recognize the value of patents. For example, Hoffman–La Roche paid Cetus Corporation $300 million for all patent rights to Taq, a thermostable polymerase used to amplify sequences of nucleotides in P.C.R (Dickson, 1994).

Many initially opposed biotechnology patents, arguing that no living organisms should be patentable. In 1980, however, the U.S. Supreme Court recognized that proteins and nucleic acids were not fundamentally different from other building blocks used to make patentable subject matter. Thus, the Court held that genetically engineered bacteria were patentable as articles of manufacture (*Diamond v. Chakrabarty,** 447 U.S. 303 [1980]). Later in 1980, the Patent and Trademark Office (PTO) granted the first patent on a technique for the production of recombinant DNA to Drs. Cohen and Boyer. By May 1988, the Patent and Trademark Office had received 5,977 biotechnology-related patent applications, and more than 8,000 by December 1989 (Fleising and Smart, 1993).

In order to obtain a patent in the United States, the applicant must show that the invention meets the following three requirements: (1) utility, (2) novelty, and (3) nonobviousness. To satisfy the *utility* requirement, an applicant must disclose a "useful process, machine, manufacturer, or composition of matter, or any new and useful improvement thereof" (Title 35 United States Code § 101). In *Brenner v. Mason,* 383 U.S. 519 (1966), the U.S. Supreme Court held that the necessary degree of utility is "substantial utility representing specific benefit in currently available form." In the biotechnology context, the PTO interpreted this to mean that applicants must demonstrate the utility of a new drug or other biotechnical product through data from human clinical trials. This created what PTO Commissioner Bruce Lehman described as a "Catch-22" situation. Companies needed large capital investment in order to conduct trials to support the patent applications, but investors were unwilling to provide such capital without the assurance that the inventions would be patentable. The PTO recently eased its requirement in hopes of addressing this problem. Now companies need only show "potential usefulness" of new biotechnology products by submitting data from less expensive animal or lab studies indicating a scientifically plausible use (Pear, 1994).

The American patent system is the only one in the world that bases patent ownership on who "first invented" the item, not who "first filed" the patent application. This is the essence of the *novelty* requirement. In order to prove novelty, an applicant must prove (1) the invention is new (not previously discovered) and (2) that the applicant is the inventor (Title 35 United States Code § 102). When more than one person seeks to patent the same subject matter, the PTO determines priority based upon who first conceived the idea and then diligently worked to reduce the idea to practice. This is especially difficult in the context of biotechnology. How does one conceive of an invention involving DNA? This issue was addressed in the recent case of *Fiers v. Revel v. Sugano,* 984 F.2d 1164 (Fed. Cir. 1993). The court held that with technology available at the time of the patent application, conception of DNA required isolation and sequencing. Technological advancements may force the court to readdress this question since there may be no "flash of conception" in the mind of a technician conducting modern high-speed sequencing.

No patent shall be granted unless the invention is *nonobvious* to one of ordinary skill in the art, at the time of invention (Title 35 United States Code § 103). In a recent decision, *In re Bell,* 991 F.2d 781 (Fed. Cir. 1993), a court of appeals addressed the requirement of nonobviousness in a dispute regarding a biotechnology patent application. A patent examiner had rejected patent claims for the nucleic acid sequence coding for a certain protein on grounds that the nucleic acid sequence would be obvious in light of prior art describing the amino acid sequence of the protein. The court reversed the patent examiner's rejection and held that a known amino acid sequence for a protein did not necessarily make the nucleotide sequence obvious because different nucleotide triplets code for the same amino acid, and thus a vast number of nucleotide sequences might code for a specific protein.

Do patents really promote the progress of science? Many scientists argue that the patentability of basic research has a detrimental effect on science. The promise of potentially large financial rewards may tempt scientists to seek patents before the results of the experiments are clear. Researchers may also be less willing to communicate and cooperate with competitive colleagues for fear of losing eventual patent rights (Milstein, 1993). Furthermore, scientific progress is moving so quickly that the patent system cannot keep up; the application process is too slow and prolongs the time in which new inventions are kept secret. The Patent and Trademark Office has been overwhelmed with applications relating to recently discovered DNA sequences. Thus, many patent applications do not disclose the identity of the protein for which the DNA codes (McCoy, 1992).

Native human DNA sequences are a product of nature and therefore unpatentable under American and most western European patent law. However, cDNAs (complementary DNAs), nucleic acid sequences that are complementary to messenger RNAs from expressed genes, do not occur naturally and are patentable articles of manufacture (Kevles and Hood, 1992). Once researchers have determined the cDNA sequence, they have an advantage over other researchers working on the same gene. It is common practice to file patent applications at the earliest possible moment in order to preserve a certain filing date. If the patent claims are skillfully worded, additional information (such as the protein the gene codes for and its function) might be added later while still preserving the original filing date priority over competitors. In this way, rights to lucrative proteins might be protected from competition by filing an application before the actual use of the protein is known. This has created a race to file patent claims in order to preclude others from trespassing on one's staked out intellectual property. However, by limiting access to the subject matter, a patent holder might inhibit the progress of science and the useful arts by keeping science's sharpest minds from working on the specific subject matter (Eisenberg, 1992).

REFERENCES: *Brenner v. Mason,* 383 U.S. 519, 534–535 (1966); *Diamond v. Chakrabarty,* 447 U.S. 303 (1980); Dickson, D. 1994. "Patent on PCR Enzymes May Reignite Old Controversy." *Nature* 372: 212; Eisenberg, Rebecca S. 1992. "Patent Rights and the Human Genome Project." In *Gene Mapping: Using Law and Ethics as Guides,* ed. George J. Annas and Sherman Elias. New York: Oxford University Press, 230–243; *Fiers v. Revel v. Sugano,* 984 F.2d 1164, 25 U.S.P.Q.2d 1601 (Fed. Cir. 1993); Fleising, U., and Smart, A. 1993. "The Development of Property Rights in Biotechnology." *Culture, Medicine and Psychiatry* 17: 43–57; *Hybritech, Inc. v. Monoclonal Antibodies, Inc.,* 802 F.2d 1367 (Fed. Cir. 1986), *cert. denied,* 480 U.S. 947 (1987); *In re Bell,* 991 F.2d 781, 26 U.S.P.Q.2d 1529 (Fed. Cir. 1993); Kevles, Daniel J., and Hood, Leroy. 1992. "Reflections." In *The Code of Codes.* Cambridge, MA: Harvard University Press, 308–335; McCoy, T. 1992. "Biomedical Process Patents: Should They Be Restricted by Ethical Limitations?" *J. Legal Medicine* 13: 501–519; Milstein, C. 1993. "Patents on Scientific Discoveries Are Unfair and Potentially Dangerous." *The Scientist* (November 1): 11; Pear, R. 1994. "U.S. Easing Rules on Biotech Patents: Clinical Trials of Drugs on

Humans Will No Longer Be Required.'' *New York Times,* December 22, B11; Title 35 United States Code.

RICHARD M. CHAPMAN

PATENT TERM EXTENSION AND "EXPERIMENTAL USE"

The Drug Price Competition and Patent Term Restoration Act of 1984 ("the Act"), Public Law 98–417, developed from a legislative attempt to balance competing interests of proprietary drug houses and generic drug manufacturers in the United States. A conflict between these interests was highlighted in *Roche Products, Inc. v. Bolar Pharmaceutical Co.,* 733 F.2d 858 (Fed. Cir.), *cert. denied,* 496 U.S. 856 (1984), where the U.S. Court of Appeals for the Federal Circuit held that regulatory testing of a patented drug by Bolar, a generic manufacturer, was not insulated from infringement liability as an "experimental use" of the drug Dalmane, the subject of a Roche-owned patent that was soon to expire. To negate the impact of the *Roche* ruling, the Act cedes to an owner of a drug patent as many as 5 years in restored patent term, with a maximum extended term of 14 years, to compensate for marketing time lost during Food and Drug Administration* (FDA) review of a New Drug Application for that drug. In return, generic manufacturers are allowed to undertake activities needed to secure an Abbreviated New Drug Application for compounds covered by another's patent, without risk of patent infringement liability. The Act thus addresses what was deemed a de facto penalty, incurred by patent owners seeking first-time regulatory approval for a patented drug, while accelerating the entry of generic equivalents upon expiration of patent coverage.

Although patent term extension is likely to prove valuable for developers of biopharmaceuticals, the Act relies on a convoluted, overly complex scheme to determine an extension of patent term, a flaw manifest in *Hoechst AG v. Quigg.* In that case the federal circuit granted a patent extension of 6.8 years, finding that none of the "limitations" of the Act covered the patented drug but acknowledging that the result probably was a "windfall" for the patent owner. Moreover, the narrow sweep of the Act leaves unresolved whether there is any practical scope to the so-called experimental use patent infringement defense, recognized in principle by U.S. jurisprudence, such that a commercial enterprise may be free to use a patented invention to create new technology.

REFERENCES: *Hoechst AG v. Quigg,* 917 F.2d 522 (1990); Lourie, Alan. 1986. "Patent Term Restoration—The First Two Years." *Journal of the Patent & Trademark Society* 68: 538–60; Wegner, Harold C. 1992. *Patent Law in Biotechnology, Chemicals & Pharmaceuticals,* §§ 355–356. New York: Stockton Press.

STEPHEN A. BENT

PAYTON V. ABBOTT LABS

Payton was a class action suit brought by approximately 4,000 women exposed to the drug diethylstilbestrol (DES). These women sued because their mothers ingested DES while pregnant and transmitted the drug to them in utero. As a result, they are at increased risk for a rare type of genital cancer as well as abnormalities of the reproductive organs. The defendants were pharmaceutical companies, including Abbott, Eli Lilly, Merck, Rexall, Squibb and Sons, and Upjohn, all of which manufactured and marketed DES as a miscarriage preventative between 1945 and 1976. The plaintiffs contended that the defendants were negligent in marketing DES and that they should be compensated for the higher risk of cancer and other abnormalities they incurred. To confuse the situation even more, most of the plaintiffs were unable to identify the specific manufacturer of the DES ingested by their mothers.

Based on precedents treating in utero injury resulting from ingestion of a drug by the mother, the court held that the plaintiffs could maintain a cause of action. The *Payton* court rejected the defendants' arguments that recovery should be denied because of the difficulty of proving causation and because of the risk of fictitious claims. The difficulties of proof or the possibility of false claims could not bar action by plaintiffs with ethically demonstrable injuries.

Although *Payton* was rendered in response to a certified question by the federal court as to whether there is a cause of action in Massachusetts for those injured by a drug prior to birth, the precedental force was expected to be substantial. According to Seksay (1983, 266), the prenatal injury holding in *Payton* results in a potential increase in liability for anyone who negligently supplies a pregnant woman with drugs or medication.

REFERENCES: *Payton v. Abbott Labs,* 83 F.R.D. 382, 386 (D. Mass. 1981); Seksay, E. H. 1983. ''Tort Law—Begetting a Cause of Action for Those Injured by a Drug Prior to Birth.'' *Suffolk University Law Review* 17: 257–268.

See also **PRENATAL INJURY TORTS.**

ROBERT H. BLANK

PERSISTENT VEGETATIVE STATE

The persistent vegetative state is a form of neurological disability characterized by eyes open unresponsiveness. It is a direct result of advances in intensive care in which patients who sustained severe brain injury are resuscitated medically but not neurologically. The vegetative state most commonly results from head trauma and anoxic brain injury due to cardiac arrest. Patients who sustain severe brain injury either awaken, die within a few days, or pass through an initial phase of deep coma. If a comatose patient survives longer than two to three weeks, he may lighten and begin to open his eyes and look randomly around the room. If the patient remains unresponsive, this phase is termed the *vegetative state.* Lay and medical professionals commonly confuse persistent coma with the vegetative state. Coma is universally defined as eyes closed unresponsiveness, whereas the vegetative state is defined as eyes open unresponsiveness.

The term *persistent vegetative state* was first coined by Drs. B. Jennett and F. Plum to define a permanent state of sleep and wake cycles without cognition.

Another name for the vegetative state is *neocortical death,* or death of structures above the brain stem and thalamus. The American Academy of Neurology (1989) defines the persistent vegetative state as a

form of eyes open permanent unconsciousness in which the patient has periods of wakefulness and physiologic sleep wake cycles, but at no time is the patient aware of himself or the environment. Neurologically, being awake, but unaware is the result of a functioning brainstem, and the total loss of cerebral cortical functioning.

It is commonly assumed that patients in a vegetative state are deeply comatose with their eyes closed, but the contrary is the rule. Patients in a vegetative state usually have their eyes open, may smile or frown, and may look about the room in roving or random fashion. Such individuals will grimace to pain, may startle when awakened, may make unrecognizable sounds, may open and close their eyes spontaneously, and may even move their limbs in response to pain. They will not track with their eyes to a bright light and may blink their eyes to a clap or bell but do not open eyes to command or follow any commands.

The vegetative state is caused by widespread neuronal injury and cell loss in the cerebral cortex, hippocampus, and thalamus, with relative sparing of the brain stem. In some cases, the cerebral cortex may be relatively intact, as was the case with Karen Ann Quinlan (see *In re Quinlan**). Because of persistent brain stem function, cardiac regulation and respiratory function are preserved. Because of preservation of the brain stem, vegetative patients do not meet the criteria for brain death,* which requires death of the cerebral cortex and brain stem. Such individuals may survive for years with basic nursing care including hygiene, prevention and treatment of bed sores, hydration, nutrition, and antibiotics. A ventilator is usually not necessary for life support, as illustrated by the cases of Karen Ann Quinlan and Nancy Cruzan (see *Cruzan v. Director, Missouri Department of Health**).

The vegetative state is defined as persistent when it has occurred for longer than one to three months. The President's Commission for the Study of Ethical Problems in its 1983 report titled *Foregoing Life Sustaining Treatment* stated that "absence of all responsiveness, vocalization, or purposive action one month after trauma makes lack of recovery virtually certain." It was commonly believed at the time of the President's Commission report that coma or the vegetative state for longer than one month precluded recovery. However, recent data from the Traumatic Coma Databank is changing this misperception. Of 140 patients who were in a vegetative state at one month after head trauma, 42 percent recovered consciousness, and 10 percent recovered independent function by one year. This has been confirmed in another study by Sazbone et al. (1990) who found that 54 percent of 134 patients in a persistent vegetative state due to head trauma awakened. Forty-nine percent were able to work in sheltered workshops, and 11 percent were able to return to normal work. Recovery may be protracted and slow, and it is difficult to reliably predict early in coma who will recover and who will not. Further, after cardiac arrest, recovery past one to three months is extremely rare. However, after head trauma, there is growing consensus that it is difficult to make a reliable diagnosis of irreversibility and persistent vegetative state before six months. Despite perceptions to the contrary, the persistent vegetative state is a rare condition.

The American Academy of Neurology has taken a similar position. Problematically, it is often difficult to confirm the diagnosis of persistent coma or the vegetative state. No laboratory test exists that definitely confirms the diagnosis. Most clinicians agree that only continued and prolonged observation and repetitive examination of the patient will reliably determine if a patient is truly in a persistent vegetative state. Recent studies indicate that the diagnosis of the vegetative state is frequently incorrect. Childs et al. (1993) reported that 37 percent of patients transferred to a rehabilitation facility with a diagnosis of coma or vegetative state were incorrectly diagnosed. Many of these patients were able to move to command, to have purposeful eye movements, to mouth or blink yes or no, and in some cases, to smile at jokes. These errors may result from confusion among physicians as to what constitutes the diagnosis of persistent vegetative state and the failure to examine patients for long durations and at repeated intervals.

The care of individuals in the persistent vegetative state has been the subject of intense legal debate. In the Clarence Herbert case (*Barber v. Superior Court*, 1983), a California appellate court ruled that withdrawal of hydration and nutrition from a comatose patient (who in reality was in a coma for only a few days) was acceptable and defined proportional treatment as that which ''has a reasonable chance of providing benefits to the patient.'' The court emphasized the benefit of treatment versus the burden. In the *Brophy* case, the Supreme Court of the Commonwealth of Massachusetts ruled that a feeding tube could be removed from a firefighter who was in a persistent vegetative state after a ruptured cerebral aneurysm. The court ruled that a patient's constitutional right to refuse treatment included the refusal of hydration and nutrition. In 1990, in the most important decision to date, the U.S. Supreme Court ruled in the case of Nancy Cruzan, a young woman who was in a persistent vegetative state for several years after a motor vehicle accident. The family wished to have a gastrostomy tube removed and feeding discontinued on the grounds that she did not wish to live in a persistent vegetative state. The state of Missouri refused to withhold feedings on the grounds that in the absence of a specific consent of the patient, a guardian could not withhold treatment. The U.S. Supreme Court upheld the state court ruling but asserted that patients have the right to refuse all means of life-sustaining treatment and defined hydration and nutrition as a treatment that could be withheld. However, it deferred to the state the right to protect human life in the absence of definitive advanced directive.

Many argue that the term *vegetative* dehumanizes such severely disabled individuals and implies a state of coma or worse. In reality, we know quite little about the nature of cognition, will, emotions, or dreams in such patients. They clearly have periods of sleep and wakefulness, and as was the case of Karen Ann Quinlan, the cerebral cortex may be functionally and anatomically preserved. Stimulation experiments by the Japanese have resulted in arousal and cognitive recovery in small numbers of patients, but the numbers are too small for concrete conclusions. There is growing research into whether such individuals can process information, and multiple centers have recorded a P300 brain potential, which is a function of arousal or cortical information processing. It is likely that with growing awareness of the potential for long-term recovery in vegetative patients after head trauma, and further research into stimulation of such severely disabled individuals, that old paradigms of the vegetative state may change.

In summary, the vegetative state is a form of neurological disability characterized by eyes open unresponsiveness. It is unique from coma but frequently confused with coma and misdiagnosed. New data, especially in the setting of head trauma, are causing clinicians to reassess the prognosis in the vegetative state.

REFERENCES: American Academy of Neurology. 1989. "Position of the American Academy of Neurology on Certain Aspects of the Care and Management of the Persistent Vegetative State." *Neurology* 39:125–126; *Barber v. Superior Court.* 1983. 195 Cal. Rpt. 484; Childs, N. L., et al. 1993. "Accuracy of Diagnosis of Persistent Vegetative State." *Neurology* 43:1465–1467; Council on Scientific Affairs and Council on Ethical and Judicial Affairs. 1990. "Persistent Vegetative State and the Decision to Withdraw or Withhold Life Support." *JAMA* 263:426–430; DeGiorgio, C. M., et al. 1993. "Predictive Value of P300 Event-Related Potentials Compared with EEG and Somatosensory Evoked Potentials in Non-traumatic Coma." *Acta Neurologica Scandinavica* 87:423–427; Jennett, B., and Plum, F. 1972. "Persistent Vegetative State After Brain Damage. A Syndrome in Search of a Name." *Lancet* 1:734–737; Levin, H. S., et al. 1991. "Vegetative State After Closed Head Injury: Traumatic Coma Data Bank Report." *Archives of Neurology* 48:580–585; Marosi, M., et al. 1993. "Event Related Potentials in Vegetative State." *Lancet* 341:1473; The Multi-Society Task Force on PVS, American Academy of Neurology. 1994. "Medical Aspects of the Persistent Vegetative State. (First of Two Parts)." *New England Journal of Medicine* 330:1499–1508; *Patricia Brophy v. New England Sinai Hosp., Inc.* 1986. 398 Mass. 417 NE 2d 626; Sazbone, et al. 1990. "Outcome in 134 Patients with Prolonged Posttraumatic Unawareness. Part 1. Parameters Determining Late Recovery of Consciousness." *Journal of Neurosurgery* 72:75–80; Shewmon, D. A., and DeGiorgio, C. M. 1989. "Early Prognosis in Anoxic Coma." *Neurologic Clinics* 7:823–843.

CHRISTOPHER M. DeGIORGIO

PLANNED PARENTHOOD V. CASEY

In April 1988, several Pennsylvania abortion providers filed suit in the U.S. District Court for the Eastern District of Pennsylvania against 1988 amendments to the Pennsylvania Abortion Control Act, arguing that they violated a woman's right to choose abortion recognized in *Roe v. Wade,* 410 U.S. 113 (1973), and reaffirmed in *Thornburgh v. American College of Obstetricians & Gynecologists,* 476 U.S. 747 (1986) (see *Roe v. Wade**). Amended again in 1989, the measures require all women seeking abortions to delay at least 24 hours after receiving mandated information from a physician, including the probable gestational age of the fetus and its development, the availability of state-funded social service programs, a list of health care facilities that can help ensure a healthy birth, and a statement that the putative father may be liable for child support; a married woman must notify her husband of her abortion choice except in very limited circumstances; a young woman must obtain the consent of a parent or obtain judicial approval prior to an abortion; and abortion providers must file detailed reports with the state. The health care providers also alleged that the law's definition of "medical emergency," which allowed for the requirements to be waived, was unconstitutionally narrow.

In August 1990, the district court issued a permanent injunction against virtually all of the contested provisions, finding that they violated a woman's fundamental right to choose abortion. On appeal, in October 1991, the U.S. Court of Appeals for the Third Circuit reversed the district court's ruling. Upholding all of the challenged abortion restrictions except husband notification, the court found that the right to choose abortion was no longer a fundamental constitutional right. Citing *Webster v. Reproductive Health Services** and *Hodgson v. Minnesota,** the appeals court held that the U.S. Supreme Court had already abandoned the key holdings of *Roe v. Wade* in those decisions. The court found that unless a law places "an absolute obstacle" or "severe limitation" on a woman's right to make reproductive decisions, it would be upheld as constitutional. The court used this analysis, instead of *Roe*'s "strict scrutiny" test, even though an "undue burden" approach had, at that time, only been adopted by Justice Sandra Day O'Connor in dissenting opinions in two abortion cases.

Appealing to the U.S. Supreme Court, plaintiffs argued that the provisions at issue should be struck down and *Roe v. Wade* reaffirmed. Recognizing that a majority of the Court in *Webster v. Reproductive Health Services** indicated a willingness to overrule *Roe* outright, many believed that *Planned Parenthood v. Casey* would be the vehicle to undo that landmark 1973 decision. In a fractured decision issued on June 29, 1992, a majority of the Supreme Court upheld all of the challenged measures, except the husband notification requirement and a related reporting mandate. Nonetheless, the opinion jointly authored by Justices O'Connor, Souter, and Kennedy, joined in part by Justices Blackmun and Stevens, reaffirmed what it deemed the central and core holding of *Roe:* (1) before fetal viability, a woman's decision to terminate her pregnancy is a liberty interest protected against undue state interference by the due process clause of the Fourteenth Amendment; (2) after viability, the state is free to restrict abortions, but exceptions must be made for pregnancies that endanger a woman's life or health; and (3) from the onset of pregnancy, the state has legitimate interests in protecting both the health of the woman and the potential life of the fetus. Throughout the decision, the Court used strong language linking reproductive choices to women's privacy, autonomy, and equality. Reiterating that bans on abortion remain unconstitutional, the opinion likened the right to choose abortion to the right to use contraceptives and characterized a woman's ability to make such basic decisions about when to bear children as "central to personal dignity and autonomy." The Court further commented that "[t]he ability of women to participate equally in the economic and social life of the Nation has been facilitated by their ability to control their reproductive lives.''

At the same time, the joint opinion significantly revised the holding in *Roe,* rejecting the trimester framework and abandoning the ''strict scrutiny'' standard for reviewing the constitutionality of abortion restrictions. Explicitly overruling portions of previous decisions that struck down abortion restrictions mirroring the Pennsylvania measures at issue in this case, the Court adopted a less protective ''undue burden'' standard: States may impose restrictions so long as they do not have the ''purpose or effect of placing a substantial obstacle in the path of a woman seeking an abortion.'' The strict scrutiny standard established for the abortion right in *Roe* had required courts to strike down any effort to interfere with a woman's ability to choose to terminate her pregnancy prior to fetal viability—unless the restriction could be shown to actually promote maternal health. In contrast, the new standard places the initial burden on women to demonstrate ''undue'' harm. Federal courts are thus directed to measure the degree to which each restriction interferes with a woman's ability to exercise her right to choose abortion. In the wake of this decision, however, the U.S. Supreme Court has refused to review challenges to abortion bans and other state laws restricting a woman's right to choose abortion.

REFERENCES: Benshoof, Janet. 1993. ''*Planned Parenthood v. Casey:* The Impact of the New Undue Burden Standard on Reproductive Health Care.'' *Journal of the American Medical Association* 269:2249. Boston Women's Health Book Collective. 1992. *The New Our Bodies Ourselves.* New York: Simon & Schuster; Friedman, Leon et al., eds. 1993. ''The Supreme Court Confronts Abortion.'' In *The Briefs, Argument, and Decision in Planned Parenthood v. Casey.* New York: Farrar, Straus and Giroux.

ANDREA MILLER

PREGNANCY DISCRIMINATION ACT

Title VII of the Civil Rights Act of 1964 included a prohibition against sex discrimination in employment, but this provision was not originally included in the act. An amendment to include sex as a protected class (along with race, religion, and national origin) was proposed by civil rights opponents in an attempt to ensure its defeat. Their tactic backfired, however, and the amended act was passed. The act, however, did not put a swift end to sex discrimination in employment, and the newly created Equal Employment Opportunity Commission (EEOC) did not pursue gender discrimination claims with any force at the outset because it did not view this part of its mission as entirely legitimate.

As the EEOC slowly began to respond to pressure and take seriously its mandate regarding sex discrimination, more subtle means of hindering women in the labor force were adopted by employers. Women were denied employment opportunity and benefits due to pregnancy, rather than simply sex. Pregnancy discrimination took many forms, including forced leave, loss of seniority, lack of medical coverage, and outright dismissal. The EEOC itself issued guidelines against pregnancy discrimination in 1972. But when women brought Title VII suits against pregnancy-based instances of discrimination, courts upheld the exclusionary policies as being gender neutral since the policies distinguished between *some women,* on the one hand, and *nonpregnant women and men,* on the other.

In *Geduldig v. Aiello* (1974), the Supreme Court upheld California's exclusion of pregnancy from disability benefits using this "pregnant and nonpregnant persons" rationale. This case was brought as an equal protection challenge, and the Court ruled that a pregnancy-based classification did not violate equal protection. The Court followed in 1976 with *General Electric v. Gilbert,* the most noted of the pregnancy discrimination cases. In *Gilbert,* a private employer's disability plan that excluded pregnancy, similar to California's policy, was also upheld, this time in the face of a Title VII challenge. The Court reasoned that it was acceptable for the company to exclude pregnancy because it only affected women and that covering it would in effect discriminate against men. It made this argument in spite of the fact that General Electric's plan did cover certain conditions unique to men, such as hair transplants and vasectomies.

Viewing these decisions as directly circumventing the intent of Title VII, a coalition of women's rights, labor, civil rights, and church groups formed to lobby Congress for redress. Named the Campaign to End Discrimination Against Pregnant Workers (CEDAPW), this was the first time that a major coalition of such interests was created, and it proved ultimately successful (Spalter-Roth and Gibbs, 1990). The movement for the Pregnancy Discrimination Act (PDA) was notable in its uniting of usually antagonistic groups; feminists were joined by "pro-life" activists who saw the *Gilbert* decision as antimotherhood.

Despite opposition from industry groups such as the Chamber of Commerce and the National Association of Manufacturers, as well as insurance companies, on October 31, 1978, Congress passed the PDA to amend Title VII to include all exclusions based on pregnancy, childbirth, or related medical conditions as sex discrimination. The impetus for the legislation was the denial of disability coverage to pregnant women; the act, however, applies to all aspects of employment, including hiring, firing, and seniority.

The PDA was first addressed by the Supreme Court in 1983 in *Newport News Shipbuilding and Dry Dock v. EEOC.* Ironically, the Court here used the act to find discrimination against men. An employer's health insurance package that gave pregnancy disability to female employees, but less coverage to the wives of male employees, was found to violate the act because "the protection it affords to married male employees is less comprehensive than the protection it affords to married female employees. . . . The pregnancy limitation in this case violates Title VII by discriminating against male employees."

The Pregnancy Discrimination Act stated that pregnancy could not be treated less favorably than other disabilities but left open the question of whether it could be treated *more* favorably. This debate was addressed by the Supreme Court in 1987 in *California Federal Savings and Loan v. Guerra.* This case concerned mandatory reinstatement of female employees returning from child-bearing leave when such reinstatement was not guaranteed to employees returning from other disabilities. In its decision, the Court essentially held that pregnancy may be treated different from other conditions if "different" equals "better" but not if it equals worse.

More recently, the PDA was invoked by the Supreme Court in *International Union, UAW v. Johnson Controls* to strike down employer "fetal protection" policies that excluded women from working in jobs considered dangerous to a developing fetus. The Court ruled that such policies were in violation of Title VII since they classified women, and restricted their employment opportunities, according to their ability to bear children.

REFERENCES: *California Federal Savings and Loan v. Guerra,* 479 U.S. 272 (1987); Civil Rights Act of 1964—Pregnancy Discrimination, Public Law 95–555; *Geduldig v. Aiello,* 417 U.S. 484 (1974); *General Electric v. Gilbert,* 429 U.S. 125 (1976); *International Union, UAW v. Johnson Controls,* 111 S. Ct. 1196 (1991); *Newport News Shipbuilding and Dry Dock v. EEOC,* 462 U.S. 669 (1983); Spalter-Roth, Roberta M., and Sheila R. Gibbs. 1990. *Improving Employment Opportunities for Women Workers: An Assessment of the Ten Year Economic and Legal Impact of the Pregnancy Discrimination Act of 1978.* Washington, D.C.: Institute for Women's Policy Research.

JULIANNA S. GONEN

PREIMPLANTATION GENETIC DIAGNOSIS

Preimplantation diagnosis involves the screening and diagnosing of genetic disease on the embryo prior to in vitro fertilization (IVF).* Even though the current success rate of IVF is a low 14 percent (Andrews et al., 1994, 82), most researchers remain optimistic regarding this experimental procedure, especially with the identification of certain fatal recessive disorders, such as Tay-Sachs disease. In fact, successful preimplantation genetic diagnosis was recently reported for a Louisiana couple carrying the Tay-Sachs gene. After four disease-free embryos were implanted into the Louisiana woman through IVF, a healthy and disease-free baby girl was delivered. However, many problems exist, and much work still needs to be done to improve the success rate and the cost of both the IVF procedure and the preimplantation genetic testing.

Researchers working in 1 of the 190 clinics nationwide with the IVF procedure will continue to face many problems if laws continue to be passed banning embryo and/or fetal research. According to Blank (1990), there are laws that ban or limit this type of research in 25 states. Additionally, he notes that laws in some of these states could prohibit reproductive-mediating technologies such as embryo donation, cryopreservation of embryos, or manipulation of the embryo. Like the prenatal diagnosis procedure being inextricably related to the ethical problems surrounding the abortion debate, the preimplantation diagnosis procedure suffers from deep ethical concerns as well. Let us examine these controversial debates.

Brigham, Rifkin, and Solt (1993) note that a host of genetic abnormalities can be determined at two weeks gestation and that fetal sex can be determined as early as three days gestation. This early identification leads to the ethical dilemma of embryo discarding due to gender. Will certain embryos be cast aside simply due to their sex? Put another way, will all male embryos be "thrown away" due to the X-linked disorders commonly found in males? Cohen and Hotz (1992) note that although other countries, such as England, Australia, Germany, and Spain, have enacted comprehensive regulatory legislation regarding the new reproductive technology regarding embryos, the United States has not. In fact, we have seen in two recent court cases, *Davis v. Davis** and *York v. Jones,** rejection of specified guidelines that could have served as possible policy directives.

Inevitably, questions regarding the legal and moral status of the embryo continue to be raised. Deep religious and philosophical questions—such as "When does human life begin?"—continue to creep into the discussion, causing monumental contention between the differing groups, with little hope for national or international consensus. Dawson (1993) outlines and describes the three major groups that are in opposition to IVF and human embryo research in general. The first group is referred to as "The Right-to-Life View." This group believes that human life should be protected at every stage, assuming that life begins at conception. The second group, named "The Official Vatican View," is against any attempts at usurping the role of God and, in essence, bans any research whatsoever on embryos or fetuses. Finally, the third group, "The Radical Feminist View," asserts that the new reproductive technology not only threatens women's freedom but also places undue burdens regarding future generations on the backs of women (see also Charo, 1993).

Aside from this complex philosophical debate, very real and pragmatic problems exist within this realm of reproductive technology. One area of concern, already mentioned, is the issue regarding spare embryos. Rowland (1992) notes that stockpiles of embryos continue to accumulate due to government policy ambiguity and inaction. Several researchers have suggested the use of consent forms delineating the disposition of excess embryos. This method could prove to be especially important for embryos that have been frozen. Edwards and Schulman (1993) report that the cryopreservation of embryos creates many opportunities for preimplantation genetic diagnosis because embryos can be frozen before or after typing. However, questions often arise regarding custody of these embryos. For example, a couple recently killed in an airplane crash left the question of the custody of their previously frozen embryos in the hands of the court. Perhaps signed consent forms regarding their embryos would have alleviated this unforeseen dilemma.

Another troubling question is, What should be done with unclaimed embryos? Cohen and Hotz (1992) report that Australia has considered putting all unclaimed frozen embryos up for adoption or donation (see also Dawson, 1993). However, there are no formal U.S. federal guidelines, policies, or federally funded research programs in place regarding this matter.

Other concerns exist regarding preimplantation genetic diagnosis. Notions of creating the perfect human call into question the definition of medical progress. Accusations of eugenics abound. And, with all of this energy oriented toward eliminating genetic disease, there is an underlying parallel thought that people with disabilities should have no place in this world.

Additionally, there are limitations to the preimplantation procedure itself. Although there has been some experimentation with noninvasive and semiinvasive methods, primarily involving a biopsy of the blastocysts, these methods are far from perfected (Andrews et al., 1994, 36). Many researchers conclude that preimplantation genetic diagnosis is still at the very early research stage, as witnessed by the countless problems encountered with the biopsy of gametes and embryos. Amidst the skepticism, however, Handyside et al. (1992) reported in *JAMA* the successful birth of an infant girl to a woman who had undergone preimplantation genetic diagnosis and IVF. The preimplantation diagnosis was for cystic fibrosis, and the baby was born disease free. Thus, with more and more successes like this one and the healthy baby delivered to the Tay-Sachs couple, perhaps future preimplantation diagnosis procedures will be available for diseases that are currently tested prenatally.

REFERENCES: Andrews, Lori B., Jane E. Fullarton, Neil A. Holtzman, and Arno G. Motulsky. 1994. *Assessing Genetic Risks: Implications for Health and Social Policy.* Washington, D.C.: National Academy Press; Blank, Robert H. 1990. *Regulating Reproduction.* New York: Columbia University Press; Brigham, John, Janet Rifkin, and Christine G. Solt. 1993. "Birth Technologies: Prenatal Diagnosis and Abortion Policy." *Politics and the Life Sciences* 12:31–44; Charo, R. Alta. 1993. "Effect of the Human Genome Initiative on Women's Rights and Reproductive Decisions." *Fetal Diagnosis and Therapy* 8 (Supp. 1):148–159; Cohen, Jacques, and Robert Lee Hotz. 1992. "Toward Policies Regarding Assisted Reproductive Technologies." In *Emerging Issues in Biomedical Policy: An Annual Review,* Vol. 1., ed. Robert H. Blank and Andrea L. Bonnicksen. New York: Columbia University Press; *Davis v. Davis.* 1990. C/A No. 180 Court of Appeals of Tenn., Eastern §, Sept. 13, 1990; Dawson, Karen. 1993. "Ethical Aspects of IVF and Human Embryo Research." In *Handbook of In Vitro Fertilization,* ed. Alan Trounson and David K. Gardner. Boca Raton: CRC Press; Edwards, R. G., and J. D. Schulman. 1993. "History of and Opportunities for Preimplantation Diagnosis." In *Preconception and Preimplantation Diagnosis of Human Genetic Disease,* ed. Robert G. Edwards. Cambridge: University Press; Handyside, Alan, John Lesko, Juan Tarin, Robert Winston, and Mark Hughes. 1992. "Birth of a Normal Girl After In Vitro Fertilization and Preimplantation Diagnostic Testing for Cystic Fibrosis." *JAMA* 327(13):

905–990; Rowland, Robyn. 1992. *Living Laboratories: Women and Reproductive Technologies.* Bloomington: Indiana University Press; *York v. Jones.* 1989. 717 F. Supp. 421.

See also **GENETIC DIAGNOSIS; HUMAN GENOME PROJECT; PRENATAL GENETIC DIAGNOSIS; PRESYMPTOMATIC GENETIC DIAGNOSIS.**

PATRICIA GAIL McVEY

PRENATAL DIAGNOSIS

Over the last two decades, there has been a continual expansion of prenatal diagnostic techniques available to women to identify fetal anomalies. Amniocentesis, chorionic villus sampling (CVS), and ultrasound/sonography have become standard clinical procedure. These techniques are now key components of clinical prenatal care and have quickly become the medical standard for certain women at risk for abnormal offspring. Of the over 3.5 million infants delivered in the United States annually, about 0.5 percent will suffer from a chromosomal abnormality, 1 percent will have a dominant or X-linked disease, 0.25 percent will have a recessive disease, and about 9 percent will have an irregularly inherited disorder. Although many genetic diseases are very rare, collectively they represent a significant cause of infant mortality. In addition, between 30 and 50 percent of hospitalized children have diseases of intrinsic origin, meaning birth defects, single-gene, and gene-influenced diseases.

In addition to questions regarding the clinical use of these procedures and the diffusion in some cases before their safety and efficacy has been fully evaluated (Oakley, 1984), prenatal diagnosis also raises questions as to what responsibilities parents have to utilize these technologies that might enhance the health of their potential children or lead to selective abortion of affected fetuses. These new capabilities in human genetic and prenatal intervention also force us to confront the issue of whether a child has a right to be born with a ''sound mind and body'' and, if so, what this requires of the pregnant woman. Finally, if we place so much emphasis on technologies designed to maximize production of ''perfect'' or ''healthy'' children, what impact will this have?

Although these technologies can enhance a woman's reproductive freedom by providing information that helps her decide how to manage the pregnancy, as with all reproductive technologies, anything that can be done voluntarily can also be coerced. Moreover, coercion can take many forms, from subtle ''pressures'' to conform to accepted medical practice and the technological imperative to legally defined duties. For instance, even though a 1984 NIH/FDA (National Institutes of Health/Food and Drug Administration) report found no clear benefit from routine use of ultrasound, at least one third of all pregnant women in the United States undergo that procedure, with some evidence of substantially higher figures.

One dilemma surrounding current use of these techniques is that while they give us the ability to reduce the incidence of genetic disease, they do so primarily by eliminating the affected fetus through selective abortion, not by treating the disease. Future developments in gene therapy might shift emphasis toward treatment, but prenatal diagnosis will continue largely to expand maternal choice only to the extent it allows the pregnant woman to terminate the pregnancy of an affected fetus. Thus, it will continue to be a policy issue congruent with abortion.

The dilemma becomes more immediate, however, if therapy is available in conjunction with the diagnosis, for instance, in the case of Rh incompatibility. In *Grodin v. Grodin* (301 N.W.2d 869 [1983]), a Michigan appellate court recognized the right of a child to sue his or her mother for failure to obtain a pregnancy test. The logic of this ruling implies that a child would also have legal recourse to sue his or her mother for failing to monitor the pregnancy and identify and correct threats to his or her health during gestation. Robertson (1983: 448) points out that "the issue in such a case would be whether the mother's failure to seek a test was negligent in light of the risks that the test posed to her and the fetus and the probability that the test would uncover a correctable defect." Technically, prenatal diagnosis could be directly mandated by state statute with criminal sanctions for women who fail to comply with the law.

Although Robertson (1983, 449) argues that state authorities could justify such a statute on public health grounds, this seems most unlikely given the absence of any national health insurance that would guarantee access of all pregnant women to such technologies. It would be most unfair and illogical to hold a pregnant woman liable for failing to utilize a medical procedure that she was unable to afford. In addition, other observers argue that the state should never intervene to override the decision of the pregnant woman (Gallagher, 1987). Lacking legislation for the use of prenatal intervention, the courts will become increasingly active in this area.

REFERENCES: Baird, P. A., I. M. Yee, and A. D. Sadovnick. 1994. "Population-Based Study of Long-Term Outcomes After Amniocentesis." *Lancet* 344(8930): 1134–1136; D'Alton, Mary E., and Alan H. De Cherney. 1993. "Prenatal Diagnosis." *New England Journal of Medicine* 328(2): 114–120; Gallagher, J. 1987. "Prenatal Invasions and Interventions: What's Wrong with Fetal Rights." *Harvard Women's Law Journal* 10: 9–58; Heckerling, P. S., and M. S. Verp. 1994. "A Cost-Effectiveness Analysis of Amniocentesis and Chorionic Villus Sampling for Prenatal Genetic Testing." *Medical Care* 32(8): 863–880; Oakley, A. 1984. *The Captured Womb: A History of the Medical Care of Pregnant Women.* Oxford: Oxford University Press; Robertson, J. A. 1983. "Procreative Liberty and the Control of Conception, Pregnancy and Childbirth." *Virginia Law Review* 69: 405–464.

See also **AMNIOCENTESIS; CHORIONIC VILLUS SAMPLING (CVS); FETAL SURGERY; FETOSCOPY; ULTRASOUND/SONOGRAPHY.**

ROBERT H. BLANK

PRENATAL GENETIC DIAGNOSIS

Over 250 genetic diseases and birth defects can be diagnosed prenatally (Nightingale and Goodman, 1990). Brigham, Rifkin, and Solt (1993) note that law relating to expanding prenatal diagnosis depends in part on the treatment of viability of the fetus. This in turn has a direct influence with regard to the diagnostic procedures used in prenatal diagnosis. Thus, there has been increased pressure to develop prenatal tests that can be performed early on in pregnancy since the treatment for most of these diseases is therapeutic abortion. The administration of these tests has far-reaching effects that should be taken into consideration with prenatal genetic diagnosis.

Listed below are eight diagnostic procedures used for testing genetic disease. The first six tests represent more of the traditional tests used, and most of these have been in place for quite some time. These tests include amniocentesis,* chorionic villus sampling (CVS),* maternal serum alpha-fetoprotein* (MSAFP), ultrasound/sonography,* and fetoscopy.* These tests are described individually and more completely in other sections of the encyclopedia.

The next two tests are tests performed genetically. Recombinant DNA testing and fetal diagnosis through maternal blood sampling represent the two most innovative categories of genetic diagnosis. These two tests demonstrate how sophisticated the technology has become, and therefore, these tests are probably more representative of future prenatal genetic diagnosis.

Recombinant DNA analysis is a new technology that isolates DNA molecules into fragments for analyzation. Recombinant DNA is made by restriction enzymes that in essence cut the DNA into fragments. These fragments can then be arranged and the nucleotide sequences studied. Nightingale and Goodman (1990) state that the most accurate form of recombinant DNA technology for diagnosing genetic diseases prenatally is via direct gene detection using a gene probe. Using this method, fetal DNA can be tested for specific genes for specific genetic disorders such as phenylketonuria (PKU), hemophilia A, sickle-cell disease, alpha$_1$-antitrypsin deficiency, autosomally inherited disorders, and thalassemia. There is a second, indirect method used in recombinant DNA analysis that is based on analyzing restriction fragment–length polymorphisms, or RFLPs. By looking at these segments or markers of DNA, healthy nucleotide patterns can be differentiated from disease patterns. Huntington's disease has been identified using RFLPs.

Fetal diagnosis through maternal blood sampling, a second prenatal genetic diagnostic test, is an experimental procedure by which fetal blood cells are sorted from the maternal cells. This new diagnosis has been enhanced through the usage of polymerase chain reaction (PCR), a process that amplifies the DNA in the fetal blood cells. Another experimental technique, called fluorescent in situ hybridization (FISH), has been utilized for this sorting process. For example, trisomic cells have been recently identified using the FISH sorting technique.

Robertson (1992) identifies two types of legal, ethical, and social problems that will arise in the intersection of genetics and prenatal diagnosis: informed consent with the ensuing malpractice considerations and access to prenatal information obtained from genetic screening. First of all, concerning informed consent, physicians informing patients of prenatal screening should include the authorization or the declination by the patient of any diagnostic test. Here we see the crucial role that genetic counseling plays with the increased onus on physicians to keep patients fully informed about their reproductive options. However, with the decision in *Rust v. Sullivan** that places limits on the content of disclosure concerning abortion in family planning programs, this area continues to be complicated with vague and conflicting, and often confusing, guidelines.

With the burden on the physician, the responsibility for omission or negligence regarding informed consent has resulted in malpractice lawsuits filed against the physician. There are basically two types of malpractice cases concerning informed consent, wrongful birth and wrongful life. We should note that these types of cases have evolved since the *Roe v. Wade** decision in 1973. In short, wrongful birth suits are those in which parents allege that their health care provider failed to provide genetic information. If the parents would have known about this genetic information, then they would have taken measures to prevent an unwanted pregnancy.

On the other hand, wrongful life suits are those claims brought by the genetically disabled children themselves. Suits for wrongful life allege that these genetic disabilities could have been known or predicted during the prenatal period. There are approximately 60 wrongful birth and wrongful life cases that have been appealed to intermediate appellate courts or to the higher supreme court levels (Wright Clayton, 1993). While parents are nearly always successful in their suits for wrongful birth, there have only been four major cases in which the child was successful in its claim for wrongful life (Wright Clayton, 1993). Both types of malpractice claims allege negligence on the part of the provider, and there are a handful of suits that have been brought due to negligence in the health care provider providing information regarding prenatal genetic diagnosis (Wright Clayton, 1993).

A second ethical, legal, and social implications (ELSI) problem has to do with access to prenatal information obtained from genetic screening and the determination of alternative decisions. We will review three issues related to this problem: mandatory screening, abortion, and the early determination of sex.

Currently, the only mandatory screening that is in place in the United States involves testing newborns for metabolic diseases such as PKU, an inherited metabolic disease that can be successfully treated through a special low-protein diet. This screening test involves testing infants *after* they are born (and *not* prenatally). However, Blank (1990) notes that we could see a return to mandated prenatal genetic screening programs in the future. In fact, there are current discussions, especially in New York, to implement mandatory screening for the HIV-II virus in all pregnant women. This issue brings to bear numerous ethical, legal, and social implications. The patient-physician relationship is grounded in confidentiality and based on trust. The issue of mandatory screening, especially for genetic diseases in which there are no treatments, challenges this notion of confidentiality and trust. Due to mandatory screening, the patient could be placed in the uncomfortable position of having to inform other family members, employers, or insurance companies of this sensitive information.

Prenatal diagnosis is closely tied to federal and state laws regarding abortion. The 1973 decisions of *Roe v. Wade* and *Doe v. Bolton* serve as a watershed in federal policy regarding women's rights and reproductive freedom. Although the *Roe* decision giving women the right to terminate a pregnancy has recently been challenged in numerous states, research in prenatal diagnosis has continued amidst the shadows of the abortion debate.

The crucial link between abortion and prenatal diagnosis is that abortion remains the only "treatment" for certain identified genetic diseases. If we continue to see states, like Louisiana, moving in the direction of placing tighter restrictions on abortion, then necessarily some prenatal diagnostic tests could become futile.

Rothenberg (1993) highlights this irony by noting the inconsistent laws and public policies among states that may fund genetic services but not abortion. Another complicating factor has to do with the interpretation of these laws. Bonnicksen (1992) cautions of the wrongful interpretation of laws that were passed with abortion in mind but that are being interpreted 10 to 20 years later with respect to in vitro fertilization (IVF)* and embryo studies. In effect, old laws address new problems and issues for which they may be inappropriate. New laws are required to deal directly with genetic testing, diagnosis, and treatment, including abortion.

Prenatal testing for the purpose of sex determination raises numerous ethical questions, especially regarding those genetic diseases that are X-linked. Prenatal gender identification to avoid genetically linked disease is widely accepted. But as Nightingale and Goodman (1990) note, the U.S. President's Commission for the Study of Ethical Problems in Medicine and Biomedical and Behavioral Research described prenatal diagnosis for the explicit reason of sexual selection as "an affront to the notion of human equality."

Other concerns exist regarding treatment. Somatic cell gene therapy is one of the new and experimental methods under consideration for genetic disease treatment. This therapy involves inserting genetically engineered cells directly into the patient's body, with the intention of correcting the disease. Concerns regarding safety guide this new treatment, whereas strong ethical concerns are raised with the discussion of germ-line therapy, in which these inserted engineered cells will be passed along to future generations (Cook-Deegan, 1994). The overall consensus seems to be that somatic gene therapy holds real promise, and the germ-line therapy should not be practiced. However, as Bonnicksen (1992) points out, some researchers claim that germ-line therapy is more cost-effective *because* the current gene pool, as well as the future gene pool, can become disease free. In sum, however, efficiency has not been a sufficient reason for germ-line therapy to prevail.

REFERENCES: Blank, Robert H. 1990. *Regulating Reproduction.* New York: Columbia University Press; Bonnicksen, Andrea L. 1992. ''Human Embryos and Genetic Testing: A Private Policy Model.'' *Politics and the Life Sciences* 11:53–62; Brigham, John, Janet Rifkin, and Christine G. Solt. 1993. ''Birth Technologies: Prenatal Diagnosis and Abortion Policy.'' *Politics and the Life Sciences* 12:31–44; Cook-Deegan, Robert Mullan. 1994. ''Germ-Line Gene Therapy: Keep the Window Open a Crack.'' *Politics and the Life Sciences* 13:217–220; *Doe v. Bolton.* 1973. 410 U.S. 179, 93 S. Ct. 739; Nightingale, Elena O., and Melissa Goodman. 1990. *Before Birth: Prenatal Testing for Genetic Disease.* Cambridge: Harvard University Press; Robertson, John. 1992. ''The Potential Impact of the Human Genome Project on Procreative Liberty.'' In *Gene Mapping: Using Law and Ethics as Guides,* ed. George J. Annas, and Sherman Elias. New York: Oxford University Press; *Roe v. Wade.* 1973. 410 U.S. 113, 93 S. Ct. 705; Rothenberg, Karen H. 1993. ''The Law's Response to Reproductive Genetic Testing: Questioning Assumptions About Choice, Causation and Control.'' *Fetal Diagnosis and Therapy* 8 (Supp. 1): 160–163; *Rust v. Sullivan.* 1991. 111 S. Ct. 1759; Wright Clayton, Ellen. 1993. ''Reproductive Genetic Testing: Regulatory and Liability Issues.'' *Fetal Diagnosis and Therapy* 8 (Supp. 1):39–59.

See also **GENETIC DIAGNOSIS; HUMAN GENOME PROJECT; PREIMPLANTATION GENETIC DIAGNOSIS; PRESYMPTOMATIC GENETIC DIAGNOSIS.**

PATRICIA GAIL McVEY

PRENATAL INJURY TORTS

In the past several decades, major changes have occurred in the body of case law surrounding the processes of birth and pregnancy. Preconception, conception, and prenatal legal actions are commonplace in part due to alterations in social values regarding birth and pregnancy. Major causes of the growing legal attention to these subjects are the recent advances in medical science that have brought about significant changes to the physiological aspects of the birth process and altered perceptions of it.

A child's right to recover from a third party for prenatal injuries, although largely unquestioned today, is a very recent judicial development. Prior to 1946, the courts largely accepted the precedence of *Dietrich v. Inhabitants of Northampton* (1884) where the Massachusetts Supreme Court disallowed recovery for negligently inflicted prenatal injuries in a wrongful death action of a child that did not survive its premature birth. In that case, a woman four to five months pregnant slipped and fell, by reason of a defect in the highway, and subsequently had a miscarriage. The plaintiff was alive when delivered but was too premature to survive. In arriving at its decision, the *Dietrich* court relied on the lack of precedent and upon the concept that the fetus was part of the mother and not a separate entity.

Despite the growing realization that *Dietrich* reasoning was faulty, it was relied upon as controlling until the U.S. District Court of D.C. dismissed it in *Bonbrest v. Kotz* (1946). In that case, infant Bette Gay Bonbrest by her father attempted to recover for injuries sustained when she was negligently removed by a physician, a clear instance of injury to a viable child. In order to distinguish itself from *Dietrich,* the court emphasized that the plaintiff was viable and capable of surviving outside the womb. The Bonbrest court reasoned that once the child demonstrated it was capable of survival outside its mother's womb, the argument that the fetus had no independent existence was inexplicable. If a child after birth is denied right of action for prenatal injuries, there is a wrong inflicted for which there is no remedy (at 141).

After *Bonbrest,* the right to recover for injuries sustained in utero gained rapid and widespread acceptance. In *Williams v. Marion Rapid Transit Co.* (1949), the Supreme Court of Ohio held that a viable fetus was a "person" within the mean of the Ohio Constitution and thus after birth could maintain an action for tortious prenatal injuries. Shortly thereafter, the Supreme Court of Minnesota (*Verkennes v. Corniea,* 1949) held that the representative of a stillborn child could maintain an action for wrongful death because it was viable at the time of the injury. Likewise, the Supreme Court of New Jersey (*Smith v. Brennan,* 1960), in a case where the infant plaintiff sustained injuries during an automobile collision while in his mother's womb, stated:

Regardless of analogies to other areas of the law, justice requires that the *principle be recognized that a child has a legal right to begin life with a sound mind and body* [italics mine]. If the wrongful conduct of another interferes with that right, and it can be established by competent proof that there is a causal connection between the wrongful interference and the harm suffered by the child when born, damages for such harm should be recoverable by the child. (at 503)

The *Smith* court concluded that the semantic argument whether an unborn child is a "person in being" is irrelevant to recovery for prenatal injury. Furthermore, the difficulty of proving fact of prenatal injury to the infant in the mother's womb is not sufficient reason for blocking all attempts to prove it (at 503).

Although there is a clear case law trend in favor of allowing a claim for prenatal injury regardless of the stage of gestation during which the injury occurred, there is far from unanimity in the courts on the question of viability. The viability rule developed originally as a means of distinguishing cases from *Dietrich,* which assumed that the fetus was part of the mother. In *Bonbrest,* the court refuted *Dietrich* by concluding that a viable fetus could sustain life independent of the mother and was, therefore, a distinct legal entity. Courts relying on *Bonbrest* thus often limited the authority of their decisions to suits involving injuries incurred after viability. For instance in *Albala v. City of New York* (1981), the Supreme Court, Appellate Division, of New York upheld the viability requirement when it refused recovery for injuries suffered by a previable fetus.

Increasingly, however, courts have either expressly renounced the viability rule or ignored it. The Georgia Supreme Court (*Hornbuckle v. Plantation Pipe Line Co.,* 1956) held that viability was not the deciding factor in a prenatal personal injuries action and that recovery for any injury suffered after the point of conception should be permitted. In another case arising out of an automobile collision, the Supreme Court of New Hampshire (*Bennett v. Hymers,* 1958) held that the fetus from the time of conception becomes a separate organism and remains so.

According to the court in *Smith v. Brennan* (1960 at 504), "Whether viable or not at the time of injury, the child sustains the same harm after birth, and therefore should be given the same opportunity for redress." In *Sylvia v. Gobeille* (1966), a Rhode Island appellate court state: "We are unable logically to conclude that a claim for injury inflicted prior to viability is any less meritorious than one sustained after." In *Wilson v. Kaiser Foundation Hospital* (1983), the California Court of Appeal, Third District, agreed with this reasoning and concluded that birth is the condition precedent that establishes the beginning of the child's rights. A tort action may be maintained if the child is born alive— whether the injury occurred before viability or after is immaterial once birth takes place. However, if the injured child is not born alive, a cause of action for prenatal injuries does not arise on its behalf because a stillborn fetus is not a person within the wrongful death statute of California (at 650).

In a further extension of this logic, some courts recently have recognized a cause of action for personal injuries that occurred prior to conception. In *Renslow v. Mennonite Hospital* (1977), a physician was held liable for injuries suffered by an infant girl as a result of a blood transfusion to the mother that occurred nine years before the child's birth. These "preconception torts" arise when a negligent act has been committed against a person not yet conceived but whose eventual existence is foreseeable (*Harbeson v. Parke-Davis,* 1983).

Although inconsistencies exist in case law as to viability, proof of causation, and so forth, a consensus now exists in all 50 states that there is a right of a child to bring common-law action for injuries suffered before birth. This unanimity has been achieved in a short span in part because new medical knowledge of the deleterious effects of particular action on the unborn permitted causation susceptible to legal proof. As in all tort action, the plaintiff must prove existence of a legal duty on the part of the defendant to conform to a specific standard of conduct for the protection of the plaintiff against unreasonable risk of injury as well as a breach of that duty by the defendant. For the breach to occur, there must be actual misfeasance—the defendant must be found to have been affirmatively negligent. Moreover, it must be proven that damage was suffered by the plaintiff and that the proximate cause of the damage was the negligence of the defendant. Legal causation may be established even though the biological processes that bring the injury about are not precisely understood. Legal cause does not need be the sole or even predominant cause of the injury. It is only required that the defendant's conduct must be a substantial or material factor in bringing about the injury—but for the defendant's negligent conduct the injury would not have occurred.

REFERENCES: *Albala v. City of New York,* 78 A.D.2d 389, 434 N.Y.S.2d 400 (1981); *Bennett v. Hymers,* 101 N.H. 483, 147 A.2d 108 (1958); *Bonbrest v. Kotz,* 65 F. Supp. 138 (D.D.C. 1946); *Dietrich v. Inhabitants of Northampton,* 138 Mass. 14 (1884); *Harbeson v. Parke-Davis,* 98 Wash. 2d 460, 656 P.2d 483 (1983); *Hornbuckle v. Plantation Pipe Line Co.,* 212 Ga. 504, 93 S.E.2d 727 (1956); *Renslow v. Mennonite Hospital,* 67 Ill. 2d 348, 367 N.E.2d 1250 (1977); *Smith v. Brennan,* 31 N.J. 353, 157 A.2d 497 (1960); *Sylvia v. Gobeille,* 101 R.I. 76, 220 A.2d 222 (1966); *Verkennes v. Corniea,* 38 N.W.2d 838 (Minn. 1949); *Williams v. Marion Rapid Transit Co.,* 87 N.E.2d 334 (Ohio 1949); *Wilson v. Kaiser Foundation Hospital,* 141 Ca. A.3d 891, 190 Cal. Rptr. 649 (1983).

See also **TORT FOR WRONGFUL LIFE.**

ROBERT H. BLANK

PRESIDENT'S COMMISSION FOR THE STUDY OF ETHICAL PROBLEMS IN MEDICINE AND BIOMEDICAL AND BEHAVIORAL RESEARCH

The President's Commission is an 11-member commission created in 1978 by the U.S. Congress to study and report on a variety of ethical problems in medicine and research (P.L. 95–622). The President's Commission, which worked from January 1980 until the end of March 1983, published 12 volumes: ten reports, the proceedings on a workshop on whistleblowing in research (*Whistleblowing in Biomedical Research,* 1982), and a guidebook for Institutional Review Boards* that oversee research with human subjects (*The Official IRB Guidebook,* 1983). The reports are *Defining Death* (1981), *Protecting Human Subjects* (1981), *Compensating for Research Injuries* (1982), *Making Health Care Decisions* (1982), *Screening and Counseling for Genetic Conditions* (1983), *Securing Access to Health Care* (1983), *Deciding to Forego Life-Sustaining Treatment* (1983), *Splicing Life* (1983), *Implementing Human Research Regulations* (1983), *Summing Up* (1983).

In some of its reports, the President's Commission made specific policy recommendations (e.g., a uniform law in *Defining Death,* laws recognizing living wills in *Making Health Care Decisions,* revised adoption laws and new laws governing sperm donors in *Screening and Counseling for Genetic Conditions*). In other reports (*Protecting Human Subjects, Compensating for Research Injuries, Implementing Human Research Regulations*), the commission concluded that policy change could best be accomplished through various administrative agencies. In many of the reports, though, the commission recommended less formal approaches to problems (e.g., changing the curriculum in medical and

nursing schools to include instruction on communicating with patients and recognizing ethical issues), offered general principles (e.g., the standard of equitable
access to health care for all), or suggested areas for further study (e.g., methods
of providing compensation to injured research subjects). In all of its publications,
the commission worked to achieve three goals: "to help clarify the issues and
highlight the facts that appear to be most relevant for informed decisionmaking;
to suggest improvements in public policy at various levels . . . ; to offer guidance
for people involved in making decisions, though not to dictate particular choices
on moral grounds" (President's Commission, 1983, 3).

The work of the President's Commission had considerable influence on public
policy formation. Its conclusions regarding the definition of death, for instance,
have been accepted in most states, as have its endorsements of living will laws.
Its recommendation that all federal departments and agencies adopt the regulations governing research with human subjects issued by the Department of
Health and Human Services (45 CFR 46) led to the development of the Common
Federal Rule for the Protection of Human Subjects.

REFERENCES: Annas, George J. 1994. "Will the Real Bioethics (Commission) Please
Stand Up?" *Hastings Center Report* 24: 19–21; Arras, J. D. 1984. "Retreat from the
Right to Health Care: The President's Commission and Access to Health Care." *Cardozo
Law Review* 6:321–346; Capron, A. M. 1983. "Looking Back at the President's Com-
mission." *Hastings Center Report* 13:7–10; Hanna, K. E., et al. 1993. "Finding a Forum
for Bioethics in U.S. Public Policy." *Politics and the Life Sciences* 12:205–219; Presi-
dent's Commission for the Study of Ethical Problems in Medicine and Biomedical and
Behavioral Research. 1983. *Summing Up*. Washington, D.C.: Government Printing Office. President's Commission reports are available through the U.S. Government Printing
Office, Washington, D.C.

DEBORAH R. MATHIEU

PRESYMPTOMATIC GENETIC DIAGNOSIS

Presymptomatic genetic diagnosis involves testing an individual for a specific
genetic disorder prior to that individual having any symptoms of the disease.
Adult-onset genetic diseases such as Huntington's disease, myotonic dystrophy,
Charcot-Marie-Tooth disease, adult polycystic kidney disease (APKD), and Alzheimer's disease are examples of genetic diseases that need special attention
with regard to identification since they do not manifest themselves until age 30
or later. Knowledge of these genes that cause or contribute to the occurrence of
adult-onset disease "permits scientists to develop tests to detect people who will
suffer the disease, before they experience symptoms," so they can benefit from
early intervention if in fact it is available (Andrews et al., 1994, 29).

As Caskey (1992) argues, genetic testing is the only alternative for accurate
presymptomatic diagnosis before the patient at risk makes reproductive decisions. For example, if an individual is diagnosed with having the Huntington's
gene, then chances are virtually 100 percent that the individual will develop this
dread disease. While there is currently no treatment available regarding Huntington's disease, knowledge of this gene would be helpful before planning a

family. This could be especially critical for those adoptees who do not have access to parental disease history. Unfortunately, this area of genetic diagnosis is not well developed. While tests are available for many single-gene disorders, tests for the more common and complex diseases are still in the developmental phase (Andrews et al., 1994).

Consequently, with regard to presymptomatic diagnosis, there are many ethical, legal, and social concerns that carry potentially negative consequences for the individual. First, although the genetic disease can be identified, it does not necessarily follow that scientists understand the gene defect. Thus, few, if any, treatment options are open to the affected individual. Research has shown that besides having these limited treatment options, heavy psychological burdens can be present in asymptomatic individuals contemplating having the presymptomatic genetic tests.

Two other primary areas of concern relate to the potential discrimination that an affected individual might suffer—and the related issue of confidentiality. Discriminatory patterns abound within the insurance industry. As Bonnicksen (1992) forewarns, being labeled as presymptomatically ill can leave an individual open to manipulation. However, according to Rothstein (1992a, 43), carriers of APKD or Huntington's disease will more than likely be covered under the Americans with Disabilities Act,* thus affording them protection from these discriminatory practices.

With regard to issues of confidentiality, Nelkin (1992) notes that genetic discrimination has been known to occur with individuals who have been presymptomatically diagnosed with a genetic disease or predisposition, even without exhibiting any manifestation of the disease. Nelkin also notes that these genetic tests can serve as gatekeepers, preventing these affected individuals from obtaining employment and insurance.

In light of this, Rothstein (1992a) notes that several state laws have been enacted to prevent this kind of broad-based genetic discrimination. According to Rothstein, Florida, Louisiana, North Carolina, New Jersey, Oregon, New York, and Wisconsin have all passed laws prohibiting genetic discrimination due to an individual having an atypical hereditary cellular or blood trait, such as sickle-cell trait or Tay-Sachs trait. If state or federal law protects individuals within the insurance industry and the employment market, will this extend into other areas of life, such as divorce proceedings (Rowland, 1992) or mortgage applications, scholarship committees, and others (Rothstein, 1992b)? These issues must be addressed as more genetic diseases become identifiable presymptomatically.

REFERENCES: Andrews, Lori B., Jane E. Fullarton, Neil A. Holtzman, and Arno G. Motulsky, eds. 1994. *Assessing Genetic Risks: Implications for Health and Social Policy.* Washington, D.C.: National Academy Press; Bonnicksen, Andrea L. 1992. "Introduction: Emerging Issues in Genetic and Reproductive Technologies." In *Emerging Issues in Biomedical Policy: An Annual Review,* Vol. 1, ed. Robert H. Blank and Andrea L. Bonnicksen. New York: Columbia University Press; Caskey, Thomas C. 1992. "Presymptomatic Genetic Diagnosis—A Worry for the United States." In *Gene Mapping: Using Law and Ethics as Guides,* ed. George J. Annas and Sherman Elias. New York: Oxford University Press; Nelkin, Dorothy. 1992. "Social Implications of Biological Tests." In *Emerging Issues in Biomedical Policy: An Annual Review,* Vol. 1, ed. Robert H. Blank and Andrea L. Bonnicksen. New York: Columbia University Press; Rothstein, Mark A. 1992a. "Genetic Discrimination in Employment and the Americans with Disabilities Act." *Houston Law Review* (Health Law Issue) 29(1):23–84; Rothstein, Mark A. 1992b. "Symposium: Legal and Ethical Issues Raised by the Human Genome Project, Forward." *Houston Law Review* (Health Law Issue) 29(1):1–6; Rowland, Robyn. 1992. *Living Laboratories: Women and Reproductive Technologies.* Bloomington: Indiana University Press.

PATRICIA GAIL McVEY

PREVALENCE AND CAUSES OF INFERTILITY

Infertility is a problem that is estimated to affect at least one in six couples in the United States. It is estimated that the sperm count of males has fallen by over 30 percent in the last five decades. Although the causes of this decline are unknown, environmental pollution appears to be a prime suspect. Whatever the cause, nearly 25 percent of all men now have sperm counts so low as to be considered by some researchers to be functionally sterile.

Similarly, the proportion of women experiencing fertility problems has increased. In 1990 the total number of American women with impaired fertility was 5.3 million, or 9.1 percent of all women aged 15 to 44, although only 43 percent of these women had ever obtained any infertility service (Wilcox and Mosher, 1993, 122). Although it appears that the rate of infertility has remained constant for the past decade, there was a substantial increase in infertility in the previous decades, and the factors that often cause infertility continue to be widely present in the United States.

The causes of infertility are complex and not fully understood, but they include environmental, heritable, pathological, and sociobehavioral factors. Some of the major factors predisposing individuals toward infertility are sexually transmitted diseases; pelvic inflammatory disease; endometriosis; smoking, environmental toxins, and drugs; strenuous exercise, poor nutrition, and stress; chemotherapy and radiation; and increased age. Many of these factors can be controlled and infertility reduced or prevented.

Approximately 40 percent of the women who suffer from involuntary sterility are infertile because of diseased fallopian tubes. The highly sensitive oviducts are easily scarred by disease or infection, thus blocking passage of the ovum to the sperm. Scarring can result from pelvic diseases or other low-level gynecological infections. Contemporary social patterns, including increased sexual contact of young women with a variety of partners, are linked with increased infertility in women. The epidemic proportions of gonorrhea and, more recently, herpes simplex II and chlamydia among young women promise to accentuate this problem. Although drug therapy and microsurgical intervention are effective in treating infertility in some instances, increasingly couples are turning toward an expanding selection of reproductive-aiding technologies.

A social pattern that has heightened public attention to infertility is the choice of many women to postpone parenting until their midthirties or beyond. Data consistently show that infertility increases with age in both men and women. U.S. data show approximately 8.7 percent infertility among women 25 to 29, 13.6 percent among those aged 30 to 34, 24.6 percent of those 35 to 39, and 27.2 percent of those 40 to 44 (OTA, 1988, 4). Although a French study that found even higher rates of infertility over age 30 sparked considerable debate, including suggestions that women might better postpone careers and concentrate on childbearing in their twenties (DeCherney and Berkowitz, 1982), this pattern is expected to persist. The availability of reproductive-assisting technologies to enable even postmenopause women to become pregnant expands the range of candidates for infertility treatment.

REFERENCES: Decherney, Alan H., and G. S. Berkowitz. 1982. "Female Fecundity and Age." *New England Journal of Medicine.* 306:424–426; Office of Technology Assessment (OTA). 1988. *Infertility: Medical and Social Choices.* Washington, D.C.: U.S. Government Printing Office; Sellors, John W., James B. Mahony, Max A. Chernesky, and Darlyne J. Rath. 1988. "Tubal Factor Infertility: An Association with Prior Chlamydial Infection and Asymptomatic Salpingitis." *Fertility and Sterility* 49(3): 451–56; Wilcox, Lynne S., and William D. Mosher. 1993. "Use of Infertility Services in the United States." *Obstetrics and Gynecology* 82(1): 122–27.

ROBERT H. BLANK

PSYCHOSURGERY

When used to repair physical damage caused by head injuries or tumors, brain surgery raises few objections. When the same techniques are used instead to correct mental and/or behavioral disorders (psychosurgery), they become highly controversial. These applications rest on the assumption that behavioral disorders have an organic base and that to treat the disorder the organic pathology must be corrected by physical intervention, not psychotherapy. This assumption is highly debatable according to critics of psychosurgery.

According to Valenstein (1986, 3), between 1948 and 1952 "tens of thousands of mutilating brain operations were performed on mentally ill men and women," including many from the United States who voluntarily underwent lobotomy. Although the practice of lobotomy was curtailed by 1960, primarily because of the availability of psychoactive drugs as an inexpensive alternative, in its wake it left many seriously brain-damaged persons.

Sophisticated stereotaxic instruments facilitate more precise placement of electrodes to specific brain targets, thus allowing for the destruction of relatively small areas of brain tissue. Electrolytic lesioning or selective cutting of nerve fibers is conducted after the region to be lesioned is localized by establishing coordinates using anatomical landmarks and X rays. In one procedure, called *stereotaxic subcaudate tractotomy,* a small, localized area of the brain is destroyed by radioactive particles inserted through small ceramic rods. The particular site varies with the nature of the disturbance. There have also been some applications using radiation, cryoprobes (freezing), or focused ultrasonic beams to destroy the tissue.

As with lobotomies, however, there is no way of predicting the consequences of these procedures either in the short or long run. According to critics, psychosurgery is a highly experimental procedure that "produces a marked deterioration in behavior, serious impairments of judgment, and other disastrous social adjustment effects" (Chorover, 1981, 291).

Although the National Commission for the Protection of Human Subjects (1976) criticized the use of psychosurgery for social or institutional control, it concluded that it might help some patients. Although it recommended prior screening of each proposed surgery by an independent Institutional Review Board* (IRB), its recommendations were never translated into federal legislation or regulations. Instead, action restricting psychosurgery has originated in state legislatures. In 1982, Oregon passed a statute that strengthened its earlier restrictions and prohibited psychosurgery in the state. California also instituted regulations that all but ended the practice. Although most states have not taken action, primarily because of the threat of liability, less than 200 psychosurgeries are performed annually in the United States.

Ironically, concurrent with the imposition of legal restraints, extensions of studies originally reported to the National Commission have been favorable to psychosurgery for certain classes of patients. Two independent research teams reported that the quality of life of between 70 and 80 percent of patients improved significantly after undergoing psychosurgery. Moreover, they found no evidence of physical; emotional, or intellectual impairment caused by surgery. Careful patient selection and use of surgery as a last resort only for those patients who fail to respond to drug therapy seem central to any future uses of psychosurgery.

Psychosurgery continues to generate policy issues on a range of levels. First is the dilemma of consent. The consent must come from the damaged organ itself, but if the damage is severe enough to warrant surgery, who can give consent for an irreversible procedure? Second is the question of therapy versus experimentation. Because every person's brain is unique, psychosurgery will always have a high degree of uncertainty and thus risk. Third is the question of assuming that deviant behavior has an organic base. If it does not, can we justify the use of organic procedures such as surgery to resolve a nonorganic problem? Are we not simply treating (i.e., controlling) the symptoms without dealing with the cause?

Psychosurgery also illustrates problems of social control. We are developing an impressive array of techniques to control or modify behavior. Each technique, however, offers opportunity for abuse and poses serious threats to individual liberty. Stigmatization associated with being labeled abnormal, constraints on freedom of choice, and the erosion of the dignity of the individual are seriously challenged by the presence of these innovations. In contrast, there is evidence that psychosurgery might be beneficial to many individuals and that for some persons it represents the only hope of leading a near-normal existence. To deny them the benefits of the technologies because we do not trust our ability as a society to set reasonable limits on their use is questionable.

REFERENCES: Chorover, Stephen L. 1981. "Psychosurgery: A Neuropsychological Perspective." In Thomas A. Mappes and Jane S. Zembaty, eds., *Biomedical Ethics*. New York: McGraw-Hill; De la Porte, C. 1993. "Technical Possibilities and Limitations of Stereotaxy." *Acta Neurochirurgica* 124(1):3–6; Harvey, P. D., R. C. Mohs, and M. Davidson. 1993. "Leukotomy and Aging in Chronic Schizophrenia: A Followup Study 40 Years After Psychosurgery." *Schizophrenia Bulletin* 19(4):723–732; Mirsky, A. F., and M. H. Orzack. 1977. "Final Report on Psychosurgery Pilot Study." In *Appendix: Psychosurgery*. Washington, D.C.: U.S. Government Printing Office; National Commission for the Protection of Human Subjects of Biomedical and Behavioral Research. 1976. *Report and Recommendations on the Use of Psychosurgery*. Washington, D.C.: U.S. Government Printing Office; Poynton, A. M. 1993. "Current State of Psychosurgery." *British Journal of Hospital Medicine* 50(7): 408–411; Teuber, H. L., S. H. Corkin, and T. E. Twitchell. 1977. "Study of Cingulotomy in Man: A Summary." In W. H. Sweet et al., eds., *Neurosurgical Treatment in Psychiatry, Pain and Epilepsy*. Baltimore: University Park Press; Valenstein, Elliott S. 1986. *Great and Desperate Cures: The Rise and Decline of Psychosurgery and Other Radical Treatments for Mental Illness*. New York: Basic Books.

See also **ELECTROCONVULSIVE TREATMENT (ECT); ELECTRONIC BRAIN STIMULATION (EBS).**

ROBERT H. BLANK

PSYCHOTROPIC DRUGS

There are three major groups of psychotropic drugs used as therapeutic agents. The first and most powerful are the antipsychotic drugs or major tranquilizers. With Food and Drug Administration* (FDA) approval of chlorpromazine (Thorazine) in 1954, the first of a group of powerful phenothiazenes was introduced to be used in the treatment of major mental illnesses such as schizophrenia and paranoia. These drugs demonstrate sedative, hypnotic, and mood-elevating effects. Although they do nothing to cure, but rather suppress the symptoms of the disease, they are effective in maintaining equilibriums for many patients. Maintenance therapy requires prolonged use generally at reduced dose levels. Discontinuance of the drug will result in return of symptoms. The major tranquilizers have also been used in treating violence. Administration, however, is complex because effects and dosage levels vary across individuals and prolonged use can have deleterious side effects.

The second major group of psychotropic drugs are the antidepressant drugs, which include amphetamines, Prozac, Ritalin, Preludin, monoamine oxidase inhibitors, and tricyclic derivatives of imipramine. Although amphetamines have little clinical value in the treatment of depression because of their very short duration, they are widely known and used. They also have considerable potential for abuse and dependency. Ritalin is a stimulant that has been found to have the opposite effect in hyperkinetic children. Because of its ability to calm hyperactive children, Ritalin has become overused in some school districts to pacify disruptive children, leading to many lawsuits (Moss, 1988). The use of drugs in schools for social control has come under considerable attack in recent decades because the effect of prolonged exposure is unknown. Ritalin has, in fact, been linked to complex changes in the central nervous system. Questions of its effects on personality development, innovative thinking capacity, and any psychological or physiological dependence are unanswered. According to Safer and Krager (1992), since 1987 use of Ritalin by schools has declined due to a negative media blitz, lawsuits threatened or initiated, and apprehension of parents and involved professionals.

The third grouping of psychoactive drugs are the antianxiety drugs or minor tranquilizers. Barbituates are the least effective antianxiety medication and have a high tendency to produce dependence, habituation, and addiction. Despite these factors and their low margin of safety, barbituates such as phenobarbital are effective in treating epilepsy. Another group of minor tranquilizers include diazepoxides such as Librium and Valium. These drugs are used effectively to control muscle spasms, hysteria in acute grief situations, and compulsion. They are less dangerous than barbituates and less addictive. Minor tranquilizers are not effective in the treatment of psychoses but are of special value in the treatment of tension and anxiety associated with situational states and stress. The long-term use of antianxiety drugs is discouraged, however, because they can produce dependence and have a tendency to be abused.

Psychotropic drugs are used because they are effective and convenient rather than because of a compelling scientific consensus as to how they help patients. The use of these drugs to produce the desired mood and mental functioning and thus influence behavior raises serious constitutional issues, especially where informed consent is problematic. In our drug-oriented society, however, psychotropic drugs are routinely welcomed to help us cope with life's problems. Drugs have become a quick fix for anxiety, depression, and social stresses of modern-day existence—though not without risk.

Recent attention has shifted to the development of nootropics, or "smart" drugs, designed to increase brain power and improve memory, concentration, and ability to learn. Although the original research on these substances centered on the goal of treating patients with premature dementias such as Alzheimer's disease, increasingly they are being touted as means of promoting mental agility in healthy persons who want to boost their intelligence. A "smart drug" industry is flourishing despite the lack of scientific evidence that these substances actually perform as performance enhancers in normal persons (Concar and Coughlin, 1993).

REFERENCES: Concar, D., and A. Coughlin. 1993. "Is There Money in Lost Memories?" *New Scientist* 1869: 20–22; Dean, N., and J. Morganthaler. 1992. *Smart Drugs and Nutrients: How to Improve Your Memory and Increase Your Intelligence Using the Latest Discoveries in Neuroscience*. Santa Cruz: B. and J. Publications; Moss, D. C. 1988. "Ritalin Under Fire: 16 Lawsuits Claim Drug Was Wrongly Prescribed." *American Bar Association Journal* 74: 19; Rose, S. 1993. "No Way to Treat a Mind." *New*

Scientist 1869: 23–26; Safer, Daniel J., and John M. Krager. 1992. "Effect of a Media Blitz and a Threatened Lawsuit on Stimulant Treatment." *Journal of the American Medical Association* 268(8): 1004–1007.

ROBERT H. BLANK

PUBLIC HEALTH SERVICE

The principal health agency of the U.S. government, the PHS is the largest public health program in the world. Its mission is to protect and advance the health of the American people. Among its many health-related responsibilities are to (1) conduct and support biomedical, behavioral, and health services research, (2) communicate research results to health professionals and to the public, (3) help provide health care and related services to medically underserved populations and to Native Americans, as well as to certain groups with special health needs (such as migrant workers, the mentally ill, and persons with substance abuse problems), (4) prevent and control diseases, (5) identify and control health hazards in the environment, (6) work with other nations and international agencies on global health problems, (7) protect subjects—human and other animal—of biomedical research, (8) promote healthy lifestyles, and (9) ensure that drugs and medical devices are safe and effective, that food is safe and wholesome, that cosmetics are harmless, and that electronic products do not expose users to dangerous amounts of radiation.

Established by the Public Health Service Act of 1944 (P.L. 78–410), the PHS is a component of the U.S. Department of Health and Human Services (DHHS, formerly the U.S. Department of Health, Education, and Welfare). The head of the PHS is the assistant secretary for health, who is appointed by the president and confirmed by the U.S. Senate. The assistant secretary for health is responsible for overseeing the PHS as well as for advising the secretary of DHHS on matters of biomedical policy. He/she is aided in these activities by the surgeon general, by deputy assistant secretaries for health, and by the heads of the eight PHS agencies.

The eight PHS agencies are the National Institutes of Health (NIH)*, the Food and Drug Administration,* the Centers for Disease Control and Prevention,* the Health Resources and Services Administration, the Substance Abuse and Mental Health Services Administration, the Agency for Toxic Substances and Disease Registry, the Indian Health Service, and the Agency for Health Care Policy and Research.*

The assistant secretary for health also oversees a variety of health-related activities carried out by staff offices within the PHS. Among the most significant of these in terms of biomedical policy are the Office of Minority Health, which works to improve health program activities addressing minority health issues; the President's Council on Physical Fitness and Sports, which works to improve the health of Americans by promoting participation in sports and regular exercise; the National AIDS Program Office, which advises the assistant secretary for health on acquired immune deficiency syndrome (AIDS) issues and serves as a liaison among the various PHS components and with other public and private organizations; the Office of Disease Prevention and Health Promotion (ODPHP); the National Toxicology Program; and the Office of Population Affairs.

The Office of Disease Prevention and Health Promotion coordinates DHHS efforts in disease prevention and health promotion, fosters the use of prevention activities by groups outside the federal government, and formulates national health goals. ODPHP also supports research on and development of disease prevention training programs and works to educate the public about prevention programs.

The goals of the National Toxicology Program are to strengthen and coordinate research and testing on toxic chemicals in order to prevent unnecessary exposure to hazards. The program involves the relevant toxicology activities of various components within the Public Health Service: the National Institute of Environmental Health Sciences* (one of the National Institutes of Health), the National Center for Toxicological Research (part of the Food and Drug Administration), and the National Institute for Occupational Safety and Health (part of the Centers for Disease Control and Prevention). Important recent contributions include an integrated array of tests designed to study a spectrum of effects for each chemical and a set of toxicology study systems designed to rapidly provide specialized toxicological information.

The mission of the Office of Population Affairs (OPA) is to promote public health and welfare by improving the family planning services and population research activities of the federal government. OPA was authorized in 1970 when Congress added Title X (P.L. 91–572) to the Public Health Service Act. Reauthorized by Congress each year, Title X provides grants to public and private not-for-profit entities who offer family planning services to low-income women, grants that have been critical in enabling persons who desire to obtain family planning care to have access to the requisite services. Although the goal of Title X is to provide individuals with the information and the means to exercise personal choice in determining the number and spacing of their children, Title X does not pay for abortions. Also funded under this program are grants for research to improve the delivery and effectiveness of family planning services, training for health care professionals, and an information and education program (through the Family Life Information Exchange).

REFERENCES: Institute of Medicine. 1991. *Research and Service Programs in the PHS: Challenges in Organization.* Washington, D.C.: National Academy Press; Mullan, F. 1989. *Plagues and Politics: The Story of the United States Public Health Service.* New York: Basic Books; Williams, R. C. 1951. *The United States Public Health Service, 1798–1950.* Richmond, VA: Whittet and Shepperson.

DEBORAH R. MATHIEU

R

RATIONING OF HEALTH CARE

Rationing of health care refers to conscious decisions to withhold certain forms of potentially beneficial medical interventions from specific patients in order to conserve and redirect scarce financial, human, or technological resources. Rationing, which concerns microlevel, individual patient–oriented parceling out, is distinguishable from the process of allocation, which involves macro- or policy-level decisions about how much resources ought to be devoted to a particular category of activity (e.g., What should be the size of the national health budget?). Rationing also should not be confused with the emerging topic of futile medical intervention; the latter offers no reasonable hope of any meaningful patient benefit and ethically should be withheld even if resources were infinite (Swanson and McCrary, 1994).

Rationing of potentially beneficial health care already occurs today (Friedman, 1994). In most instances, it is accomplished through implicit, unacknowledged means such as discrimination in access against the uninsured (rationing by price), geographical distribution of medical resources (rationing by quantity), restrictive eligibility criteria for persons or services (e.g., not paying for "experimental" treatments), waiting lists and other devices that weed out patients, and physician recommendations against particular treatments on the grounds that they are "medically inappropriate" for the particular patient. The "medically contraindicated" device for thinly disguising rationing practice is especially common in the British National Health Service, where physician choices must be made and executed within the confines of a fixed total health budget but in which a dollar saved on Patient A thereby becomes available for the care of Patient B (Hope, Sprigings, and Crisp, 1993).

Many participants in the health system reform debate currently engulfing the United States contend that the present implicit, and hence ad hoc and unaccountable, practice of health care rationing is morally objectionable. These critics argue for a public acknowledgment of rationing practice that is achieved through enunciation and application of explicit criteria arrived at and enforced through an open, politically accountable process. This explicit approach to the rationing dilemma is reflected in the state of Oregon's recent attempt to prioritize specific health services under its Medicaid program and to utilize its finite Medicaid funds only to pay for those services near the top of the priority list (Nagel, 1992).

A number of specific criteria have been suggested for use under an explicit health care rationing scheme. As noted, Oregon's unique approach has been to focus on particular forms of treatment, considering all persons (or at least all Medicaid recipients) as equal within any particular treatment category. Another treatment-focused approach would transform the prevailing logic of medical progress from an emphasis on developing and providing high-technology life-preserving rescue interventions toward availability of more humane caring interventions (Callahan, 1990). The majority of commentators have suggested rationing schemes based on characteristics of the persons applying for treatment. These suggested personal criteria include: medical need (distinguished from mere desire), likelihood of benefit, lottery, first-come-first-served, and social worth. Perhaps the most controversial proposals have centered on use of chronological age as a categorical "bright line" test for limiting certain forms of expensive medical treatment (Callahan, 1987). Strong opposition to age-based rationing proposals cite, among other things, the practical and moral appropriateness of considering important, relevant individual differences among older persons rather than lumping them together indiscriminately for deprivation of resources (Binstock and Post, 1991).

A fundamental question raised by any rationing scheme is, Who will actually create the criteria that result in limiting treatment to particular potential patients? Possible candidates for the rationer role include the government (legislatively or through agency bureaucracies), private insurance companies and corporate benefits managers, health care institutions, and physicians at the bedside. Additionally, some suggest that consumers themselves can serve as responsible, effective rationers if individuals are encouraged to execute advance planning documents such as living wills and physicians are encouraged to respect patient preferences for limiting aggressive treatment near the end of life (Singer and Lowy, 1992).

Several analysts argue that the enormous amount of waste and inefficiency now found in the American health care system could be eliminated through a combination of aggressive outcomes research, delivery system reform such as more emphasis on prepaid managed care, and provider respect for patients' autonomous choices near the end of life. If this were done, the argument continues, enough money would be saved that rationing would become unnecessary. This viewpoint is not generally accepted as consistent with the economic realities, even though numerous ethical (e.g., irreparable damage to the physician/patient relationship) and pragmatic (e.g., there is no certainty that the resources conserved would be put to better use than they are at present) qualms with rationing have been raised. There does exist a consensus, though, that rationing ought to occur only for just cause, that is, as a last resort. Other broadly agreed upon ethical guidelines are that the rationing process should involve public participation and consensus building, serve the common good, and not unfairly discriminate on the basis of irrelevant personal characteristics.

REFERENCES: Binstock, Robert H., and Stephen G. Post, eds. 1991. *Too Old for Health Care?* Baltimore: Johns Hopkins University Press; Callahan, Daniel. 1987. *Setting Limits: Medical Goals for an Aging Society.* New York: Simon & Schuster; Callahan, Daniel. 1990. *What Kind of Life: The Limits of Medical Progress.* New York: Simon & Schuster; Friedman, Emily. 1994. "Money Isn't Everything: Nonfinancial Barriers to Access." *Journal of the American Medical Association* 271:1535–1538; Hope, Tony, David Springings, and Roger Crisp. 1993. " 'Not Clinically Indicated': Patients' Interests or Resource Allocation?" *British Medical Journal* 306:379–381; Nagel, Jack H. 1992. "Combining Deliberation and Fair Representation in Community Health Decisions." *University of Pennsylvania Law Review* 140:1965–1985; Singer, Peter A., and Frederick H. Lowy. 1992. "Rationing, Patient Preferences, and Cost of Care at the End of Life." *Archives of Internal Medicine* 152:478–480; Swanson, Jeffrey W., and S. Van McCrary. 1994. "Doing All They Can: Physicians Who Deny Medical Futility." *Journal of Law, Medicine & Ethics* 22:318–326.

MARSHALL B. KAPP

RECOMBINANT DNA ADVISORY COMMITTEE OF THE NATIONAL INSTITUTES OF HEALTH

The Recombinant DNA Advisory Committee (RAC) was formed by the director of the National Institutes of Health (NIH)* on October 7, 1974. Such a committee had been recommended by the National Academy of Sciences (NAS)* (Berg et al., 1974) after considering concerns about potential biohazards of genetic engineering raised at the June 1973 Gordon Conference (Singer and Soll, 1973). The *Charter* of the RAC states, "The goal of the Committee [RAC] is to investigate the current state of knowledge and technology regarding DNA recombinants, their survival in nature, and transferability to other organisms; to recommend guidelines for the conduct of recombinant DNA experiments; and to recommend programs to assess the possibility of spread of specific DNA recombinants and the possible hazards to the public health and to the environment. This Committee is a technical committee, established to look at a specific problem" (39 *Fed. Reg.* 39306 [1974]). The RAC met for the first time, February 28, 1975, the day after the Asilomar conference on biohazards ended (Krimsky, 1982, 350).

Today, the RAC is composed of 25 voting members. The *1994 Guidelines for Research Involving Recombinant DNA Molecules (Guidelines)* (59 *Fed. Reg.* 34496 [1994]) require that at least 14 be selected from authorities knowledgeable in scientific fields and at least 6 be "persons knowledgeable in applicable law, standards of professional conduct and practice, public attitudes, the environment, public health, occupational health, or related fields" (Section IV-C-2). Nonvoting representatives from interested federal agencies may participate. The RAC is responsible for advising the director on major actions as listed in Section IV-C-1-b-(1) of the *Guidelines*.

The RAC developed the *Guidelines* as required by the *Charter*. The first version of the *Guidelines* was published in 41 *Fed. Reg.* 27902 (1976). The *Guidelines* are developed, modified, and administered by the RAC for the secretary "to specify practices for constructing and handling (i) recombinant deoxyribonucleic acid (DNA) molecules and (ii) organisms and viruses containing recombinant DNA molecules" (Section I-A). The *Guidelines* apply to "all recombinant DNA research within the United States (U.S.) or its territories" (Section I-C-1-a) and to some experiments done abroad (Section I-C-1-b). Some experiments are reviewable by other federal agencies (Section I-A-1). Recombinant DNA is defined as "either (i) molecules that are constructed outside living cells by joining natural or synthetic DNA segments to DNA molecules that can replicate in a living cell, or (ii) molecules that result from the replication of those described in (i) above" but excludes certain synthetic DNAs and transposable elements (Section I-B).

The *Guidelines* are intended to be amended to consider advances in the research of recombinant DNA. Section IV-A states, "The NIH Guidelines will never be complete or final since all conceivable experiments involving recombinant DNA cannot be foreseen." Certain experiments assessed as posing no significant risk may be exempted from compliance with the *Guidelines* (Section III-E-6).

The *Guidelines* classify experiments based on their assessed biohazard. Based on this classification, experiments may (1) require specific review by the RAC on a case-by-case basis and approval by the NIH and the Institutional Biosafety Committee (IBC) before initiation of the experiment, or (2) require NIH's Office of Recombinant DNA Activities and IBC approval before initiation, or (3) require IBC approval before initiation of the experiment, or (4) require IBC notification at the time of initiation of the experiment, or (5) be exempt from the *Guidelines* (Section III).

Appendix G establishes standard microbiological practices and four levels of physical containment that can be required of recombinant DNA experiments. Biological containment levels are set by Appendix I. Microorganisms are ranked based on hazard in Appendix B. Different levels of physical and biological containment are combined, along with constant use of standard practices, to establish the desired level of containment based on the assessed experimental biohazard. Institutions to which the *Guidelines* apply must establish an IBC (Section IV-B-1-b). Institutions conducting BL3 or BL4 physical containment level experiments (Section IV-B-3-b) or certain large-scale research or production activities (Section IV-B-3-a) are required to appoint a biosafety officer. Physical and biological containment of plants and animals is now regulated in Appendixes P and Q, respectively.

The *Guidelines'* authority is limited to recombinant DNA research conducted at institutions receiving NIH funding for recombinant DNA research (Section I-C-1-a). The most severe sanction the RAC can impose is termination of all NIH funding for recombinant DNA research at the violator's institution. The RAC is not a regulatory body and depends on self-enforcement by the regulated community (Section IV-A). Compliance of commercial entities with the *Guidelines* is encouraged but strictly voluntary (Section IV-E-1). Note, however, some local laws have made the *Guidelines* binding on recombinant DNA research within their jurisdiction (Krimsky, 1982, 294–311). Also, the standard of care a commercial entity will be held to in a tort action probably will be established by the *Guidelines* (Palmer, 1994, 297). Finally, the *Guidelines'* definition of recombinant DNA does not apply to DNA molecules constructed inside living cells by techniques such as cell fusion, conjugation, and transposition.

The issue of whether the *Guidelines* are federal rules has been avoided by observance of the notice (by publishing proposed major actions in the *Federal Register*) and comment requirements of the Administrative Procedure Act (5 U.S.C. § 4332(C) 1993). RAC-recommended and director-approved actions are published in the *Recombinant DNA Technical Bulletin*. Limiting the *Guidelines'* applicability to recipients of federal funding and to "possible hazards to the public health and to the environment" (*Charter*) deemphasizes constitutional issues of First Amendment rights of researchers to conduct research.

The history of the RAC can be classified into four phases. During the first phase the probability and magnitude of the risks of genetic engineering were unknown. Before the creation of the RAC, scientists proceeded with extreme caution in the face of these unknowns by calling for a voluntary moratorium on certain recombinant DNA experiments (Berg et al., 1974). After creation of the RAC, the 1976 *Guidelines* placed explicit bans on some classes of recombinant DNA experiments (41 *Fed. Reg.* 27902, 27914–15 [1976]). Thus, unknown risk was dealt with by absolutely avoiding it. During this first phase, the RAC was primarily concerned with ensuring that adequate precautions were taken against an accidental release of genetically engineered microorganisms (GEMs) from research laboratories conducting permissible experiments.

The second phase of the RAC's history began with the approval of risk assessment experiments confined to the laboratory. An experiment to assess the risk that recombinant DNA in bacteria might transfer to the bacteria's animal host was challenged as banned under the 1976 *Guidelines* in *Mack v. Califano*, 447 F. Supp. 668 (D.D.C. 1978). The district court deferred to the RAC's finding that this experiment was not unreasonably risky. Later risk assessment experiments were interpreted as showing recombinant DNA was not inherently dangerous.

The *Guidelines* were amended to eliminate the bans and allowed NIH approval of reasonably risky experiments. The third phase of the RAC's history began in 1983. The director, acting on the advice of the RAC, issued an approval of a deliberate release of GEMs into the environment by Dr. Steven Lindow of the University of California at Berkeley. Deliberate releases had been subject to a ban in the 1976 *Guidelines* (41 *Fed. Reg* 27902, 27915 [1976]). This approval was enjoined by the district court for the District of Columbia in *Foundation on Economic Trends v. Heckler*, 587 F. Supp. 753 (D.D.C. 1984) and the injunction upheld in *Foundation on Economic Trends v. Heckler*, 756 F.2d. 143 (D.C. Cir. 1985). Both courts enjoined the experiment due to the NIH's procedural failure to consider adequately the environmental impact of dispersal of the released GEMs from the application site. However, the circuit court overturned the district court's injunction of NIH approval of all deliberate release experiments.

A deliberate release experiment by a licensee of Dr. Lindow's technology was the subject of a court challenge in *Foundation on Economic Trends v. Thomas*, 637 F. Supp. 25 (D.D.C. 1986). The procedurally proper substantive assessment by the Environmental Protection Agency (EPA) that the risk was reasonable was upheld by the district court. The EPA used the RAC's experience in reaching this assessment. Review of deliberate releases is now conducted mostly by the EPA and the U.S. Department of Agriculture (USDA) (59 *Fed. Reg.* 34472, 34473 [1994]).

The RAC is now dealing with use of recombinant DNA in human gene therapy. The RAC formed the now-disbanded Working Group on Human Gene Therapy to respond to *Splicing Life* (President's Commission, 1983). This Working Group developed a document now known as *Points to Consider in the Design and Submission of Protocols for the Transfer of Recombinant DNA into the Genome of One or More Human Subjects (Points to Consider)* (*Guidelines*, Appendix M, as amended by 59 *Fed. Reg.* 40170 [1994]). *Points to Consider* provides "guidance in preparing proposals for NIH consideration under Section III-A-2 [Major Actions] and III-B-2 [Minor Actions]" (59 *Fed. Reg* 34496, 34528). All such proposals are considered on a case-by-case basis. Most recombinant DNA experiments in human subjects will not be considered by the RAC until approved by the local IBC and the Institutional Review Board (IRB)*. Appendixes M-V and M-VI allow use of a compassionate plea. Proposals for germ-line alterations will not be considered at present (59 *Fed. Reg* 34496, 34529). As seen in the RAC's prior phases, this leaves open the possibility of future consideration. One researcher now views "the RAC [as] restricted to evaluating the ethical and social implications of proposed methods and clinical designs, while a critical evaluation of the technical aspects of the protocol is left to the FDA" (Ledley, 1994, 286). Another observer notes the *Charter* makes no reference to "the broad social or ethical issues," however (Krimsky, 1982, 155).

The RAC was the model for other federal science advisory committees. These committees include the Biotechnology Science Advisory Committee (BSAC) of the EPA, the Scientific Advisory Committee of the National Science Foundation (NSF),* and the Agricultural Biotechnology Research Advisory Committee (ABRAC) of the USDA. These committees have taken the burden of regulating commercial recombinant DNA application off the RAC, allowing it to focus on its initial and primary goal of advising the director on regulation of recombinant DNA technology as applied by basic research. Also, since the RAC only has jurisdiction over experiments funded by the NIH, the BSAC and ABRAC are the proper authorities to advise EPA and USDA on regulation of commercial application of recombinant DNA technology.

Finally, the NIH both promotes and regulates recombinant DNA research through the RAC. Some doubt the rigor with which the NIH will regulate (Fogelman, 1987, 211).

REFERENCES: Berg, Paul, et al. 1974. "Potential Biohazards of Recombinant DNA Molecules." *Science* 183: 303; Fogelman, Valerie M. 1987. "Article: Regulating Science: An Evaluation of the Regulation of Biotechnology Research." *Envtl. L.* 17: 183–273; Krimsky, Sheldon. 1982. *Genetic Alchemy.* Cambridge, MA: MIT Press; Ledley, Fred. 1994. "Designing Clinical Trials of Somatic Gene Therapy." In *Gene Therapy for Neoplastic Diseases,* ed. Brian E. Huber and John S. Lazo. New York: Annals of the New York Academy of Sciences; Palmer, Julie G. 1994. "Human Gene Therapy: Suggestions for Avoiding Liability." In *Gene Therapy for Neoplastic Diseases,* ed. Brian E. Huber and John S. Lazo. New York: Annals of the New York Academy of Sciences; Singer, Maxine, and Soll, Dieter. 1973. "Guidelines for DNA Hybrid Molecules." *Science* 181: 1114; President's Commission for the Study of Ethical Problems in Medicine and Biomedical and Behavorial Research. 1983. *Splicing Life.* Washington, D.C.: U.S. Government Printing Office.

MICHAEL D. HINDS

REFUSAL OF LIFE-SUSTAINING MEDICAL TREATMENT

Since *In re Quinlan** (1976) (when the New Jersey Supreme Court authorized the removal of a ventilator from Karen Ann Quinlan, who was in a coma), many courts have held that the United States Constitution, through the right of privacy, guarantees to individuals a fundamental right to reject medical treatment, including medical treatment without which they will die. Some courts have explicitly characterized this as a "right to die."

The right to refuse medical treatment has roots in both the common-law right to be free from invasion of one's bodily integrity and the notion of battery, which is a rejection of unwanted touching. Judge (later Justice) Cardozo explained in *Schloendorff v. Society of New York Hospital* (1914): "Every human being of adult years and sound mind has a right to determine what should be done with his own body; and a surgeon who performs an operation without his patient's consent commits an assault, for which he is liable in damages." Thus, the right to refuse medical treatment is grounded in the notion that medical treatment without the patient's consent constitutes a battery of the patient.

There are three primary ways in which life-sustaining medical treatment may be refused: (1) Competent patients may refuse consent to treatment; (2) patients may execute a living will to refuse certain medical treatments after the patient becomes incompetent; and (3) a surrogate decision maker may refuse treatment on behalf of an incompetent patient under the authority of a durable power of attorney for health care, by means of which the previously competent patient appointed a substitute to make health care decisions for him when he is no longer competent to do so.

First, competent patients may make an informed refusal of life-sustaining treatment. While a refusal of medical treatment may be motivated by a specific intent to die, it is often motivated by other considerations, such as the patient's assessment of the comparative benefits, burdens, and risks of accepting and foregoing the treatment. For example, if a form of medical treatment holds the uncertain prospect of extending life, but has a high degree of probability of being painful and debilitating, a patient might conclude that the possibility of benefit was simply not worth the burdens of treatment. Life-sustaining treatments that have been refused include ventilation, tube feeding,* resuscitation, dialysis, surgery, blood transfusions (usually for religious reasons), and antibiotics.

Second, competent patients may refuse life-sustaining treatment by executing a living will. A living will, usually authorized by state statute, is a written document that indicates the conditions under which a person refuses most or all forms of life-sustaining medical treatment or care. It becomes effective when a person loses the ability to make informed consent or informed refusal decisions regarding life-sustaining medical treatment. Living will statutes* usually require a determination of terminal illness or other irreversible life-threatening condition. Living wills usually state a preference to refuse all life-sustaining medical treatment with the exception of comfort care and sometimes the provision of appropriate nutrition and hydration. By contrast, some states (e.g., Indiana) and private organizations (e.g., National Right to Life Committee, Inc.*) have prepared life-prolonging procedures declarations or will-to-live forms. These forms state that the patient desires all reasonable life-sustaining procedures and provides space so that the patient may explicitly list any treatments they wish to refuse. All 50 states and the District of Columbia now have living will statutes. The circumstances under which life-sustaining treatment may be withdrawn and the nature of the treatment or care involved vary considerably among the states.

Third, competent patients may also execute a durable power of attorney for health care, a declaration by the patient that selects a person or persons to make health care decisions when they have become incompetent to make their own decisions. They may also contain instructions as to what life-sustaining medical treatments the patient wishes to receive or refuse. As of 1992, 32 states had durable power of attorney statutes.

In 1990, Congress enacted as part of the Omnibus Budget Reconciliation Act of 1990 the Patient Self Determination Act (PSDA). The PSDA requires health care providers to inform their patients upon admission to a health care facility about their right to accept or refuse medical or surgical treatment. The PSDA applies to any hospital, skilled nursing facility, home health care agency, hospice, and health maintenance organization that serves recipients of Medicare or Medicaid. These providers must document in every patient's medical records whether the patient has signed a living will or other advance directive. The PSDA also obligates the providers to follow applicable state law on advance directives.

If a patient is incompetent (e.g., unconscious, mentally retarded, or brain injured) and has not previously executed an advance directive, it may be necessary to petition a court for an order establishing a guardianship over the patient. That guardian would then be empowered to make health care decisions for the patient. Some states have laws providing for surrogate decision makers (e.g., spouse, adult child, parent, sibling, religious superior) for incompetent patients who have not executed an advance directive. Persons authorized by statute to make health care decisions for another would not be required to obtain a guardianship.

Four state interests have been identified by various state courts that may be asserted in opposition to a patient's refusal of life-sustaining medical treatment: (1) the preservation of life; (2) protecting the interests of third parties (e.g., dependent family members); (3) prevention of suicide; and (4) maintaining the ethical integrity of the medical profession where termination of treatment would violate a professional ethical standard. When any one of these qualified state interests is successfully asserted, a court may order a health care provider to continue care despite a patient's or patient representative's refusal of life-sustaining medical treatment.

The United States Supreme Court, in *Cruzan v. Missouri Dept. of Health* (1990), the only treatment refusal case to reach the nation's highest Court, held that no fundamental right to refuse life-sustaining medical treatment can be asserted by a third party (e.g., spouse or other family member, attorney in fact, or guardian). Instead, guardians and other decision makers have an affirmative duty to consent to life-sustaining medical care for their wards. Only two exceptions release the decision maker from this duty. First, the ward may have rejected the treatment in advance through a specific informed refusal (e.g., a living will). Or second, the ward is burdened by extreme pain from the treatment. The Supreme Court held that the existence of either of these exceptions must be proved by clear and convincing evidence before a court may authorize that such life-sustaining treatment be withheld.

REFERENCES: Avila, Daniel. 1993. "Medical Treatment Rights of Older Persons and Persons with Disabilities: 1991–92 Developments." *Issues in Law & Medicine* 8:429–66; Avila, Daniel. 1994. "Medical Treatment Rights of Older Persons and Persons with Disabilities: 1992–93 Developments." *Issues in Law & Medicine* 9:345–60; *In re Quinlan,* 70 N.J. 10, 335 A.2d 647, *cert. denied sub nom. Garzer v. New Jersey,* 429 U.S. 922 (1976); National Legal Center Staff. 1992. "Medical Treatment Rights of Older Persons and Persons with Disabilities: 1991 Developments." *Issues in Law & Medicine* 7:407–28; Patient Self Determination Act, 42 U.S.C. §§ 1395i-3 (c) (1) (E), 1395l (r),

1395cc (a) (1) (Q), 1395cc (f) (1), 1395bbb (a) (6), 1396 (m) (1) (A), 1396aa (a) (57) and (58), 1396a (w), and 1396r (c) (2) (E) (Supp. 1991); *Schloendorff v. Society of New York Hospital,* 211 N.Y. 125, 105 N.E. 92 (1914).

BARRY A. BOSTROM

REGULATORY CLEARANCE OF BIOPHARMACEUTICAL PRODUCTS

The U.S. Food and Drug Administration* in 1981 approved Eli Lilly's Humulin (human insulin), the first drug for human use that was manufactured via recombinant DNA technology. Nearly four years passed before Genentech's Protropin, a human growth hormone product for treating growth failure in children due to inadequate endogenous growth hormone secretion, became the second FDA-certified biopharmaceutical and the first marketed by one of the new "biotechnology" companies. The generally slow pace of FDA clearance of other human biopharmaceuticals—alpha interferon to treat Kaposi's sarcoma (1985), tissue plasminogen activator to counteract clotting associated with heart attack (1987), erythropoietin to promote replenishment of red blood cells in kidney dialysis patients (1989), interleukin-2 to treat metastatic renal cell carcinoma (1992), among others—prompted calls for reform that led in 1993 to the FDA's imposing a schedule of user fees, for funding of additional reviewers at the FDA's Center for Biologics Evaluation and Research (CBER), streamlining the certification process for biologics. The tremendous impact of the drug-regulatory scheme on the overall health of the U.S. biopharmaceutical sector was illustrated in 1993, when negative findings by FDA advisory groups undercut commercial prospects for Centocor, Xoma, and Synergen (all concerning monoclonal antibodies to combat sepsis) and for MedImmune (drug against respiratory syncytial virus).

REFERENCES: Shamel, Roger E. 1994. "Trends in Biopharmaceutical Product Development and Commercialization." *Genetic Engineering News* 14(1):6; Southerland, Daniel. "MedImmune Continues Slide After FDA Vote." *The Washington Post,* December 4, 1993, at C1; Sugawara, Sandra. "Centocor Tries to Dust Off Its Fallen 'Star': Biotech Firm's Future Is Threatened After FDA Demands More Tests on Premier Drug." *The Washington Post,* June 7, 1992, at H1.

STEPHEN A. BENT

REGULATORY CONTEXT OF WORKPLACE HAZARDS

Reproductive hazards in the workplace potentially can be regulated by a variety of federal agencies. Part of the regulatory confusion today results from jurisdictional conflict among these agencies. There are three appropriate sources of regulation: the Occupational Safety and Health Act (OSH Act), the Toxic Substances Control Act (TSCA), and Title VII of the Civil Rights Act.

The OSH Act was passed in 1970 in response to the black lung disease movement and pressure from labor unions for protection from workplace hazards. The purpose of the OSH Act is "to assure so far as possible every working man and woman in the Nation safe and healthful working conditions'' (29 U.S.C. Sec. 6516, 970). The OSH Act gives the secretary of labor various mechanisms for regulating workplace safety and health including a broad general duty clause that provides that each employer ''shall furnish to each of his employees employment and a place of employment which are free from recognized hazards that are causing or are likely to cause death or serious physical harm to his employees'' (29 U.S.C. Sec. 654 [1]).

In 1978, the Occupational Safety and Health Administration (OSHA) promulgated the lead standard, which, among other things, called for periodic blood tests for all workers exposed to lead, required medical removal of workers found to have blood lead levels exceeding standard acceptable levels, and mandated job protection with full pay and benefits upon removal for up to 18 months (29 C.F.R. 1910. 1025, 1984). Importantly, OSHA expressly rejected the notion that its lead standard should be different for men and women. Despite this clear statement, the Lead Industries Association, which represented all industries affected by the lead standard, continued to support only the exclusion of fertile women. Furthermore, it filed a lawsuit against OSHA challenging its rule-making procedures, the substantive provisions of the standard, and the evidence used to frame the standard. It charged that the lead standard was set too low and that OSHA had exceeded its statutory authority in adopting the medical removal requirement.

In 1980, OSHA reiterated its view that all exclusionary policies such as the Fetal Protection Policies (FPPs) imposed against pregnant women undermine the principle that the workplace should be a safe environment for all persons. Instead of discriminating against women of childbearing age or coercing them into ending their fertility, exposure standards should be set that recognize such vulnerability. In other words, OSHA argued that high-risk industries should not be able to reduce their liability for damage awards by excluding classes of workers. Moreover, no worker should be forced to sacrifice her reproductive right to privacy in order to hold her job. OSHA became embroiled in the case involving American Cyanamid's exclusionary policy that resulted in five women being sterilized at the Willow Island, West Virginia, plant in order to keep their jobs. After considerable administrative litigation, in April 1981, the Occupational Safety and Health Review Commission dismissed OSHA's citation against American Cyanamid's Fetus Protection Policy, concluding that as a matter of law the hazard alleged by the secretary was not intended by Congress to be included under the OSH Act.

The case eventually ended up in federal court (*Oil, Chemical and Atomic Workers v. American Cyanamid Co.,* 1984) and was heard by the Circuit Court for the District of Columbia. Although the court admitted that the women who were sterilized in order to keep their jobs at the Willow Island plant ''were put to a most unhappy choice'' (at 450), it held that the ''language of [OSHA] cannot be stretched so far as to hold that the sterilization option of the fetus protection policy is a 'hazard' of 'employment' under the general duty clause'' (at 445). Furthermore, it stated that "the general duty clause does not apply to a policy as contrasted with a physical condition of the workplace" (at 448).

Although OSHA has authority under the OSH Act to set and enforce standards, perform inspections, and monitor industry compliance, court-imposed restrictions along with political interference and perennial staffing and funding shortfalls have limited OSHA's effectiveness. For instance, it has been stripped of its power to make surprise inspections and must obtain a court order to investigate a complaint. Moreover, OSHA itself has stated that inconclusive scientific evidence and its lack of jurisdiction over protection of the fetus make the agency's limited role in that area appropriate (OSHA, 1987).

The Equal Employment Opportunity Commission (EEOC) was created as the administrative agency to enforce the provisions of Title VII, the primary basis for federal court actions on sex discrimination in the workplace. The EEOC has 90 days to act on any complaint of discrimination. It can investigate and either dismiss the complaint or find cause for the complaint and then attempt to conciliate between the parties. If the employer cannot or will not settle the case, the claimant has a right to sue in federal court. In theory, then, the OSH Act and the EEOC acting under Title VII together should be able to mandate a safe and healthy workplace for all employees without discrimination. Like OSHA, however, the EEOC has not taken a vigorous role in the debate over FPPs.

According to a majority staff report of the House Committee on Education and Labor (1990), the EEOC abdicated its enforcement responsibilities during the 1980s in terms of both individual case handling and interpretive guidance. The EEOC's decision, under Chairman Clarence Thomas, not to make a determination for complaints of discrimination resulting from FPPs represented an "entombment" of charges and helped keep exclusionary policies off the public agenda for a decade (Committee, 1990, 10). Although the commission made attempts to resolve these charges in 1989, most of the cases closed were "resolved" for administrative reasons, such as a failure to locate the claimant, rather than on the merits. Over 100 charges were filed with the EEOC, and most challenged employer practices and policies that were facially discriminatory. The rationale given by EEOC was that it was unable to resolve these complex charges on a case-by-case basis because it lacked a comprehensive policy directive. According to the majority staff report, however, the failure to establish a comprehensive policy directive was of the EEOC's own doing (Committee, 1990, 17).

In 1988, the EEOC issued its first policy guidance on reproductive and fetal hazards. The policy guidance declared that any practice that denies employment opportunities to one sex because of reproductive or fetal hazard, without similarly barring the other sex, is unlawful under Title VII. The EEOC, however, recognized the application of the less stringent business necessity defense in fetal liability cases, although it stated that employers invoking the defense must demonstrate that there is a substantial risk of harm to the fetus, that the risk is transmitted only through women, and that there are no less restrictive alternatives to excluding women from the workplace. Any such denial of employment must be justified by objective, scientific evidence, which the EEOC recognized as difficult given the inconclusiveness of much of the research on fetal hazards.

In January 1990, the EEOC published additional policy guidance in reaction to the Seventh Circuit Court's decision in *Johnson Controls* (see *United Auto Workers v. Johnson Controls*). The EEOC rejected the court's finding for placing the burden of proof on the employee. Because fetal protection cases involve facially discriminatory policies, the burden of proof must be on the employer to prove that its policy is a business necessity rather than on the plaintiff to prove that it is not. Moreover, the commission found that the significantly more narrow bona fide occupational qualification (BFOQ) is a better approach than business necessity to Fetal Protection Policies. Therefore, in cases it handled after 1990, the EEOC required employers to prove that protection of fetuses from risk is reasonably necessary to the normal operation of their businesses and that the exclusionary policy is reasonably necessary to implement the protections.

A third regulatory strategy would be to use Environmental Protection Agency (EPA) powers under the Toxic Substances Control Act to regulate fetal hazards in the workplace. TSCA is a comprehensive statute that deals exclusively with toxicants. It provides a mechanism for the systematic testing of potential toxicants to determine whether they present a risk of injury to human health or the environment and provides a means to control the production or use of those substances that present an unreasonable risk of injury. TSCA requires chemical producers, processors, and distributors to report to the EPA all information that indicates that a substance presents a substantial risk. Moreover, the statutory threshold for triggering EPA action is low in that the information need only indicate that there "may be a reasonable basis" to conclude the toxin is hazardous (15 U.S.C. Sec. 2603 [f2]). Despite the clear intention of Congress that TSCA be used to regulate reproductive hazards, the EPA has not generally exercised its authority to control suspected teratogens or mutagens.

REFERENCES: Blank, Robert H. 1993. *Fetal Protection in the Workplace: Women's Rights, Business Interests and the Unborn.* New York: Columbia University Press; Equal Employment Opportunity Commission. 1988. "Policy Guidance on Reproductive and Fetal Hazards." 193 *Daily Labor Report* D-1; Maschke, Karen J. 1993. "From the Workplace to the Delivery Room: Protecting the Fetus in the Post-*Roe* Era." *Politics and the Life Sciences* 12(1): 53–60; Occupational Safety and Health Administration (OSHA). 1987. "Federal Response or Legal Recourse Limited on Issue of Reproductive Hazards in the Workplace." 123 *Daily Labor Report* (BNA) A-11; *Oil, Chemical and Atomic Workers v. American Cyanamid Co.,* 741 F.2d 444 (D.C. Cir. 1984); OSHA. 1990. 18 *Daily Labor Report* (BNA) D-1; Samuels, Suzanne U. 1993. "To Furnish a Workplace Free from Recognized Hazards: OSHA, State Occupational Safety and Health Agencies." *Politics and the Life Sciences* 12(2): 243–54; U.S., Congress, House Committee on Education and Labor. 1990. *A Report on the EEOC, Title VII and Workplace Fetal Protection Policies in the 1980s.* Washington, D.C.: Government Printing Office.

See also **UNITED AUTO WORKERS V. JOHNSON CONTROLS.**

ROBERT H. BLANK

REPRODUCTIVE-ASSISTING SERVICES: INSURANCE COVERAGE

There are no comprehensive data on the proportion of assisted reproduction costs paid out of pocket as compared to that reimbursed by private insurers, but an increasing number of carriers provide routine coverage for in vitro fertilization (IVF) and other reproductive-aiding treatment if it is medically indicated (Toth, Washington, and Davies, 1987). For instance, employees under Blue Cross/Blue Shield in Delaware have an option to purchase IVF coverage (no minimum waiting period, $24,000 lifetime maximum). Furthermore, the Prudential medical insurance programs nationwide recognize infertility as an illness and routinely cover virtually all related services, including artificial insemination—husband (AIH) and IVF, as long as the services conform to American College of Obstetricians and Gynecologists (ACOG) standards and are determined to be medically necessary. Many group insurance plans, however, do not cover IVF, usually on grounds that it is experimental. This inconsistency in coverage of IVF from one plan to the next has led to efforts by groups to lobby for state legislation that mandates third-party coverage.

To date, the courts have given mixed signals regarding insurance coverage. In *Witcraft v. Sundstrand Health and Disability Group Benefit Plan* (1988), for instance, the Iowa Supreme Court held that the dysfunctioning of the insured's reproductive organs was an illness. Since the plan covered "expenses relating to" illness, the court held the claim for IVF expenses valid. Also see *Egert v. Connecticut General Life Insurance* (1990) where the claim was withheld. In *Kinzie v. Physician's Liability Insurance Company* (1987), however, an Oklahoma appellate court denied recovery on grounds that IVF is elective and was not required to cure or preserve the insured's health. Moreover, the court did not deem it medically necessary to a woman's health to give birth to a child.

At least six states (Arkansas, Connecticut, Hawaii, Maryland, Massachusetts, and Texas) have adopted legislation mandating insurance carriers operating in their states to either provide coverage for IVF and related services or to offer such a package. Massachusetts, for example, enacted legislation (Act H. 3721, 1987) that requires all insurance plans that cover pregnancy-related benefits provide coverage for medically indicated expenses of diagnosis and treatment of infertility to the same extent that benefits are provided for other pregnancy-related procedures. Under the regulations promulgated under this act and in effect as of January 6, 1988, insurers must provide benefits for all nonexperimental infertility procedures (211 C.M.R. 37.01–37.11). These include, but are not limited to, artificial insemination (AI), IVF, and other procedures recognized as nonexperimental by the American Fertility Society (AFS) or other infertility experts recognized by the State Commissioner of Insurance. Surrogacy, reversal of voluntary sterilization, and procurement of donor eggs and sperm are specifically excluded from coverage in the regulations. The insurers may establish reasonable eligibility requirements, which are to be made available to the insured.

Despite this legislative activity, most states have no policy concerning third-party coverage for assisted reproduction services. In the absence of state mandates, the majority of health insurance plans and health maintenance organizations (HMOs) specifically exclude coverage for IVF. Its potentially high cost and its low success rate, combined with its perception as a procedure of uncertain benefit to the few at the expense of many, continues to deter many insurers from entering this market.

Although expansion of insurance coverage for fertility treatment will expand accessibility, for those women without insurance, such steps will be futile. There is little evidence that Medicaid recipients or the millions of women without health insurance will have access to IVF even though, on average, poor women have a higher prevalence of infertility than middle-class women. Whatever happens with private insurance, there has been little activity by the states or by Congress to fund assisted reproduction and is unlikely to be so in times of continued budget scarcity.

REFERENCES: *Egert v. Connecticut General Life Insurance,* 900 F.2d 1032 (7th Cir. 1990); Ingram, John Dwight. 1993. ''Should In Vitro Fertilization Be Covered by Medical Expense Reimbursement Plans?'' *American Journal of Family Law* 7: 103–108; *Kinzie v. Physician's Liability Insurance Company,* 750 P.2d 1140 (Okla. Ct. App. 1987); Toth C., D. Washington, and O. Davies. 1987. ''Reimbursement for In Vitro Fertilization: A Survey of HIAA Companies.'' *Research and Statistical Bulletin.* Washington, D.C.: Health Insurance Association of America; *Witcraft v. Sundstrand Health and Disability Group Benefit Plan,* 420 N.W.2d 785 (Iowa 1988).

See also **IN VITRO FERTILIZATION (IVF); REPRODUCTIVE TECHNOLOGIES: REGULATIONS AND GUIDELINES.**

ROBERT H. BLANK

REPRODUCTIVE TECHNOLOGIES: REGULATIONS AND GUIDELINES

The proliferation of reproductive-assisting services, the trend toward commercialization of these services, and the potential conflicts among the many parties to these new reproduction methods raise concerns over regulation. Largely, the issues surrounding these innovations have been handled by case law only when legal conflicts, primarily over custody, have arisen. Although Congress has held many hearings on reproductive-assisting technologies, they have not led to a national policy.

In 1987 and 1988, four separate House subcommittees held preliminary hearings on various aspects of reproductive technology. The Select Committee on Children, Youth, and Families took testimony from a wide range of experts on reproductive technology to explore the medical, legal, and ethical issues, with a particular focus on their implications for children and families. Also in 1987, the Subcommittee on Civil Service held hearings on the Federal Employee Family-Building Act (H.R. 2852), which would address inequities in access to reproductive technology by requiring all insurance carriers offering obstetric coverage under the federal employee health benefits program to provide benefits for "family-building" procedures, including in vitro fertilization (IVF).* With a similar focus, the Subcommittee on Human Resources and Intergovernmental Relations of the House Committee on Government Operations began hearings on the federal role in the prevention and treatment of infertility and the effects of the roadblock on funding IVF research and infertility services.

The hearings on consumer protection issues involving IVF clinics, held by the Subcommittee on Regulation and Business Opportunities of the House Committee on Small Business, hold the most promise of eventual action to address specifically the question of regulation. These hearings were motivated by Chairman Wyden's (D. Ore.) concern with the lack of adequate state regulation. Due to the de facto moratorium on federal funding of IVF research, and the resulting lack of accountability and control that normally accompany it, Congressman Wyden felt that some effort to institute federal oversight is necessary. The hearings emphasized two areas of essential action: dissemination of information to consumers and regulation.

Similarly, interest in the regulation of donor insemination (DI) services was sparked by an Office of Technology Assessment (1988) report that showed that many practitioners were doing little to protect recipients from genetic disorders or infectious diseases. In introducing the report, Senator Albert Gore (D. Tenn.) stated that "it is appalling that something as basic and essential as testing anonymous donors for the AIDs virus is not routinely done." He warned that if the Food and Drug Administration* did not take appropriate steps to regulate screening and testing of donor semen, Congress would. Senator Gore introduced a bill to establish a national data bank to store the medical and genetic history of all donors. In addition to ensuring that children of DI have access to these data, the national registry could function to monitor the frequency of the use of each donor and regulate DI services.

Despite this appearance on the national agenda in the late 1980s, regulation of infertility services, such that it is, has largely rested in the states through their authority to protect the health and their power to regulate familial relations, medical practice, licensing health personnel and facilities, and contracts. As a result, regulation of assisted reproductive services is inconsistent and at times contradictory from one state to the next. Although statutes have helped clarify the legal landscape of DI in some states, many state legislatures have yet to address even the basic issues concerning screening requirements, the legal status of the various parties, and questions of access both to the services and to information.

As one moves from DI that has been practiced for a century to more recent and provocative innovations such as IVF and gamete intrafallopian transfer (GIFT), statutory regulation becomes more scarce. Of the current laws, most only indirectly affect IVF. Several statutes (i.e., Pennsylvania) have recordkeeping and reporting provisions but largely defer to professional guidelines of the American Fertility Society (AFS) and the American College of Obstetricians and Gynecologists (ACOG).

In many ways, public policymakers have deferred to professional organizations to develop and apply guidelines for assisted reproductive services. The two most active organizations on promulgating relevant standards of practice are the AFS and the American Association of Tissue Banks (AATB). Since 1986, the AFS has prepared sets of ethical guidelines for governing these technologies, issued position papers on insurance coverage of infertility services, and published revised procedures for conducting DI, IVF, GIFT, and other relevant services. Most recently, it has published guidelines for therapeutic donor insemination, oocyte donation, and minimal genetic screening for gamete donors.

Although the standards promulgated by professional organizations are valuable and provide some control over the use of these technologies, the problem with guidelines as opposed to regulations is that there is no legal authority behind the guidelines to ensure compliance. Instead of force of law, association guidelines rely on creditation privileges and ethical sanctions. There is little to stop the establishment of nonsanctioned cryobanks,* fertility clinics, or DI/IVF/ GIFT services. Although lack of compliance by nonmember businesses carries some risk, in the emerging lucrative commercial fertility industry, voluntary guidelines alone might not be sufficient to protect all parties. One strategy for the states is to restrict practice of these services to those facilities that comply with AFS/ACOG/AATB guidelines along the lines of the 1986 Louisiana statute. Another strategy would be to use these guidelines as a framework for shaping public policy.

To date, the United States has not moved toward establishing a national policy on reproductive technologies and is unlikely to do so. The United Kingdom's Statutory Licensing Authority, which regulates reproductive services, might serve as a useful regulatory model for consideration. Also, the extensive reports of the Canadian Royal Commission on New Reproductive Technologies provide a valuable framework for establishing a regulatory framework.

REFERENCES: American Fertility Society. 1993. "Guidelines for Therapeutic Donor Insemination: Sperm." *Fertility and Sterility* 59(2): 1s–4s; American Fertility Society. 1993. "Minimum Genetic Screening for Gamete Donors." *Fertility and Sterility* 59(2): 95; Blank, Robert H. 1990. *Regulating Reproduction.* New York: Columbia University Press; Bonnicksen, Andrea L. 1992. "Human Embryos and Genetic Testing: A Private Policy Model." *Politics and the Life Sciences* 11(1): 53–62; Canadian Royal Commission on New Reproductive Technologies. 1993. *Proceed with Care.* Ottawa: Minister of Government Services; Gunning, Jennifer, and Veronica English. 1993. *Human In Vitro Fertilization: A Case Study in the Regulation of Medical Intervention.* Aldershot, England: Dartmouth Publishing Company, Ltd.; Office of Technology/Assessment. 1988. *Infertility: Medical and Social Choices.* Washington, D.C.: Government Printing Office.

ROBERT H. BLANK

ROE V. WADE

In March 1970, "Jane Roe," an unmarried pregnant woman who wished to terminate her pregnancy, challenged the Texas criminal abortion statutes, which prohibited abortions except "an abortion procured or attempted by medical advice for the purpose of saving the life of the mother." Filing in the U.S. District Court for the Northern District of Texas on behalf of herself and other women similarly situated, Jane Roe (a pseudonym) asserted that the law was unconstitutional under the First, Fourth, Fifth, Ninth, and Fourteenth Amendments to the U.S. Constitution. Later that year, the district court held that because the challenged law was vague and overbroad, it violated the Ninth and Fourteenth Amendments. Specifically, the court found that the "fundamental right of single women and married persons to choose whether to have children is protected by the Ninth Amendment, through the Fourteenth Amendment." This decision was then appealed directly to the U.S. Supreme Court, which heard arguments twice, in December 1971 and October 1972, before issuing its decision on January 22, 1973 (410 U.S. 113).

In a 7–2 opinion written by Justice Harry Blackmun, the Supreme Court recognized for the first time that the fundamental right to privacy encompasses a woman's right to terminate a pregnancy. Although no explicit "right to privacy" exists within the text of the U.S. Constitution, the Court has long held that such a fundamental right protects citizens against governmental intrusion in such intimate family matters as procreation, childrearing, marriage, and contraceptive choice. In striking down the Texas abortion prohibition, the Court extended this "zone of privacy" to encompass a woman's right to decide whether to bear children, viewing this right as arising from its previous decisions.

Moreover, the recognition of this right as fundamental meant that laws or regulations that interfere with reproductive decisions must be judged under the "strict scrutiny" standard. Under this legal test, the challenged measure can be justified only if the government can prove a "compelling interest"—the most important of the reasons the government can give for interfering with a person's liberty. Second, the measure must be designed to achieve only the legitimate interest(s) asserted by the state. In the abortion context, the Court found that the state's interests included maintaining proper medical standards, protecting the life and health of the pregnant woman, and protecting potential life. However, these interests become "compelling" at different points during the pregnancy.

The majority explicitly refused to recognize the fetus as a "person" for the purposes of the Fourteenth Amendment, which includes a guarantee that no person shall be deprived of "life" without "due process of law." Moreover, the Court rejected the state's argument that its adoption of the view that life begins at conception justified the prohibition on abortion. Nonetheless, the majority opinion acknowledged the need to strike a balance between a pregnant woman's right to privacy and the state's interests in potential human life. To this end, the Court established a framework under which the state's interest in potential life did not become "compelling" until after the point of viability— the point in pregnancy when the fetus is capable of independent survival, usually between the twenty-fourth and twenty-eighth week of gestation. During the first trimester of pregnancy, "the attending physician, in consultation with his patient, is free to determine, without regulation by the State, that, in his medical judgment, the patient's pregnancy should be terminated." After the first trimester but prior to viability, a state could only impose restrictions on abortion if the measures were necessary to protect a woman's health and were the least restrictive means of doing so. Even after viability, the Court found that the state's compelling interest in protecting potential life could not be promoted at the expense of a woman's life or health.

Roe was decided along with *Doe v. Bolton,* 410 U.S. 179 (1972), a challenge to a Georgia statute that criminalized abortions except when a pregnancy would endanger the woman's life or "seriously and permanently injure her health," the fetus would "very likely be born with grave, permanent, and irremediable mental or physical defect," or the pregnancy was the result of rape. The abortion could only be performed in a hospital after a number of other requirements had been met, including written certification of the extenuating circumstances by at least three physicians and prior approval of a hospital committee. In a 7–2 opinion issued with *Roe,* the Court found the Georgia law to be unconstitutional but recognized that the right to choose abortion is not "absolute." Specifically, in affirming a lower court decision striking down the certification requirements, the Court held that the physician's best medical judgment concerning the necessity of an abortion includes "all factors—physical, emotional, psychological, familial, and the woman's age—relevant to the well-being of the patient."

Immediately following the decisions in *Roe* and *Doe,* abortion opponents pressured state legislatures and the federal government to impose restrictions on the provision of abortion services. These individuals and organizations hoped to chip away at the right to privacy through the political process with an end goal of eliminating the legal right through court action. From the mid-1970s to the mid-1980s, legal advocates for women were forced to challenge restrictive state laws, ultimately seeking review by the U.S. Supreme Court. Finding that certain laws imposed unconstitutional limitations on a woman's right to privacy, the Court struck down:

- Husband consent for a married woman's abortion (*Planned Parenthood v. Danforth,* 428 U.S. 52 [1976]);

- Requirements that a woman receive from her physician state-approved information discouraging abortion and that the procedure be delayed at least 24 hours (*City of*

Akron v. Akron Center for Reproductive Health, 462 U.S. 416 [1983] and *Thornburgh v. American College of Obstetricians & Gynecologists,* 476 U.S. 747 [1986]);

• Filing of detailed reports on all abortions performed (*Thornburgh v. American College of Obstetricians & Gynecologists,* 476 U.S. 747 [1986]);

• Mandating that post-first-trimester abortions be performed only in hospitals (*City of Akron v. Akron Center for Reproductive Health,* 462 U.S. 416 [1983]);

• Requiring that the fetus's life and health be preserved at all stages of pregnancy and prohibiting a commonly used method of second-trimester abortion (*Planned Parenthood v. Danforth,* 428 U.S. 52 [1976]);

• Requiring the use of techniques most likely to result in a live birth when a fetus is or may be viable (*Colautti v. Franklin,* 439 U.S. 379 [1979]);

• Mandating that a physician performing a postviability abortion use the method most likely to preserve the life of the fetus, and have a second physician present to "save" the fetus (*Thornburgh v. American College of Obstetricians & Gynecologists,* 476 U.S. 747 [1986]).

During the same period, however, decisions by the Supreme Court began to erode the right to choose for low-income women (see *Harris v. McRae,** 448 U.S. 297 [1980]) and young women (see *Hodgson v. Minnesota,** 497 U.S. 417 [1990]). By the late 1980s and early 1990s, as evidenced in its decisions in *Webster v. Reproductive Health Services,** 492 U.S. 490 (1989), and *Planned Parenthood v. Casey,** 112 S. Ct. 2791 (1992), the Court turned away from *Roe*'s fundamental protection for the abortion choice for adult women, adopting a less protective standard for measuring the constitutionality of abortion laws.

REFERENCES: Bonavoglia, Angela. 1991. *The Choices We Made.* New York: Random House; Cates, Williard, Jr., and Rochat, Roger W. 1976. "Illegal Abortions in the United States: 1972–1974." 8 *Family Planning Perspective 86;* Davis, Flora. 1991. *Moving the Mountain: The Women's Movement in America Since 1960.* New York: Simon & Schuster; Faux, Marian. 1988. *Roe v. Wade: The Untold Story of the Landmark Supreme Court Decision that Made Abortion Legal.* New York: New American Library; Garrow, David J. 1994. *Liberty and Sexuality: The Right to Privacy and the Making of Roe v. Wade.* New York: Macmillan; Luker, Kristen. 1984. *Abortion and the Politics of Motherhood.* Berkeley: University of California Press; Miller, Patricia G. 1993. *The Worst of Times.* New York: HarperCollins; Mohr, James. 1978. *Abortion in America: The Origins and Evolution of National Policy, 1800–1900.* New York: Oxford University Press; Polgar, Steven, and Fried, Ellen S. 1976. "The Bad Old Days: Clandestine Abortions Among the Poor in New York City Before Liberalization of the Abortion Law." 3 *Family Planning Perspective* 125; Weddington, Sarah. 1992. *A Question of Choice.* New York: G. P. Putnam's Sons.

ANDREA MILLER

RU-486

RU-486 (Mifepristone) was developed in 1980 by Dr. Etienne-Emile Baulieu for the French pharmaceutical company Roussel Uclaf. Original efficacy for inducing early abortions averaged 80 to 85 percent. In 1984, RU-486 was tested in combination with Sulprostone, an intramuscular prostaglandin, and efficacy increased to greater than 95 percent, which compared favorably with surgical abortions performed during the earliest weeks of pregnancy. In 1988, RU-486, in combination with Sulprostone, was approved for use in France as an abortifacient. In 1991, approval was given to use RU-486 in combination with an oral prostaglandin, Misoprostol, which made the process simpler and safer. To date, over 100,000 women in 20 countries have used RU-486 for voluntary terminations of pregnancy.

RU-486 provides women with the option of a nonsurgical means of terminating an unwanted pregnancy. This eliminates the risks related to surgery, including anesthetic complications, cervical damage, perforation, and infection. It can be administered to a woman as soon as she knows that she is pregnant and wants to have an abortion and is currently being administered through the ninth week of pregnancy. Studies have found that the blood loss and pain from an RU-486 abortion are no greater than from a surgical abortion.

The major disadvantages of RU-486 include incomplete abortion in 2 to 3 percent of cases and noninterruption of pregnancy in 1 percent of cases. These women then require follow-up surgical abortions. About 1 percent of women experience heavy bleeding that requires further treatment. Another drawback to RU-486 is its administration. Currently, a woman must be screened by her physician to determine if there are any contraindications to the use of RU-486. If not, she is given tablets that she must take in the presence of the health care providers. (In those countries in which there is a waiting period, the woman must leave and return for the tablets after the waiting period has expired.) Two days later, the woman returns to receive the prostaglandin. (Now that the prostaglandin is in tablet form, a woman should be able to receive both pills at the initial visit and be instructed when to take the progesterone tablets. To date, women are being required to get the tablets at separate visits for closer medical supervision.) A final appointment is required several days later to ensure that the abortion is complete. Bleeding may last 7 to 12 days.

There have been three reported significant cardiovascular complications including one death reported following RU-486. All three patients received Sulprostone, which is known to have cardiovascular effects even when given separately from RU-486. No serious cardiovascular complications have been reported with Misoprostol, which has been used for other purposes as well. The safety of RU-486 compares favorably with other forms of abortions and with childbirth itself.

Minor side effects from RU-486 include bleeding, abdominal pain, and cramping. The change in prostaglandins has reduced significantly the side effects attributed to the prostaglandins, including nausea, vomiting, and diarrhea.

In addition to its role as an abortifacient, RU-486 has other potential uses including the control of Cushing's syndrome, the treatment of meningiomas, certain breast cancers, endometriosis, and fibroids and its use as a form of postcoital contraception. It is also being tested as an adjuvant treatment to difficult deliveries as a way to avoid cesarean sections and to treat certain other conditions that may be hormonally sensitive, including eating disorders, osteoporosis, and certain types of glaucoma.

Introduction of RU-486 into the United States has been full of obstacles. In June 1989, RU-486 was placed on an "import alert" list, meaning that it could not be brought into this country for personal use. The ban was challenged in court by Leona Benten in July 1992 but was not invalidated (*Benten v. Kessler*, 1992). Roussel chose not to apply to the Food and Drug Administration (FDA) for licensure because of protests and threats of boycotts against Roussel and its German parent company, Hoechst A.G. Instead, in April 1993, Roussel agreed to grant a license to Population Council, a nonprofit U.S. organization that would select a U.S. manufacturer for Mifepristone, sponsor an application to the FDA, and manage a large clinical trial. It took over a year to work out the licensure details. Finally, in October 1994, Population Council began testing RU-486 in various sites. The tests are likely to continue through mid-1995, after which Population Council will seek final FDA approval (Lewin, 1995, A1).

REFERENCES: Baulieu, Etienne-Emile. 1989. "RU-486 as an Antiprogesterone Steroid." *Journal of the American Medical Association* 262(13): 1808–14; *Benten v. Kessler*, 112 S. Ct. 2929 (1992); Klitsch, Michael. 1991. "Antiprogestins and the Abortion Controversy: A Progress Report." *Family Planning Perspectives* 23(6): 275–82; Lewin, Tamar. 1995. "Clinical Trials Giving Glimpses of Abortion Pill." *The New York Times*, January 30, 1995, A1, A11; a special 1992 issue of the *Journal of Law, Medicine, and Health Care* (now *Journal of Law, Medicine and Ethics*) was devoted to RU-486: *Antiprogestin Drugs: Ethical, Legal, and Medical Issues* 20(3).

LAINIE FRIEDMAN ROSS

RUST V. SULLIVAN

Several New York–area family planning providers filed two suits in February 1988 to prevent enforcement of newly promulgated regulations restricting the actions of grantees receiving family planning funds under Title X of the Public Health Service Act. The regulations at issue prohibit recipients from providing counseling about or referrals for abortions and from engaging in activities that "encourage, promote or advocate abortion as a method of family planning"; grantees that provided abortions with nonfederal funds were also required to keep these activities "physically and financially separate" from their Title X project. Plaintiffs asserted that the measures, dubbed the "gag rule," violated the First Amendment rights of health care providers and patients, restricted a woman's right to privacy in violation of the Fifth Amendment, and did not comport with the language or history of the Title X program. One month later, the U.S. District Court for the Southern District of New York granted a preliminary injunction against the restrictions. However, in June of the same year, the court granted a summary judgment request by the Department of Health and Human Services (HHS) and dismissed the case. Plaintiffs appealed to the U.S. Court of Appeals for the Second Circuit, which ruled in 1989. In its opinion, the appellate court deferred to the HHS interpretation of the Title X statute and went on to find that the new regulations did not impermissibly infringe on the fundamental rights of speech or privacy.

In a 5–4 decision on May 23, 1991 (500 U.S. 173), the U.S. Supreme Court upheld the regulations, finding that they violated neither the language of the federal statute authorizing Title X nor the U.S. Constitution's guarantees of freedom of speech and the right to privacy. Specifically, the majority held that the ban on speech about abortion does not constitute viewpoint discrimination or impinge upon the doctor-patient relationship. The Court stated that "the government is exercising the authority it possesses . . . to subsidize family planning services which will lead to conception and childbirth, and declining to 'promote or encourage abortion.' " Echoing its rulings in the context of abortion coverage under Medicaid (see *Harris v. McRae**), the Court asserted that "the difficulty that a woman encounters when a Title X project does not provide abortion counseling or referral leaves her in no different position . . . [and] with the same choices as if the government had chosen not to fund family planning services at all."

ANDREA MILLER

S

SELECTIVE TERMINATION OF MULTIPLE FETUSES

Selective termination is a prenatal intervention to reduce the number of fetuses in a pregnancy. Usually it entails an injection of potassium chloride into the heart of the fetus (or fetuses) to be killed. In some cases, selective termination has been carried out in multiple pregnancies where one of the fetuses has been diagnosed through ultrasound as abnormal. More frequently, it is used in the first trimester to reduce the number of fetuses a woman is carrying in order to reduce the risk of preterm delivery to the woman and the remaining fetuses.

One of the risks of fertility drugs to induce ovulation and transfers of multiple embryos in in vitro fertilization (IVF) is the heightened probability of gestations with three or more fetuses. In one study, for instance, at the time of the procedure, 88 women had triplets, 89 had quadruplets, 16 had quintuplets, and 7 had from six to nine fetuses. These pregnancies were reduced to 189 sets of twins, 5 sets of triplets, and 6 single births, with no increase in the incidence of intrauterine growth retardation over that anticipated in a population of twins (Berkowitz et al., 1993). Although selective termination has been shown to be effective in reducing maternal risk and risk to the surviving infants, because it does so by selectively aborting fetuses, it is inextricably linked to the continuing controversy over abortion.

REFERENCES: Berkowitz, R. L., Lauren Lynch, Robert Lapinski, and Paul Bergh. 1993. "First-Trimester Transabdominal Multifetal Pregnancy Reduction: A Report of Two Hundred Completed Cases." *American Journal of Obstetrics and Gynecology* 169: 17–21; Callahan, Tamara L., Janet E. Hall, Susan L. Ettner, et al. 1994. "The Economic Impact of Multiple-Gestation Pregnancies and the Contribution of Assisted-Reproduction Techniques to Their Incidence." *New England Journal of Medicine* 33(4): 244–249; Luke, Barbara. 1994. "The Changing Pattern of Multiple Births in the United States: Maternal and Infant Characteristics, 1973 and 1990." *Obstetrics and Gynecology* 84(1): 101–106; Nijs, Marine, et al. 1993. "Prevention of Multiple Pregnancies in an In Vitro

Fertilization Program." *Fertility and Sterility* 59(6): 1245–1250; Zaner, R. M., and M. D. Fox. 1993. "Selective Termination and Moral Risk: Choices and Responsibility." In R. H. Blank and A. L. Bonnicksen, eds., *Emerging Issues in Biomedical Policy.* Vol. 2. New York: Columbia University Press.

See also **IN VITRO FERTILIZATION (IVF); PRENATAL DIAGNOSIS.**

ROBERT H. BLANK

SEX PRESELECTION

There has long been interest in preselecting the sex of one's progeny and use of a wide variety of nonscientific approaches. In recent years, techniques have been developed that allow for increasingly reliable means of achieving this goal. Although preference for a particular gender is less clear in the United States than in many other countries, the availability of sex preselection techniques combined with the trend toward one- and two-child families will undoubtedly produce a broad demand. Data also indicate a preference for a son as the first-born and a daughter as the second in two-children families.

Although estimates vary as to when sex preselection will become widely available for humans, sex selection kits already have been marketed in the United States in 1986 by Pro-Care Industries, Ltd., under the name Gender Choice. These "child-selection kits" sold for $49.95 and contained directions, thermometers, and paraphernalia for monitoring vaginal mucus. The kits, available in pink and blue, were withdrawn in 1987 when the Food and Drug Administration* (FDA) declared that some of the implied claims on the packages and advertisements had not been substantiated.

The approaches that appear to offer the best chances of success in human application at present are based on the fact that each sperm cell carries either an X chromosome or a Y chromosome and that sex of the progeny is determined by which type of sperm fertilizes the egg. The goal of sex preselection is to control which type of sperm fertilizes a particular egg. To aid reaching this objective, some recently discovered characteristics of these two types of sperm are invaluable. First, in any male ejaculation there are more Y-bearing sperm than X-bearing sperm. In addition to being more numerous, Y-bearing sperm are smaller and less dense and move faster than their X-bearing counterparts. Conversely, the Y-bearing sperm die sooner and are more readily slowed down by normal acidic secretions of the vagina. However, they are less inhibited than the X-bearing sperm by the alkaline environment of the uterus, once past the vagina.

With this new knowledge about the characteristics of sperm, most sex preselection research is aimed at developing accurate and reliable sperm separation techniques. Techniques currently being used to do this include various sedimentation processes, centrifugation, and electrophoresis. Once the desired sperm concentrations are isolated, they are inseminated into the recipient woman's uterus using artificial insemination* techniques. Gametrics Ltd franchised an albumin density gradient method patented by Ronald Ericsson, based on the assumption that Y-bearing sperm swim faster than X-bearing. Gametrics Ltd reports that its franchised centers have a success rate of 86 percent for male selection and 74 percent for female selection.

At least 70 clinics in the United States currently are using variations of the sperm separation procedure to select sex-specific sperm. Although most fertility clinics are primarily experienced in choosing Y-bearing or male-producing sperm, several are working with both sex chromosomes. Furthermore, a 1988 survey found that 14 percent of donor insemination (DI) practitioners regularly offer sperm separation for preconception sex selection (Office of Technology Assessment, 1988, 41). In addition to overcoming infertility problems, this combined procedure offers the couple an opportunity to select the sex of their progeny with a high degree of accuracy.

REFERENCES: Beernink, F. J., W. P. Dmowski, and R. J. Ericsson. 1993. "Sex Preselection Through Albumin Separation of Sperm." *Fertility and Sterility* 59(2): 382–386; Carson, Sandra Ann. 1988. "Sex Selection: The Ultimate in Family Planning." *Fertility and Sterility* 50(1): 16–19; Office of Technology Assessment. 1988. *Artificial Insemination: Practice in the United States.* Washington, D.C.: U.S. Government Printing Office; Rogerson, P. A. 1991. "The Effects of Sex Preselection on the Sex Ratio of Families." *Journal of Heredity* 82(3): 239–243; Veit, Christina R., and Raphael Jewelawicz. 1988. "Gender Preselection: Facts and Myths." *Fertility and Sterility* 49(6): 937–940; Walker, M. K., and G. K. Conner. 1993. "Fetal Sex Preference of Second-Trimester Gravidas." *Journal of Nurse Midwifery* 38(2): 110–113.

ROBERT H. BLANK

SPIRITUAL HEALING OF MINOR CHILDREN

There is an important and continuing debate in the United States regarding whether or not parents may refuse conventional medical care for their minor children and rely instead on prayer as a form of spiritual healing. To date, five cases have reached state supreme courts. None have reached the U.S. Supreme Court.

The issues are complex, particularly in a society that constitutionally guarantees the right to freely practice religion. The United States was founded by immigrants fleeing religious persecution, and the Constitution is clear in its intent to prohibit such persecution. As of 1995, most states have clauses in their child abuse and neglect statutes that allow parents to rely on spiritual healing in lieu of conventional medical care. Some would argue that these exemptions protect constitutionally based freedom of religion, while others argue that they violate the constitutional prohibition of government establishment of religion.

A related issue is whether or not the exemption statutes shield parents from prosecution on child abuse, neglect, or manslaughter charges. The basic question revolves around the issue of whether or not fair notice has been given to these parents that they may in fact be liable for prosecution if their child dies or is seriously injured. This issue has been raised in every case to reach the state supreme court level.

Although less prominent as a litigation issue, concerns about equal protection also arise. A parent who relies on spiritual healing may avoid prosecution or conviction based on the spiritual exemption clauses, whereas a parent who refuses conventional medical care for other reasons such as a disagreement with the physician or a belief that the treatment is futile or harmful may be prosecuted. A second equal protection issue involves the children directly. The child of a parent relying on spiritual healing may be denied conventional medical care while other children receive such medical care.

As of 1995, five cases have been decided by state supreme courts; most involved Christian Science parents. In 1984, Laurie Grouard Walker was charged with involuntary manslaughter and felony child endangerment after her four-year-old daughter, Shauntay, died from meningitis. Shauntay had not received conventional medical care. Laurie Walker moved for dismissal of the charges, arguing that her conduct was protected by the spiritual exemption clause found in the California statutes and that she had therefore not received fair notice that her conduct could be criminal. The California Supreme Court found for the state, arguing that parents do not have a right to the free exercise of religion if it endangers a child's life. Walker appealed to the U.S. Supreme Court, which refused certiorari. Subsequently, Walker was convicted of manslaughter in 1990, and the conviction was upheld by the California Court of Appeal.

Another case also arose in 1984 with the death of 26-day-old Joel Hall. Joel did not receive conventional medical care, and the autopsy revealed that he died of pneumonia. His parents, members of the Faith Assembly, were convicted of reckless homicide and neglect of a dependent. On appeal, the Indiana Supreme Court found that prayer (as provided in the state's spiritual exemption clause) was not permitted as a defense when child neglect results in death. Therefore, the homicide conviction was upheld. The child neglect conviction was overturned on technical issues.

On May 9, 1989, 11-year-old Ian Lundman died from diabetic ketoacidosis in Independence, Minnesota. He had not received conventional medical care. Ian's biological parents were divorced, he lived with his mother and stepfather, Kathleen and William McKown, both practicing Christian Scientists. Ian's biological father, Douglass Lundman, had left the Christian Science Church as an adult and was living in another state at the time of Ian's death. The McKowns were subsequently indicted by the Hennepin County grand jury with second-degree manslaughter and for aiding and abetting each other in causing the death of Ian. The trial court subsequently dismissed the indictments, finding no probable cause that the McKowns were grossly negligent (the standard for a manslaughter charge) and that the spiritual exemption clause in the Minnesota statutes protected them from prosecution because they had not received fair notice that their conduct was potentially criminal. Both the Minnesota Court of Appeals and the Minnesota State Supreme Court upheld the trial court's dismissal. Douglass Lundman subsequently won a substantial civil award against his former wife, her husband, church officials, and the church itself.

William and Christine Hermanson were convicted in 1986 for child abuse and third-degree murder after their seven-year-old daughter, Amy, died from juvenile diabetes. No conventional medical care was provided. The Florida Court of Appeals affirmed the trial court decision; however, the Florida Supreme Court reversed the trial court conviction in 1989 because Florida statutes include a spiritual exemption clause, and therefore the parents had not had fair notice that their conduct could be criminal.

In 1990, David and Ginger Twitchell were convicted of involuntary manslaughter for the death of their two-year-old son from an obstructed bowel. On appeal in 1993, the Supreme Judicial Court of Massachusetts found that parents have a duty to seek medical care and that the spiritual exemption clause in the Massachusetts statutes does not protect parents from prosecution when they fail to provide medical care for their children. Despite this finding, it overturned the Twitchells' convictions because the state attorney general had previously issued an opinion indicating that parents who relied on the spiritual exemption clause could not be prosecuted.

REFERENCES: *Commonwealth v. Twitchell*, 617 N.Ed.2d 609 (Mass. 1993); *Hermanson v. State*, 604 So.2d 775 (Fla. 1992); Merrick, Janna C. 1994. "Christian Science Healing of Minor Children: Spiritual Exemption Statutes, First Amendment Rights, and Fair Notice." *Issues in Law and Medicine* 10(3): 321–342; *State v. McKown*, 475 N.W.2d 63 (Minn. 1991); *Walker v. Superior Court*, 673 P.2d 852 (Cal. 1989).

JANNA C. MERRICK

STATUTORY HEALTH CARE STATUTES

Statutory health care surrogate statutes provide for a succession for adult persons who, in order of priority, may make health care decisions for an incompetent person who has not appointed such a surrogate. By 1994, 33 states and the District of Columbia had enacted such statutes. Alaska, Alabama, Delaware, Hawaii, Kansas, Kentucky, Massachusetts, Michigan, Minnesota, New Hampshire, New Jersey, Ohio, Oklahoma, Pennsylvania, Rhode Island, Tennessee, and Wisconsin have no such statute. New York's law is limited to decisions relating to do-not-resuscitate orders.

The succession of statutory surrogates generally proceeds, in order of priority, as guardian, spouse, adult child, parent, adult sibling, and close friend. Some statutes provide that an attending physician may act as surrogate if no other surrogate is willing or able to act. Typically, the statutes provide that the decision of the majority of any class prevails but are silent on how to resolve a dispute in which there is no majority.

The decision-making authority of the statutory surrogate is broad, governing all health care decisions to be made for the incompetent adult person in all circumstances, subject only to the requirement that the surrogate act in accord with the known wishes of the person or, if the person's wishes are unknown, in the person's best interest. As such, the authority of the statutory surrogate is comparable to that of a surrogate appointed by the person; it is greater than the decision-making authority implemented through a statutorily authorized "living will," which generally governs only the forgoing of life-sustaining treatment for a person with a terminal condition or, in some states, in a persistent vegetative state.*

Statutory health care statutes attempt to mirror health care providers' customary practice of family consultation, to avoid the need to secure appointment of a guardian with authority to make health care decisions, and to provide for a decision-making mechanism for incompetent persons who have neither appointed a surrogate nor executed a living will. They also provide a mechanism for decision making on matters beyond the scope of whatever specific instructions made in a living will or in some other manner. The broad scope of the statutory surrogate's decision-making authority and the somewhat arbitrary nature of surrogate classes and priorities between them, however, obviously make execution of an instrument appointing a surrogate or execution of a living will preferable. However relatively cumbersome, guardianship might sometimes be preferable in order to provide more direct judicial oversight over decision making and because guardianship law generally provides that anyone might challenge a guardian's decisions opposed to the wishes or best interest of the person. Statutory health care statutes generally provide that only interested persons have standing to challenge the decisions of a statutory surrogate—a class usually limited to those in the statutory designated classes and the person's health care providers.

REFERENCES: Alan Meisel. 1989, 1994. *The Right to Die*. New York: Wiley Law Publications; *Right to Die Law Digest*. Various issues.

THOMAS J. MARZEN

STERILIZATION—INVOLUNTARY

There are two distinct meanings for the term *involuntary* as applied to sterilization. The first refers to sterilizations that are not voluntary because the subject is legally incompetent to exercise informed consent. The parents of a mentally retarded woman who petition the court for permission to have their daughter sterilized are attempting to substitute their consent for hers. These involuntary sterilizations are always problematic because it is difficult to determine what the subject would choose if she or he was capable of informed consent.

The second form of involuntary sterilization might best be defined as compulsory. In this situation, a person who is legally capable of informed consent is coerced to be sterilized against his or her wishes. Eugenic sterilization, punitive sterilization, and sterilization of unwilling women on public assistance are examples of this more insidious form of involuntary sterilization.

Sterilization legislation in the early twentieth century was motivated primarily by medical theories that postulated that mental illness and other social ills could be alleviated if only "undesirables" were sterilized. Although such eugenic theories fell into disrepute, as of 1991, 21 states had statutes providing for involuntary sterilization of some type.

Four states permit involuntary sterilization of institutionalized persons only, while 17 permit it on persons in the community as well as those in institutions. Persons addressed usually include the mentally retarded or mentally ill and in a few states epileptics. The Delaware statute authorizes sterilization of habitual criminals. In those states that permit only institutionalized persons to be sterilized, usually the institution's superintendent is the official who is required to initiate the request. In 14 states, parents or legal guardians can initiate sterilization proceedings, and in Virginia, a spouse or "next friend" also has that authority.

Although all but seven states require a hearing prior to sterilization, actual procedures vary considerably from state to state. Four states require only an administrative hearing usually conducted by the director of the state department with jurisdiction over public institutions. Nine states require a full judicial hearing prior to the performance of sterilization. They provide for a formal hearing, the right to counsel, the right to be present and cross examine witnesses, and a right to a full record of all testimony, both written and oral. Eight states permit substituted consent by a parent, guardian, and in several states, a spouse of the person to be sterilized.

These more recent sterilization laws clearly demonstrate the move away from eugenic rationale and toward other justifications. Only four states refer to eugenic or hereditary grounds for sterilization, and three of these include other grounds as well. Increasingly, the states refer to "the inability to care for and support children," the "best interests of the person," or the "welfare of society" as statutory standards for sterilization.

Despite the renewed interest of some state legislatures to adapt sterilization statutes, the most conspicuous activity to date is concentrated in the courts. Court activity regarding involuntary sterilization centers on two issues: Are the specific statutory schemes of the states constitutional, and in the absence of express statutory authorization, do the courts have equitable jurisdiction to approve sterilization petitions for persons who are incompetent? The court response to the first question is generally a qualified yes. Although there is no uniform response from the courts on the second question, the trend is toward allowing such orders within strict parameters.

The courts tend to agree that involuntary sterilization statutes are constitutional in the precedent of *Buck v. Bell** (1927) in which the Supreme Court upheld eugenic sterilization under Oliver Wendell Holmes's dictum that "three generations of imbeciles are enough." They have been active over the years, however, in narrowing that precedent through rulings that specific statutes lack necessary due process elements such as the right to counsel, a hearing, or appeal. In these cases, the courts usually leave it up to the legislature to rewrite laws to ensure both procedural and substantive protections to the targets of sterilization. In *Lulos v. State* (1990) an Indiana appellate court held that a guardian's petition for sterilization of an incompetent adult should be granted upon "clear and convincing evidence that judicially appointed guardian filed petition in good faith and that sterilization is in best interests of incompetent adult."

In *North Carolina Association for Retarded Children v. State of North Carolina* (1976), a U.S. district court left standing the right of state legislatures to enact sterilization laws, but only within narrow circumstances. The court explicitly dismissed eugenic bases for mandating sterilization. It noted that there was considerable agreement of medical opinion that sterilization might be desirable in extreme cases as a last resort. Sterilization might be warranted in cases of clearly identifiable genetic defects with "significant probability" that offspring will inherit that defect. Also, if a mentally retarded person would be incapable of discharging the responsibility of parenthood because of an inability to create a nondetrimental environment for his/her progeny, cause for sterilization might be established. Other indications for sterilization, the court noted, include the inability of a person to understand that the natural consequences of sexual activity is a child, a desire not to have children combined with the inability to use other forms of birth control, and in rare and unusual cases, medical determination that sterilization is in the best interests of either the mentally retarded person, the state, or both.

Using a somewhat different rationale, the Oregon Court of Appeals (*Cook v. State of Oregon,* 1972) approved sterilization of a 17-year-old girl on grounds it would be a burden to the state if she were to have children. Because of her incapacity to care for any children, they would most likely be neglected and become wards of the state. The court ruled that since she could not be an adequate parent, it was proper to sterilize her. The Oregon statute that authorized involuntary sterilization was viewed as constitutional by the court. In *Motes v. Hall City Department of Family and Children Services* (1983), however, a Georgia court declared that the state statute providing for involuntary sterilization of mentally incompetent persons was unconstitutional because it denies those persons the right to procreate.

Until 1980, with very few exceptions, courts ruled that they had no authorization to order permanent sterilization of incompetent persons without an express legislative grant of such power. Although the signals coming from the courts are not always in accord or unequivocal, there is an evolving acceptance of what until recently was perceived by most courts as a legislative role; courts are recognizing jurisdiction in sterilization of those persons incapable of consenting for themselves.

In 1985, the Supreme Court of California (*Conservatorship of Valerie N.*) invoked the jurisprudence of fundamental rights to invalidate a California statute that prohibited the sterilization of mentally retarded persons. In a long opinion with heated dissent by Chief Justice Bird, the court argued that the statute "impermissibly deprives" developmentally disabled persons of privacy and liberty interests protected by federal and state constitutions. By withholding sterilization from an incompetent woman, the statute deprived her of her only realistic opportunity for contraception and, consequently, restricted her chances for self-fulfillment. "Since the right to elect sterilization as a method of contraception is generally available to adult women, restriction on that right must be justified by a compelling state interest" (at 761).

This growing court acceptance of jurisdiction over involuntary sterilization is accompanied, however, with a hesitation to order permanent sterilization procedures except in the most extreme cases. Other high court rulings finding jurisdiction in such cases include the supreme courts of Alaska (*In re C.D.M.,* 1981), Colorado (*In re A.W.,* 1982), Iowa (*In re Guardian of Matejski,* 1988), New Hampshire (*In re Penny N.,* 1980), New Jersey (*In re Grady,* 1981), Washington (*In re Hayes,* 1980), and Wisconsin (*In re Guardian of Eberhardy,* 1981).

It is crucial to reiterate that while there is a growing tendency of the courts to accept the principle of equitable power over involuntary sterilization in the absence of authorizing statutes, there is a hesitancy to order irreversible sterilization except under extreme circumstances.

REFERENCES: Blank, Robert H. 1991. *Fertility Control.* Westport, CT: Greenwood Press; Blank, Robert H., and Janna C. Merrick. 1995. *Human Reproduction, Emerging Technologies, and Conflicting Rights.* Washington, D.C.: Congressional Quarterly Press; *Buck v. Bell,* 274 U.S. 200 (1927); *Conservatorship of Valerie N.,* 707 P.2d 760 (Cal. 1985); *Cook v. State of Oregon,* 495 P.2d 768 (1972); *In re A.W.,* 637 P.2d 366 (Col. 1982); *In re C.D.M.,* 627 P.2d 607 (Alaska 1981); *In re Grady,* 426 A.2d 467 (N.J. 1981); *In re Guardian of Eberhardy,* 307 N.W.2d 881 (Wis. 1981); *In re Guardian of Matejski,* 419 N.W.2d 576 (Iowa 1988); *In re Hayes,* 608 P.2d 637 (Wash. 1980); *In re Penny N.,* 414 A.2d 541 (N.H. 1980); Kaplan, Lawrence J., and Rosemarie Tong. 1994. *Controlling Our Reproductive Destiny.* Cambridge: MIT Press; *Lulos v. State,* 548 N.E.2d 173 (Ind. App. 3 Dist. 1990); *Motes v. Hall City Department of Family and Children Services,* 306 S.E.2d 260 (Ga. 1983); *North Carolina Association for Retarded Children v. State of North Carolina,* 420 F. Supp. 459 (M.D. N.C. 1976).

See also **BUCK V. BELL; STERILIZATION—VOLUNTARY.**

ROBERT H. BLANK

STERILIZATION—VOLUNTARY

The vast majority of sterilizations performed in the United States are classified as voluntary fertility control procedures based on individual choice. The development of less intrusive, safe, and effective sterilization procedures, combined with changes in attitude of the medical profession and the general public, led to substantial effort during the 1960s and 1970s to facilitate access to sterilization by those who wanted to terminate their fertility.

After a long process of court challenges that gradually eliminated a variety of restrictions, voluntary sterilization is legal in all 50 states. Despite significant action toward legalizing voluntary sterilization in the 1960s, a variety of restrictions remained, resulting in inequities in access to the procedure. The age-parity formula, which stated that the woman's age times the number of her live children had to equal 100 or 120, for instance, eliminated many women who had few or no living children. Other restrictions included the need for consultation with at least one other physician, consent of the spouse, and performance of sterilization only in a licensed hospital.

In response to these many legal uncertainties, a number of states have recently enacted voluntary sterilization statutes. Although variation in states' efforts to regulate voluntary sterilization continues to be confusing, most of the specific requirements fall into one of four categories: age requirements; a waiting period (usually 30 days) between time of consent and the procedure; consent of spouse; second-opinion consultation.

In addition to these legislative actions, a series of court challenges successfully have struck down the most constraining legal restrictions. In *Hathaway v. Worcester City Hospital* (1973), a U.S. court of appeals held that the refusal of a city hospital to permit its facilities to be used for sterilization operations violated the constitutional rights of a woman who wanted a tubal ligation for contraceptive purposes. Similarly, in *Avila v. New York City Health and Hospital Corporation* (1987), the supreme court, Bronx County, ruled that an institution receiving federal funds and performing sterilizations may not arbitrarily prevent a mentally competent and freely consenting individual from having the operation.

Action by other courts has eliminated additional constraints on access to sterilization. In *Ponter v. Ponter* (1975), the New Jersey Supreme Court granted Mrs. Ponter's right to be sterilized despite her husband's objections. In a related case involving age restrictions (*Carey v. Population Services International*, 1977), the Supreme Court implied that personal autonomy over contraception protected the right to sterilization as well. By invalidating New Jersey's statutory limitation on a minor's access to contraceptives, the court extended this right to all forms of birth control, presumably including sterilization.

Although these statutes and court decisions have clarified the legal right to obtain a sterilization for fertility control in some jurisdictions, impediments to the widespread availability of voluntary sterilization remain. Although publicly supported hospitals cannot refuse to perform sterilizations, in most states they still can establish their own policies regarding waiting periods, consultation, and spousal consent. Furthermore, the Church Amendment (named after its sponsor, Senator Frank Church of Idaho) to the Hill-Burton Act gives private hospitals the right to limit sterilization on moral or religious grounds.

Physicians and clinics can also impose their own restrictions on whom they consider eligible, thus making voluntary sterilization difficult to obtain in some locales. Some physicians, especially those in states that have not addressed the question of minors, require that the patient be over 21, married, and have spousal or parental consent. Others impose waiting periods ranging from 72 hours to 30 days (the same as the waiting period for all federally funded sterilizations) in order to minimize the possibility that a person might change his or her mind after the procedure is completed.

A further complicating factor is confusion in insurance coverage. Although many policies treat contraceptive sterilization as a medical procedure despite its motivation, others discriminate between medically indicated and elective sterilization and reimburse only the former. Other policies specifically exclude coverage of nontherapeutic sterilization. This consideration might discourage or even preclude voluntary sterilization for those individuals with limited monetary resources. Although Medicaid provides recourse in some states for those who qualify, about a quarter of the states do not include coverage for elective sterilization.

REFERENCES: *Avila v. New York City Health and Hospital Corporation,* 518 N.Y.S.2d 574, 136 Misc. 2d 76 (N.Y. 1987); Blank, Robert H. 1991. *Fertility Control.* Westport, CT: Greenwood Press; *Carey v. Population Services International,* 431 U.S. 678 (1977); *Hathaway v. Worchester City Hospital,* 475 F.2d 701 (1st. Cir. 1973); Kaplan, Lawrence J., and Rosemarie Tong. 1994. *Controlling Our Reproductive Destiny.* Cambridge: MIT Press, 111–138; *Ponter v. Ponter,* 135 N.J. Super 50, 342 A.2d 574 (1975).

See also **STERILIZATION—INVOLUNTARY.**

ROBERT H. BLANK

SUBDERMAL HORMONAL IMPLANTS (SHIs)

Subdermal hormonal implants are rods or capsules that contain a contraceptive steroid. Two types of SHIs are currently being developed. Norplant-2 has two capsules that provide three years of contraceptive protection. Capronor, a biodegradable implant, has one capsule that lasts 18 months. The only Food and Drug Administration* (FDA)–approved form of SHI is Norplant. Developed by the Population Council, it consists of six rods made of Silastic, a type of silicone rubber. Each rod is 34 millimeters (mm) long and 2.4 mm in diameter, and each contains 34 milligrams (mg) of levonorgestrel, a synthetic progestogen, which gradually permeates the walls of the rods and enters the body over a five-year period. The rods are implanted subdermally (under the skin) inside the upper arm or forearm in a 15-minute surgical procedure using local anesthetic. Norplant is 99 percent effective in preventing conception, and like all progestogens, it works by inhibiting ovulation and by thickening the cervical mucus, making it less penetrable by sperm. Since the rods are not biodegradable, they must be removed after five years. If they are not removed, the risk of pregnancy increases each year beyond the implant's five-year life span.

The Population Council began its research on Norplant in 1966. Since then, the implant system has been used in clinical studies and field trials by 50,000 women in 44 countries, including three sites in the United States. In 1983, Norplant was granted regulatory approval in Finland and was on the market in 15 countries when the FDA granted the implant marketing approval in December 1990. Since then, the Population Council has licensed Wyeth-Ayerst Laboratories to market Norplant in the United States, over 26,000 clinicians have been trained to perform insertions and removals, and 600,000 women have received the implant (Forrest, Darroch, and Kaeser, 1993). Outside the United States, the

Population Council licensed Leiras, a Finnish pharmaceutical firm, to sell Norplant to the U.S. Agency for International Development and the United States Population Fund, which distribute the implant to Third World family planning programs. Family planning clinics have welcomed Norplant, because of the problems they encounter in educating and gaining compliance from women who use contraceptive techniques that require daily self-administration or partner cooperation. Women choose Norplant because it is more reliable and effortless to use and provides a reversible method of birth control with no permanent adverse effect on fertility.

The FDA's approval has, however, left serious questions about Norplant unanswered because some of the studies failed to follow research protocol criteria and included women who were not adequately examined and gave Norplant to pregnant women and lactating women. Other studies did not sufficiently explain why so many women were lost to follow-up and others died. The research also failed to dispel fears about the implant's safety by giving only passing attention to the risks of ovarian cysts and ectopic pregnancy. Studies of progestogens have suggested that women who become pregnant should have the implant removed because of an increased risk of congenital abnormalities, including heart and limb defects, but these findings were not confirmed by research on Norplant. The Population Council submitted limited short-term studies of children who breast feed while their mothers were on Norplant, but so far, no research addresses the implant's long-term effects for children. Nor are there any long-term studies that directly address Norplant's risks of breast, endometrial, ovarian, and cervical cancer.

At the same time, the Norplant research has documented that women have adverse reactions from implant use. Irregular menstrual bleeding, intermenstrual spotting, prolonged episodes of bleeding (more than ten days per cycle), and spotting and amenorrhea occur. During the first year of use, 27.6 percent of women have experienced irregular bleeding, including heavy and prolonged bleeding. Women have also reported pain at the implant site and other adverse reactions common to hormonal contraceptives including headache, nervousness, nausea, dizziness, depression, appetite changes, dermatitis, acne, weight gain, fatigue, and weakness. These side effects have led 15 to 19 percent of women to have the implant removed, citing, most frequently, irregular bleeding, headaches, mood changes, and weight gain. Overall, however, the major reason, cited by 9 percent of women in the first year, was menstrual problems similar to those associated with progestogen-only methods (Bardin, 1990, 98).

Voluntary use is a critical factor, given the Norplant's long-acting character and the need to surgically remove the rods if women desire to become pregnant or suffer side effects from its use. Voluntary use requires an informed choice at the time of implantation, but studies suggest that informed consent may vary considerably. Continued Norplant use is directly linked to the extent of counseling women receive about the implant's side effects when Norplant is inserted. Voluntary use also requires that women be able to have the implant removed "whenever they want, for whatever reason, without encountering perceived or actual barriers" (Forrest, Darroch, and Kaeser, 1993, 131). Yet Norplant removal may be especially problematic for Third World women who live in rural areas, far from a nearby clinic. In the United States, where clinics are more readily accessible, women may have a financial barrier to their voluntary use of the implant.

Norplant is sold to medical providers for $365. The physician's fee brings the cost for insertion to $500 to 550. When $150 is added to remove the implant, the total average cost is $700. Still, the implant is competitive with the oral contraceptive pill, which costs about $1,500 for a five-year period. In the short run, however, Norplant's high initial cost makes it difficult to acquire without private insurance. Fifty percent of women who use Norplant are covered by Medicaid. Others who cannot afford the implant and are not eligible through Medicaid may receive it through the Norplant Foundation, a nonprofit organization, established by Wyeth-Ayerst, and through family planning clinics, mostly funded by the Public Health Service Act's Title X. Still, the implant's limited availability through the Norplant Foundation and its high initial cost to family planning clinics may well mean that it will not be available to many low-income women ineligible for Medicaid.

Norplant has become especially controversial because it is viewed as a means to address a myriad of social ills. As an instrument of social policy, the implant has been touted as a cure for teen pregnancy, welfare dependency, and drug-addicted mothers. These efforts at social engineering have generated a debate over the power of government to regulate the fertility and coerce the reproductive choices of teenagers and poor women and women of color.

Norplant use to control teenage pregnancy has raised the issue as to whether the implant will become a license for promiscuity and whether schools may only encourage its use by providing contraceptive counseling and distributing the implant to their students. These school programs acquire racial overtones when Norplant is provided to inner-city minority teenagers. Yet its advocates reply that the implant permits girls to avoid teenage motherhood, complete high school, and even college without becoming pregnant. Counseling is necessary, they argue, because sexually active girls who use Norplant are less likely to use condoms, and Norplant use without a condom does not protect a woman against sexually transmitted diseases including acquired immunodeficiency syndrome (AIDS).

Norplant's use by women who are eligible to receive the implant through Medicaid, some 50 percent of all users, has raised the question as to whether it should be used to control the cost of public assistance. Advocates argue that since all state governments cover the cost of providing the implant to women who are eligible through Medicaid and government is expected to support the children of the poor, the implant is one way to reduce welfare costs. To that end, state legislators have introduced bills to encourage or require the use of the implant to control welfare costs and to address the growing social problems of drug abuse and child neglect and abuse. Some of these bills have provided financial incentives to encourage low-income women and substance abusers to use the implant. Others have mandated its use as a condition of receiving public assistance and as a condition of probation for women, capable of becoming pregnant, who have been convicted of felony drug offense or whose babies are born with fetal alcohol syndrome.* So far, none of these bills have become law.

Norplant's mandatory use raises the fear of forced contraception. Critics argue that Norplant is the closest thing to sterilization, the second-most popular form of voluntary birth control after the pill, and that public officials have tried to impose the implant on women who have the least power in society. Conditioning the amount of a woman's welfare payment or her probation in a case of child abuse or neglect on her use of Norplant is highly controversial because it may require a woman to waive her fundamental constitutional right to procreate. Norplant's use to address the problems of child abuse and neglect came to national attention when Darlene Johnson, a welfare mother, was convicted of felony child abuse and ordered to use the implant for three years as a condition of probation (*People v. Johnson,* 1991). On appeal, the state argued that the condition was reasonably related to its goal of rehabilitation and its compelling interest in protecting the welfare of unconceived children. In response, Johnson's attorney claimed that the order exceeded the trial court's discretion and violated her constitutional right to procreate. Yet the appellate court never resolved these arguments because her case was dismissed when she violated another condition of her probation and was sent to jail. As a consequence, the *Johnson* case pointedly raised, but did not resolve, the question of Norplant's use as a probation condition. In a wider ambit, the case also raised a critical question about the use of any long-acting contraceptive as a mandatory biomedical tool to repair our social problems.

REFERENCES: Arthur, Stacey L. 1992. "The Norplant Prescription: Birth Control, Woman Control, or Crime Control." *UCLA Law Review* 40: 1–101; Bardin, C. Wayne. 1990. "Norplant Contraceptive Implants." *Obstetrics and Gynecology Report* 2: 96–102; Forrest, Jacquelin Darroch, and Lisa Kaeser. 1993. "Questions of Balance: Issues Emerging from the Introduction of the Hormonal Implant." *Family Planning Perspectives* 25: 127–32; Kaeser, Lisa. 1994. "Public Funding and Policies for Provision of the Contraceptive Implant, Fiscal Year 1992." *Family Planning Perspectives* 26: 11–16; *People v. Johnson,* No. 29390 (Sup. Ct. Tulare Co.), No. F015316 (Cal. App. 5th Dist.), filed but not decided, April 25, 1991; Persels, Jim. 1992. "The Norplant Condition: Protecting the Unborn or Violating Fundamental Rights." *Journal of Legal Medicine* 13: 237–62; Samuels, S. E., and M. D. Smith, eds. 1992. *Dimensions of New Contraceptives: Norplant and Poor Women.* Palo Alto: Henry J. Kaiser Family Foundation; U.S. Food and Drug Administration. Fertility and Maternal Health Drugs Advisory Committee. April 27, 1989. *Transcript of Minutes [of Its Public Hearing on Norplant].* Rockville, MD: Food and Drug Administration.

WILLIAM C. GREEN

SUBSTITUTED JUDGMENT

The term *substituted judgment* refers generally to decisions made on behalf of incompetent persons. The basic notion is that when, for reasons of mental disability, a person cannot make personal choices, some third party or parties can make those choices on the person's behalf. As a legal term of art, "substituted judgment" refers particularly to making and implementing a decision in the way that the incompetent person "would have" done. The doctrine appears regularly in the context of the refusal of life-sustaining medical treatment.

The legal doctrine of substituted judgment arose, in the Anglo-American tradition, in the context of property law. Courts articulated the doctrine as far back as the early nineteenth century (*Ex parte Whitbread*, 1816) as a means of asserting judicial control over the disposition of the estate of an incompetent person. In the late 1960s, courts began borrowing this doctrine from property law and applying it to decisions regarding the physical person of the incompetent individual. This extension of the doctrine of substituted judgment first appeared in the context of organ donations (*Strunk*, 1969) and then later the refusal of life-sustaining treatment (*Saikewicz*, 1977), sterilization (*Valerie N.*, 1985), and abortion (*Doe*, 1987).

There are currently a variety of mechanisms for exercising substituted judgment on behalf of incompetent persons. Some courts exercise the power themselves (*Saikewicz*, 1977) or authorize its exercise by private parties such as family members (*Quinlan*, 1976). Some state statutes authorize relatives, physicians, and others to make substituted judgments. Other statutes authorize individuals, while competent, to appoint others ("designated power of attorney") or provide instructions ("living will" or "advance directive") in the event of future incompetency.

Proponents of substituted judgment in its various forms typically frame the issue as one of preserving and effectuating the decisional rights of the person who is incompetent. Proponents also offer substituted judgment as a means of discontinuing assertedly unwarranted or unhelpful treatment when the patient is unable personally to decline consent.

Opponents of substituted judgment typically criticize the potential for abuse of helpless individuals. According to the critics, genuine personal decisions are by their nature incapable of delegation to, or assertion by, third parties. Substituted judgment, in this view, more likely authorizes third parties to implement their own preferences at the expense of the incompetent person's well-being.

REFERENCES: *Cruzan v. Director, Mo. Dep't of Health*, 497 U.S. 261 (1990); *DeGrella v. Elston*, 858 S.W.2d 698 (Ky. 1993); *Ex parte Whitbread in re Hinde, a Lunatic*, 35 Eng. Rep. 878 (1816); L. Harmon. 1990. "Falling Off the Vine: Legal Fictions and the Doctrine of Substituted Judgment." *Yale Law Journal* 100: 1; *In re Conservatorship of Valerie N.*, 40 Cal. 3d 143, 707 P.2d 760, 219 Cal. Rptr. 387 (1985); *In re Doe*, 533 A.2d 523 (R.I. 1987) (per curiam); *In re Quinlan*, 70 N.J. 10, 355 A.2d 647, *cert. denied*, 429 U.S. 922 (1976); S. Schultz, W. Swartz, and J. Appelbaum. 1977. "Deciding Right-to-Die Cases Involving Incompetent Patients: Jones v. Saikewicz.'' *Suffolk University Law Review* 11: 936; *Strunk v. Strunk*, 445 S.W.2d 145 (Ky. 1969); *Superintendent of Belchertown State School v. Saikewicz*, 373 Mass. 728, 370 N.E.2d 417 (1977).

WALTER M. WEBER

SUPERINTENDENT OF BELCHERTOWN STATE SCHOOL V. SAIKEWICZ

In 1977, a court applied for the first time the ''substituted judgment''* doctrine to a case involving a surrogate request to withhold a patient's life-sustaining medical treatment. The patient, Joseph Saikewicz, had an acute form of leukemia requiring chemotherapy. His physicians recommended against treatment because of its limited prospects for success and a high risk of negative side effects. Saikewicz was 67 years old and had severe mental retardation. Because of his lifelong mental disabilities, Saikewicz was never capable of making his own medical decisions. Officials from the facility where Saikewicz resided petitioned the Massachusetts courts to appoint a guardian for the purpose of obtaining chemotherapy on Saikewicz's behalf. The question of whether treatment should be withheld and on what basis was ultimately addressed by the Massachusetts Supreme Judicial Court.

The facility had argued that because Saikewicz's views were unknowable, then the courts must apply a ''reasonable person'' test to determine whether treatment should be provided. The facility pointed to public opinion polls indicating that competent persons diagnosed with cancer would consent to chemotherapy despite its burdens because of the possibility of prolonged life and concluded that based on these data a reasonable person in Saikewicz's circumstances would consent to treatment.

The Massachusetts high court disagreed. In a unanimous decision, the court ruled that treatment could be withheld under a theory of substituted judgment. Rather than determining what most people would do in the circumstances, the court considered ''the primary test [to be] subjective in nature—that is, the goal is to determine with as much accuracy as possible the wants and needs of the individual involved.'' According to the court, the appropriate basis for a surrogate decision would not be the likely judgment of reasonable persons but the likely judgment of Saikewicz, ''if [he] were competent, but taking into account [his] present and future incompetency . . . as one of the factors which would necessarily enter into the decision-making process of [a] competent person.''

Thus, for example, in this case the surrogate decision maker had to consider whether Saikewicz was intellectually capable of understanding why he would be subjected to intrusive treatment. Unlike the general population of reasonable persons who would choose chemotherapy because they were capable of understanding that the burdens should be endured in order to prolong life, Saikewicz permanently lacked such understanding. His physicians testified that he likely would have resisted out of fear any painful intervention required to administer treatment. Thus, treatment could be refused on his behalf by ''substituting'' the surrogate's estimation of his likely judgment in place of any objective and contrary judgment by others in favor of life.

The substituted judgment approach has been adopted by many courts and ethicists as the preferred means for making surrogate decisions for presently incapacitated patients. Most authorities, however, reject this approach in cases involving never-competent patients or once-competent patients who failed to issue advance directives while competent. In these latter cases, the idea that the patient is making the decision would be a legal fiction having no basis in fact. REFERENCE: *Superintendent of Belchertown State School v. Saikewicz,* 370 N.E.2d 417 (Mass. 1977).

DANIEL AVILA

SURGEON GENERAL

The Office of the Surgeon General of the U.S. Public Health Service* (PHS) is responsible for managing the Health Service Corps, a uniformed service corps composed of approximately 6,000 commissioned officers who respond to medical emergencies and serve in medically underserved areas. The surgeon general also advises the federal government and the nation's population on disease prevention, health maintenance, and health hazards, focusing on such areas as acquired immunodeficiency syndrome (AIDS) prevention, alcohol abuse, nutrition, and aging. In addition, the surgeon general participates in international health activities, represents the PHS on various boards, interfaces with several governmental departments, and oversees the PHS offices of minority health, women's health, and population affairs. The office is responsible for researching and writing several reports, including the annual report on smoking and public health.

The Office of the Surgeon General dates back to the nineteenth century when Congress established the Public Health Service Commissioned Corps with the surgeon general in command. The surgeon general headed the PHS until 1968 when a reorganization put the service under the leadership of the assistant secretary for health. The surgeon general was retained as a deputy to the assistant secretary with responsibility for advising and assisting on professional medical matters. The positions of assistant secretary for health and surgeon general were combined into a single position in 1977 but separated again in 1981; since then the surgeon general has reported to the assistant secretary for health.

REFERENCES: Furman, B. 1973. *A Profile of the United States Public Health Service, 1798–1948.* Washington, D.C.: U.S. Department of Health, Education, and Welfare; Mullan, F. 1989. *Plagues and Politics: The Story of the United States Public Health Service.* New York: Basic Books; Voelker, R. 1993. "New Surgeon General Has Expanded Role." *American Medical News* 36 (36): 1.

ANA MARIA LOPEZ

SURROGACY CONTRACTS: THE IMPACT ON WOMEN'S RIGHTS

Surrogacy occurs when a woman agrees to become pregnant, usually by artificial insemination,* with a contracting man's sperm. The woman agrees that when the baby is born, she will give the child to the contracting man, sever her rights as biological mother, and often free the man's wife to adopt the child. In this type of surrogacy, the contracting man is also the genetic father and, therefore, has some legal claim on the child from the beginning.

Calling the gestating and birth mother a "surrogate" is actually misleading since the so-called surrogate or substitute is really the biological mother or, at a minimum, the gestating and birth mother (if the embryo is from an implant), and the contracting or adopting wife of the genetic father is the actual surrogate. There can be instances where the contracting man is not the biological father— for instance, if the semen in the artificial insemination is from an anonymous sperm donor. Surrogacy involving donated eggs* or embryo transfer further complicates matters. Here there is the possibility of the birth mother having no genetic connection to the baby (although the mother gestated and labored and birthed the child).

Egg donation and embryo transfer also could lead to the possibility of Third World women or poor women of color the world over gestating a fetus and birthing a baby completely genetically unrelated to them. These women would cost less for their services, and their countries might not regulate these practices very well. The potential abuses of these poor women are grave.

Surrogacy is a very old practice. There is reference to it in the biblical story of Abraham who deliberately fathered a child with his wife Sarah's maid, and with Sarah's permission, since Sarah herself was barren. What is new about surrogacy is how it is being formalized into contract law and the different permutations of it possible, given artificial insemination, egg donation, embryo transfer, and the like.

Questions involving what people may barter for in the open market are raised when a surrogacy contract somehow ends up in court. Should the courts uphold these contracts between consenting adults, or is there something involved here that should be outside the bounds of mere contract enforcement? Many of these issues were brought to public attention and debate by a surrogacy arrangement that went sour, the 1987 *Baby M* case.

In *Baby M,* a birth mother changed her mind about giving up the baby, and the contractual couple sued to have the original terms of the surrogate contract upheld in court. In April 1987 a New Jersey trial judge ruled that Baby M should become the child of the contracting couple; the judge severed the birth mother's claims to the child and did not allow her any visitation. In February 1988, the New Jersey Supreme Court ruled the Baby M surrogacy contract illegal because it resembled baby selling. The court recognized the birth mother's maternal rights while granting custody to the contractual and genetic father.

Surrogacy arrangements bring up many issues about gender politics and the possible impact these policies could have on women. Since women usually have less money than men, have lower salaries, and have fewer options, the potential for exploitation in the name of "choice" is troublesome. Motherhood is also deeply influenced by our culture. The idea of women being paid to have a baby, and then give it away, raises ethical, moral, and cultural issues about women's role in society, the relationship of children to their genetic parents, the impact these arrangements will have on the children involved, and questions of power and class.

As some feminist scholars have noted, equating the male experience of genetic parenthood to the woman's, comparing men's abilities to separate out their sperm from their bodies, sell it (as in sperm banks for artificial insemination), or pass it on to a "surrogate" mother to women's "equal opportunity" to do the same through surrogacy, imposes male experience as the universal. The gestalt of maternity—women's psychological as well as physical experiences— is compartmentalized and devalued by defining childbirth in discontinuous terms (a "rented womb") rather than as the woman's linear experience of maternity. Other feminists, though, see surrogacy as an opportunity for women, and attempts to restrict it as patronizing and paternalistic.

REFERENCES: Andrews, Lori B. 1989. *Between Strangers: Surrogate Mothers, Expectant Fathers, and Brave New Babies.* New York: Harper & Row; Field, Martha A. 1988. *Surrogate Motherhood.* Cambridge, MA: Harvard University Press; *In the Matter of BABY M, A Pseudonym for an Actual Person,* 217 N.J. Super. 313, 525 A.2d 1128 (March 31, 1987); *In the Matter of BABY M, A Pseudonym for an Actual Person,* 109 N.J. 396, 537 A.2d 1227 (February 3, 1988); Rae, Scott B. 1994. *The Ethics of Commercial Surrogate Motherhood: Brave New Families?* Westport, CT: Praeger Publishers; Ragone, Helena. 1994. *Surrogate Motherhood: Conception in the Heart.* Boulder, CO: Westview Press; *Reproductive Laws for the 1990s.* 1989. Edited by Nadine Taub and Sherrill Cohen. Clifton, NJ: Humana Press; Shalev, Carmel. 1989. *Birth Power: The Case for Surrogacy.* New Haven: Yale University Press; *Surrogate Motherhood: Politics and Privacy.* (1990). Edited by Larry Gostin. Bloomington: Indiana University Press; Woliver, Laura R. 1991. "The Influence of Technology on the Politics of Motherhood: An Overview of the United States." *Women's Studies International Forum* 14 (5): 479–490.

LAURA R. WOLIVER

SURROGATE PARENTING V. COM. EX REL. ARMSTRONG

The Louisville *Courier Journal* requested an opinion from the attorney general of Kentucky on the legality of an advertisement that was printed in a November 1979 issue of the newspaper. The advertisement involved a search for a surrogate. The attorney general subsequently issued an opinion in January 1981 (OAG 81–18) that surrogate motherhood contracts were illegal and unenforceable. Additionally, the statement declared that surrogate motherhood violated a public policy against baby buying and state statutes involving adoption (Philips and Philips, 1980–1981).

A suit was then filed by the attorney general in March 1981. The suit involved a move by the attorney general of Kentucky to have the charter of Surrogate Parenting Associates, Inc. (SPA) revoked, based on grounds of "abuse and misuse of its corporate powers detrimental to the interest and welfare of the state and its citizens" (*Surrogate Parenting v. Com. Ex Rel. Armstrong,* 1986, 210). The suit alleged that the procedures followed by SPA in making surrogate motherhood arrangements violated three Kentucky statutes: KRS 199.590(2), which prohibits the sale, purchase, or the procurement for sale or purchase, of children for adoption; KRS 199.601(2), "which prohibits filing a petition for voluntary termination of parental rights prior to five (5) days after the birth of a child" (at 210); and KRS 199.590(5), which specifies that a consent for adoption is not valid if it is given prior to five days after the birth of a child. Franklin Circuit Court ruled in favor of the SPA, declaring that their activities did not violate state statutes and did not constitute an abuse of corporate power. They held that the fact that the wife of the biological father might eventually adopt the child did not automatically place surrogate motherhood under the adoption statutes. The appellate court reversed this decision, ruling that adoption of the baby by the biological father's wife was predicated on the relinquishment of parental rights by the biological mother. Therefore, agreement to relinquish parental rights made prior to conception was prohibited by KRS 199.590(5). The Supreme Court of Kentucky in February 1986 reversed the decision of the court of appeals and affirmed the judgment of the Franklin Circuit Court. The suit was dismissed.

SPA is an organization that facilitates surrogate motherhood arrangements involving artificial insemination* of a surrogate with the semen of a man who will be the biological and social father of the child. The procedure followed by SPA in these arrangements includes the signing of a contract by the biological father and the surrogate mother. The contract specifies that following the birth of the child the mother will relinquish parental rights to the child, thus allowing the father to assume custody. The biological father agrees to pay a fee to the surrogate for her "services" and to pay legal, medical, and additional costs associated with the surrogacy arrangement. The wife of the biological father is not a party to the contract, but the relinquishing of parental rights by the surrogate mother allows the wife to subsequently adopt the child as a stepparent.

The Kentucky Supreme Court agreed with the ruling of the circuit court that the statute prohibiting purchase of a child for adoption, KRS 199.590(2), was not violated by this agreement. The parties involved in the surrogate motherhood contract were both biological parents of the child; thus, it was not necessary for the child to be adopted. The arrangement only stipulates that the wife may adopt the child as a stepparent. The Kentucky Supreme Court also held that the surrogate motherhood arrangement did not violate the intent of the statute, which is to prevent pregnant women from being financially coerced into giving up their child. Because the agreement of custody occurs before conception, the surrogate motherhood arrangement is fundamentally different from that of adoption of a child of an unwed mother. It is more similar to artificial insemination. The Kentucky Supreme Court rejected an argument by the attorney general that a 1984 amendment to KRS 199.590, which specifically states that the statute does not prohibit in vitro fertilization (IVF),* by failing to include surrogate motherhood in its exclusion, does prohibit surrogate motherhood by implication.

The Kentucky Supreme Court also rejected the argument that relinquishment of parental rights by the mother is required in the arrangement primarily to allow the wife of the biological father to adopt. Relinquishment of parental rights in surrogate motherhood arrangements is accomplished so that custody of the child will be facilitated. The Kentucky Supreme Court agreed with SPA that the contract was voidable, not illegal, and void. Thus, the relinquishment of parental rights and consent to adopt stipulated in the contract and made prior to conception are unenforceable under Kentucky law. Recognition of the mother's right to revoke surrender of custody and relinquishment of parental rights is stipulated in the SPA contract. SPA, by recognizing the right of the surrogate mother to change her mind, does not violate KRS 199.601(2) or 199.500(5).

The Kentucky state constitution delegates separation of powers, empowering the legislation to stipulate public policy related to health and welfare. The Kentucky Supreme Court viewed the major question of this case to be whether or not the legislature "had spoken" on surrogate motherhood or whether present laws should be interpreted as covering surrogate motherhood. The Kentucky Supreme Court concluded that the legislature had not spoken on surrogate motherhood. They called for legislation to decide public policy in this area and affirmed that surrogate motherhood arrangements as conducted by SPA are not prohibited by present Kentucky legislation.

Surrogate Parenting v. Com. Ex Rel. Armstrong was cited in *Matter of Adoption of Baby Girl L.J.* (505 N.Y.S.2d 813 [Sur. 1986]) in support of the court's conclusion that surrogate motherhood did not violate New York adoption statutes that were similar to the adoption statutes of Kentucky and that surrogate motherhood contracts are voidable but not void and unenforceable (Barbaruolo, 1993). This case was also cited in a dissenting opinion in *Com. v. Wasson* (Ky., 842 S.W.2d 487 [1992]) as properly recognizing the authority of the legislature, not the judiciary, to determine public policy applying to health and welfare.

REFERENCES: Barbaruolo, Paula M. 1993. "The Public Policy Considerations of Surrogate Motherhood Contracts: An Analysis of Three Jurisdictions." *Albany Law Journal of Science and Technology* 3: 39–77; *Com. v. Wasson* (1992) Ky., 842 S.W.2d 487; *Matter of Adoption of Baby Girl L.J.* (1986), 505 N.Y.S.2d 813 (Sur. 1986); Philips, John W., and Susan D. Philips. 1980–1981. "In Defense of Surrogate Parenting: A Critical Analysis of the Recent Kentucky Experience." *Kentucky Law Journal* 69: 877–931; *Surrogate Parenting v. Com. Ex Rel. Armstrong* (1986) Ky., 704 S.W.2d 209.

CHERYLON ROBINSON

T

TECHNOLOGY ASSESSMENT IN BIOMEDICINE

Assessment of biomedical technology has received considerable attention both in the public and private sectors. At least 45 organizations are involved in biomedical technology assessment, the most prominent of which are the Clinical Efficacy Assessment Project (American College of Physicians); the Diagnostic and Therapeutic Technology Assessment Program (American Medical Association [AMA]); the Medical Necessity and Technology Evaluation and Coverage Programs (Blue Cross/Blue Shield); and the Hospital Technology Service Program (American Hospital Association). In addition, many medical professional societies, health provider organizations, nonprofit health-related organizations, university health institutes, and manufacturers of drugs and medical devices have formal or informal capacities for evaluation and assessment.

Impetus for government involvement in health technology assessment came from a 1976 Office of Technology Assessment (OTA) report that concluded that assessment should be made before costly new medical technologies and procedures were put into general use. This report called for the establishment of formal mechanisms for accomplishing that task and played a part in the program of the National Institutes of Health (NIH)* designed to develop a consensus on technical issues. The short-lived National Center for Health Care Technology (NCHCT) was an attempt to strengthen and centralize efforts to assess health care technologies. After NCHCT's demise in 1981, the OTA reiterated the importance to the nation of a rational and systematic approach to medical technology assessment. "The most important policy need is to bring forth a rational, systematic approach from the present multiplicity of agencies and activities to promote and coordinate medical technology" (OTA, 1982, 18).

In 1984, Congress enacted legislation signed by President Ronald Reagan (Public Law 98–551) that revised the existing National Center for Health Services Research and broadened its mandate for assessing new technology to include not only considerations of safety and efficacy but, as appropriate, cost-effectiveness. The new name of the center became the National Center for Health Services Research/Health Care Technology Assessment (NCHSR/ HCTA). This law also established a council to advise the secretary of the Department of Health and Human Services (DHHS) and the director of the center about health care technology assessment, and it instituted a Council on Health Care Technology under the sponsorship of the National Academy of Sciences (NAS),* with partial governmental support.

The latter provision implemented a recommendation by the Institute of Medicine* (IOM) that proposed creation of a private/public organization to assess medical technology as part of the institute. In the legislation as passed, the council is charged with promoting technology assessment and identifying obsolete or inappropriately applied health care technologies. It has responsibility for establishing a clearinghouse for information on health care technologies and assessments as well as coordinating and commissioning assessments of specific technologies. DHHS was authorized to award the NAS up to $500,000 to cover two thirds of the costs for planning and establishing the council. Operational funds match $1 of federal grant money with at least twice that amount from private sources.

The initiation of the council was delayed due to the need for sufficient long-term private support, opposition from the AMA, and some initial constitutional problems with the authorizing legislation. In addition to the problem of soliciting funds and cooperation from groups in the private sector concerned with the results of technology assessment, there was the question of the degree of cooperation the council would receive from federal agencies. Without such cooperation, the council would be unable to implement its mandate to establish a clearinghouse. Also, there remained questions as to whether a council under the aegis of the IOM, and therefore dependent on support by private sector interested parties, could render unbiased assessments.

In 1989, Congress concluded that this joint public-private sector effort was not fulfilling the perceived needs. As a result, it renamed NCHSR/HCTA the Agency for Health Care Policy and Research* and expanded its role to provide federal leadership in medical technology assessment. One of the initial charges to the new agency was to select a priority-setting process for selecting technologies for assessment.

Another privately sponsored effort to establish a broad framework for decision making on the issues that will confront the health sector into the next century is the Health Policy Agenda (HPA) for the American People. Initiated by the AMA in 1982, it represented the combined effort of 172 private and public organizations working together to provide a broad health care policy framework while simultaneously safeguarding the essential elements of individual decision making. Phase I of the two-phase project produced 159 principles and 41 issues covering a wide spectrum of health concerns. During phase II, which began in late 1984, policy proposals consistent with these principles were developed in response to the issues. At a press conference on February 23, 1987, HPA unveiled its report. Among its position statements, the report concluded: "Society must come to grips with the moral and ethical questions posed by rapid developments in health care technology—who should have access to this technology, under what circumstances should technology be applied or withdrawn, and the respective roles of providers and patients in reaching these decisions." Throughout its deliberations, HPA placed emphasis on consensus building across the wide array of groups participating in the project. As with other such efforts, it is questionable whether HPA had any lasting policy impact.

A clear example of the difficulties inherent in establishing an unbiased national assessment program is the Prospective Payment Assessment Commission (ProPAC) that was established by the legislation that imposed a prospective payment system for Medicare. ProPAC was included in the legislation because of concern that the Health Care Financing Administration and DHHS, in their quest to contain costs, would not pay adequate attention to technological advances if they increased costs. In order to check this perceived bias, ProPAC members are appointed by the congressional OTA, even though it also advises DHHS in the executive branch.

In congruence with congressional intent, ProPAC members vowed in 1985 to take an unbiased approach toward technology assessment. They suggested that adjustments may be required in the financial incentives created by prospective payments to encourage adoption of more costly but quality-enhancing technologies. Presently, the diagnostic related groupings* (DRGs) system encourages adoption of cost-reducing technologies but discourages cost-raising ones. Unbiased assessment, however, will likely result in recommendations to use some technologies that will increase costs and thus run counter to current efforts to cut the costs of Medicare. Because of this inherent conflict in values, it is probable that recommendations by ProPAC to introduce beneficial, but costly, technologies into the DRG system will be rejected, thereby throwing this entire assessment enterprise into question.

ProPAC was also charged by Congress with conducting or sponsoring original assessments of medical technology that are necessary to advise the secretary of DHHS about reimbursement rates for DRGs. Not surprisingly, little funding for that task was forthcoming. As a result, ProPAC was forced to rely primarily on published literature and existing assessments as it develops recommendations about the incorporation of new medical technologies into the prospective payment system. Although it can emphasize those appraisals that it regards as the most appropriate and fair, the lack of resources to produce original assessments weakens its role in the policymaking process. To the extent that the allocation and, ultimately, rationing of health care will be based on technology assessment, the lack of coherent and nonpolitical assessment mechanisms put into question any such efforts.

In 1982, the OTA concluded that emerging drugs and medical devices are adequately and appropriately identified and tested but that emerging medical and surgical procedures are not. "The most pressing need is for some routine mechanism, e.g., the reimbursement system, to identify new procedures before they are adopted" (OTA, 1982, 17). Unlike other substantive areas, the reimbursement system, rather than a regulatory agency, may be the prime candidate for assessment because coverage and payment decisions by the government have become critical factors in the diffusion of medical technologies.

Despite the fact that the OTA's critical assessment of the assessment process for medical procedures is a decade old, its observations remain relevant today. No class of medical technology is adequately evaluated on a continuing basis for either cost-effectiveness or social or ethical implications. Despite efforts at technology assessment (TA) described above, there is no single organization whose mission it is to ensure that medical and surgical procedures are fully assessed before their widespread use.

Furthermore, the synthesis phase of TA continued to be weak at best. Research evidence regarding the safety, efficacy, and effectiveness of emerging technologies is seldom analyzed systematically and objectively. As evidenced by the expansion of Medicare coverage for heart and liver transplantations and funding of acquired immunodeficiency syndrome (AIDS) research and treatment, reimbursement and regulatory decisions continue to be under the heavy influence of the political climate and clearly reflect a value system mired in the technological imperative.

The strong predisposition in U.S. society against precluding or even slowing development of potentially life-saving technologies makes biomedicine a particularly sensitive area for critical TA. Moreover, the unrealistic dependence of the public on a technological fix to health problems, and the search for quick cures at the expense of prevention and health promotion in the United States, explains the reluctance of Congress to deny funding even for unproven biomedical innovations. Any attempts to stop or slow development of particular biomedical innovations face vehement criticism from those individuals, interest groups, and economic interests that have a personal stake in continued funding. "Admiration for the new technology assessment is not universal. Many practicing physicians believe it will further erode their ability to practice as they deem best; similarly, medical researchers, pharmaceutical manufacturers, and producers of medical devices fear that it will inhibit the development and diffusion of new forms of technology" (Fuchs and Garber, 1990, 673).

The result of these value preferences is an almost universal failure of TA in this area to recommend against development of questionable techniques such as the artificial heart* or to reassess older technologies and consider discontinuing their use (Banta and Thacker, 1990, 236). Part of this problem might stem from an inherent difficulty of TA to deal with futuristic problems. Whether because of short-term political pressures, the difficulty of forecasting long-term problems, or some combination of both, the time frame of TA continues to be limited to the near future. Moreover, the strong preference of the public and leaders for more and more advanced biomedical interventions makes any attempts to restrict their development politically unattractive. The burden these technologies may place on future generations and the negative consequences that might accompany them are thus minimized or absent from most assessments.

REFERENCES: Banta, H. David, and Stephen B. Thacker. 1990. "The Case for Reassessment of Health Care Technology." *Journal of the American Medical Association* 264(2): 235–39; Fuchs, Victor R., and Alan M. Garber. 1990. "The New Technology Assessment." *New England Journal of Medicine* 323(10): 673–77; McDonough, Paul G. 1992. "The Need for Technology Assessment in the Reproductive Sciences." *American Journal of Obstetrics and Gynecology* 166(4): 1082–90; Office of Technology Assessment (OTA). 1982. *Strategies for Medical Technology Assessment.* Washington, D.C.: U.S. Government Printing Office; Schwartz, William B. 1994. "In the Pipeline: A Wave of Valuable Medical Technology." *Health Affairs* (Summer): 70–79.

ROBERT H. BLANK

TORT FOR WRONGFUL LIFE

Tort for wrongful life is a suit brought on behalf of an affected infant, most commonly against a physician or other health professional who, it is alleged, negligently failed to inform the parents of the possibility of their producing a severely ill child, thereby preventing a parental choice in avoiding conception or birth of the child. The unique aspect of such suits is the assumption that a life has evolved that should not have. If not for the negligence of the defendant, the child plaintiff would never have been born. Although the term *wrongful life* has been applied to a variety of situations, including those where parents are suing for damages to the child, it is more precise to limit wrongful life action to that brought solely by the affected child. Most recent suits for wrongful life have been brought on behalf of children with severe mental or physical defects and ask for monetary damages to be awarded on the basis of the children's very existence, as compared to their nonexistence. Wrongful life suits differ from traditional negligence actions in that the harm here is in being born, even though compensation ultimately is asked in the form of monetary damages.

Legal questions surrounding wrongful life action center on whether the defendant has a legal cognizable duty to the infant plaintiff, even though the plaintiff was not born or in some cases even conceived at the time of the defendant's allegedly negligent act. There is considerable disagreement, however, over whether the plaintiff is harmed by the defendant's negligence and, if so, how such damages can be measured. A question that the courts traditionally have been unwilling to face is whether or not the infant plaintiff is damaged by being born with defects when the only alternative is nonexistence. The plaintiff here must successfully argue that he or she would have been better off never born. On public policy grounds, which have been interpreted by many legal observers as always favoring life over nonexistence, most courts have asserted that the plaintiff cannot be harmed by his or her birth.

Prior to the late 1970s, the courts unanimously refused to recognize the possibility of a cause of action for wrongful life. In *Gleitman v. Cosgrove* (1967), the New Jersey Supreme Court declared that the preciousness of human life, no matter how burdened, outweighs the need for recovery by the infant. In 1980, however, a California appeals court (*Curlender v. Bio-Science Laboratories*) agreed that a Tay-Sachs infant was entitled to seek recovery for an alleged wrongful life. In 1981, the New Jersey Supreme Court (*Schroeder v. Perkel*) agreed with *Curlender* and allowed a plaintiff born with cystic fibrosis to collect for his "wrongful," "diminished" life. For other supporting cases, see *Procanik v. Cillo* (1984) and *Harbeson v. Parke-Davis* (1983).

Many courts, however, refuse to recognize wrongful life actions. In *Sienieniec v. Lutheran General Hospital,* the Illinois Supreme Court held that a child born with hemophilia could not maintain a wrongful life action against physicians allegedly negligent in failing to advise, counsel, or test his or her parents during the mother's pregnancy concerning the risk that the fetus would have hemophilia. According to the court, recognition of a legal right not to be born, rather than to live with hemophilia, was contrary to public policy.

Similarly, in *Ellis v. Sherman* (1984), the Pennsylvania Superior Court affirmed a lower court's refusal to recognize an infant's cause of action for wrongful life. This case involved the failure of an obstetrician to diagnose the manifestations of neurofibromatosis, a hereditary disorder that the father exhibited. Moreover, in *Di Natale v. Lieberman,* the Florida Appellate Court denied a cause of action for wrongful life because of the difficulty in assessing damages for being born, while in *Dorlin v. Providence Hospital* and *Nelson v. Krusen* (1982), the child's claim for wrongful life was rejected because the assessment of damages would be too speculative.

In response to court actions for wrongful life, at least six states (Idaho, Montana, Minnesota, Missouri, South Dakota, and Utah) have enacted measures limiting or prohibiting actions brought by, or on behalf of, infant plaintiffs for wrongful life. The 1982 Minnesota statute, for example, prescribes such tort actions, stating: "No person shall maintain a cause of action or receive an award of damages on behalf of himself based on the claim that but for the negligent conduct of another, he would have been aborted." California law prohibits children from bringing wrongful life actions against parents, but it does imply that such actions against third parties should be recognized.

REFERENCES: Botkin, J. R. 1988. "The Legal Concept of Wrongful Life." *Journal of the American Medical Association* 259(10): 1541–1545; *Curlender v. Bio-Science Laboratories,* 165 Cal. Rptr. 477 (1980); *Di Natale v. Lieberman,* 409 So.2d 512 (Fla. 1982); *Ellis v. Sherman,* No. J26052 (Pa. 1984); *Gleitman v. Cosgrove,* 49 N.J. 22, 227 A.2d 689 (1967); *Harbeson v. Parke-Davis,* 98 Wash. 2d 460 (1983); *Nelson v. Krusen,* 6355. W2d 582 (Tex. 1982); *Procanik v. Cillo,* 97 N.J. 339, 478 A.2d 755 (1984); *Procanik v. Cillo,* N.J. Sup. Ct. No. A-89 (1984); *Schroeder v. Perkel,* 87 N.J. 53 (S.C.N.J. 1981); *Sienieniec v. Lutheran General Hospital,* 512 NE. 2d 691 (Ill. 1987).

See also **PRENATAL DIAGNOSIS.**

ROBERT H. BLANK

TUBE FEEDING

A "feeding tube" is used most commonly to provide nutrition and hydration to an individual who is unable to take food and water orally. Feeding tubes have been used since 1822 but were perfected in the early 1970s. There are four basic types of feeding tubes: (1) a nasogastric tube (inserted through the nostril and threaded into the stomach; (2) a gastrostomy tube (inserted into the stomach directly through the abdominal wall); (3) a jejunostomy tube (placed through the abdominal wall into the jejunum, the first part of the small intestine after the stomach); and (4) a gastrostomy "button" (a skin-level one-way valve implanted on an outpatient basis under a local anesthetic that replaces the jejunostomy tube and the gastrostomy tube. The gastrostomy button allows a feeding tube to be inserted and removed from the stomach at will.

Feeding tubes must be distinguished from nasogastric tubes used medically to evacuate the stomach in the postoperative patient or patients with gastrointestinal bleeding. These latter devices are often large-bore and made of relatively inflexible rubber, which makes them uncomfortable when used for more than 12 hours. In contrast, feeding tubes are usually the diameter of a broom straw, or of a 50-pound test fishing line. Feeding tubes could more properly be termed "feeding lines," but the description of the device as a "tube" is a pervasive carry-over from the older, more crudely designed delivery systems.

Nasogastric feeding tubes are used for the intermediate-term management of nutrition and hydration of postoperative patients, trauma victims, stroke victims, respirator-dependent patients, patients who are near death, and in a variety of illnesses where intravenous access is a problem. Gastrostomy and jejunostomy tubes and the gastrostomy button are used for long-term management in a variety of central nervous system injuries or diseases (such as stroke or tumor) and in any patient who cannot reasonably be expected to recover the ability to take food by mouth. The feedings given through these tubes are carefully formulated, full-liquid, nutritionally complete supplements. These supplements are commercially available in several combinations that recognize the needs of the particular patient (e.g., the diabetic patient or the lactose-intolerant patient). The cost of a nutritionally complete daily liquid feeding plan including administration is less than the average cost of a conventional diet.

Patients who receive long-term nutrition and hydration through a feeding tube tolerate the procedure well, with remarkably few complications. Since the daily cost of the feedings is not a significant factor, maintenance of a patient by a feeding tube is not physically or financially burdensome. Despite the fact that some courts have accepted the argument that a feeding tube is burdensome, there is little scientific foundation to this claim. The "burdensome" part of such appeals (if in fact there is a burden) is in reality found in the emotional pain the family may feel when observing a loved one unable to act independently. It is often difficult for an adult child to deal with childlike dependency of an elderly parent.

REFERENCES: May, William E., et al. 1987. "Feeding and Hydrating the Permanently

Unconscious and Other Vulnerable Persons." *Issues in Law and Medicine* 3: 203–217; McCarrick, Pat Milmoe. 1992. "Active Euthanasia and Assisted Suicide." *The National Center for Bioethics Literature: Scope Note* 18: 1–17; McCarrick, Pat Milmoe. 1992. "Withholding or Withdrawing Nutrition or Hydration." *The National Reference Center for Bioethics Literature: Scope Note* 7: 1–17; Orentlichner, David. 1989. "Physician Participation in Assisted Suicide." *Journal of the American Medical Association* 262: 1844–1845; Pankratz, Robert C. 1992. "A Response to the Death Debate." *Christian Medical Dental Society Journal* 23: 12–15; Schiedermayer, David. 1994. *Putting the Soul Back in Medicine.* Grand Rapids, MI: Baker Books; Schiedermayer, David. 1994. "Why Am I Still Tube Feeding Mrs. Johnson?" *Long-term Care Forum* 4: 1–15; Shewmon, D. Alan. 1987. "Active Voluntary Euthanasia: A Needless Pandora's Box." *Issues in Law and Medicine* 3: 219–244.

CURTIS E. HARRIS

TUSKEGEE SYPHILIS STUDY

In 1972, the public learned about the federally funded syphilis study conducted in Tuskegee, Alabama, which has since come to symbolize unethical research using human subjects. This was not an isolated incident, nor was it the first to come to light; the atrocities of the Nazi doctors during World War II had been highly publicized, and in the late 1960s, Henry Beecher and Henry Pappworth published their criticisms of hundreds of unethical experiments. The Tuskegee study stands out, though, because it endured for decades and involved hundreds of innocent victims.

The study was carried out by researchers in the U.S. Department of Health, Education, and Welfare (now the Department of Health and Human Services). It began in 1932 in an area of the United States where the incidence of syphilis was the highest. The research subjects were all African-American males in the late stages of syphilis (usually not infectious); men with early, infectious syphilis were screened out, as were women and children. The point was to study the natural progression of the disease when left untreated.

Over the 30 years of the study, approximately 600 African-American men were recruited to be subjects. Most of them were led to believe that they would receive free medical care. The men's syphilis remained untreated, however, even after the discovery of penicillin in 1943. Researchers even took steps to ensure that local physicians did not treat the subjects. It is estimated that 28 of the participants died as a result of nontreatment, and a further 100 suffered disabilities such as blindness and insanity. In addition, the men were not told that they had syphilis; they were not told they were being studied instead of treated; they were not told that treatment was available; and they were enticed to undergo painful spinal taps for nontherapeutic purposes.

The Tuskegee study came to the public's attention after a young researcher alerted a journalist friend. Her story on the subject ran in the *New York Times* and other newspapers in the summer of 1972, effectively ending the study. In response, the Department of Health and Human Welfare appointed a panel to investigate the Tuskegee study, and two years later, Congress passed the National Research Act (P.L. 93–348), which established the National Commission to address ethical issues in the conduct of research involving human subjects. The commission articulated three requirements for proceeding with research involving human subjects: the subject must give his/her informed and voluntary consent; the benefits of the research must outweigh the risks; and the selection of subjects must be fair. All of these requirements have been codified into federal regulations (45 CFR 46, 21 CFR 50 & 56), in an attempt to ensure that research like the Tuskegee study—which violated the most fundamental rights of its subjects—will not happen again.

REFERENCES: Beecher, Henry. 1966. "Ethics and Clinical Research." *New England Journal of Medicine* 274: 1354–1369; Frankel, M. S. 1975. "The Development of Policy Guidelines Governing Human Experimentation in the United States." *Ethics in Science and Medicine* 2: 43–59; Jones, J. H. 1981. *Bad Blood: The Tuskegee Syphilis Experiment.* New York: Free Press; Pappworth, M. H. 1968. *Human Guinea Pigs.* Boston: Beacon Press; Pence, Gregory E. 1990. *Classic Cases in Medical Ethics.* New York: McGraw-Hill; Thomas, S. B., and Quinn, S. C. 1991. "The Tuskegee Syphilis Study, 1932 to 1972." *American Journal of Public Health* 81: 1498.

ERIC M. MESLIN and DEBORAH R. MATHIEU

U

ULTRASOUND/SONOGRAPHY

Ultrasound and sonography are prenatal diagnostic procedures using high-frequency nonionizing, nonelectromagnetic sound waves directed into the abdomen of the pregnant woman to gain an echovisual image of the fetus, uterus, placenta, and other inner structures. It is a noninvasive technology that is painless for the woman and reduces the need for X-ray scanning procedures. Extensive studies have found no harmful long- or short-term hazards to the fetus from diagnostic sonography (Office of Medical Applications of Research, 1984). Its routine use, however, should be weighted against false-positive or -negative diagnoses and the considerable monetary investment involving screening large numbers of low-risk pregnancies. Moreover, one study of over 15,000 low-risk pregnant women found that routine ultrasound screening did not improve perinatal outcome when compared to its selective use on the basis of clinical judgment (Ewigman et al., 1993).

In addition to its use in conjunction with amniocentesis to determine fetal position, fetal age, and amniotic fluid volume, ultrasound can also be used to observe fetal development and movement as well as detect some musculoskeletal malformations and major organ disorders. More sophisticated devices can show images of fetal organs, such as the ventricles and intestines, and, in some cases, identify Down syndrome fetuses. Ultrasound is also essential in conjunction with fetoscopy* or placental aspiration and in fetal surgery. Finally, in conjunction with ultrasound, magnetic resonance imaging (MRI) has the potential to provide detailed diagnosis of nervous system abnormalities and other internal fetal problems.

REFERENCES: Berkowitz, Richard L. 1993. "Should Every Pregnant Woman Undergo Ultrasonography?" *New England Journal of Medicine* 329(12): 874–875; Bronshtein, M., E. Z. Zimmer, L. M. Gerlis, et al. 1993. "Early Ultrasound Diagnosis of Fetal Congenital Heart Defects in High-Risk and Low-Risk Pregnancies." *Obstetrics and Gy-*

necology 82(2): 225–229; Ewigman, B. G., J. P. Crane, F. D. Frigoletto, et al. 1993. "Effect of Prenatal Ultrasound Screening on Perinatal Outcome." *New England Journal of Medicine* 329(12): 821–827; Office of Medical Applications of Research, National Institutes of Health. 1984. "The Use of Diagnostic Ultrasound Imaging During Pregnancy." *Journal of the American Medical Association* 252: 649–672; Smith, Ramada S., and Signey F. Bottoms. 1993. "Ultrasonographic Prediction of Neonatal Survival in Extremely Low-Birth-Weight Infants." *American Journal of Obstetrics and Gynecology* 169(3): 490–493.

See also **PRENATAL DIAGNOSIS.**

ROBERT H. BLANK

UNIFORM ANATOMICAL GIFT ACT

Passed by the U.S. Congress in 1968 and adopted in all 50 states, the UAGA was designed to enable individuals to make anatomical bequests for a variety of purposes, especially to medical schools and for organ, tissue, and cornea transplantation (8A U.L.A. 19 [1994]). The act, which relies on the values of voluntary choice and altruism, provides that (1) anyone over the age of 18 may give all or part of his/her body to education, research, or transplant; (2) the gift may be authorized by a card carried by the individual or by written or verbally recorded communication; (3) anatomical gifts made by deceased individuals cannot be revoked by next of kin; (4) in the absence of a clear objection by the deceased, the next of kin may make a donation on behalf of the deceased; (5) there must be no disagreement among the next of kin regarding the decision to donate the deceased individual's body or organs. To ensure that decisions to donate are made voluntarily and altruistically, subsequent federal legislation explicitly prohibited the sale of organs (P.L. 98–507).

Because the UAGA had not been utilized to the extent hoped, in 1987 various amendments were enacted to simplify the making of anatomical gifts and to require that the donor's intentions be followed. The amendments included provisions requiring physicians to ask the families of newly dead patients to donate the organs, requiring hospital personnel to ask patients about their willingness to donate their organs, increasing efforts to search for documentation of a gift or next of kin if there is no indication of the patient's wishes, and simplifying gift requests by no longer requiring witnesses.

The most common way that people express their interest in donation is via an organ donor card. Forty-five states and the District of Columbia allow people to indicate their donor status on their driver's license. Recently, some states, such as Texas, have begun to require that people choose whether or not they want to be a donor when obtaining a driver's license (so-called mandated choice). The reported proportion of persons who actually have completed a donor card varies from 8 to 37 percent. While donor cards are rarely found at the time of death, they do serve to promote a family's awareness of their loved one's wishes regarding donation. This information is felt to be critical to the family's decision to donate. Ironically, while the UAGA stresses that the deceased's wishes are controlling, almost all physicians continue to ask the family's permission for the organs and will not take the organs if the family refuses—even if the deceased had signed a donor card.

REFERENCES: American Medical Association. 1994. "Strategies for Cadaveric Organ Procurement." *Journal of the American Medical Association* 272:809–12; Jeddoloh, N. P. 1976. "The Uniform Anatomical Gift Act and a Statutory Definition of Death." *Transplantation Proceedings* 8(Supp. 1):245–49; Lee, P. P., and Kissner, P. 1986. "Organ Donation and the Uniform Anatomical Gift Act." *Surgery* 100:867–75; Overcase, T. D., et al. 1984. "Problems in the Identification of Potential Organ Donors: Misconceptions and Fallacies Associated with Donor Cards." *Journal of the American Medical Association* 251:1559–62; Sutton, E. C. 1990. "The Revised Uniform Anatomical Gift Act: An Analysis." *The Medical Staff Counselor* 4:37–41.

LAURA A. SIMINOFF, ROBERT M. ARNOLD, and MOLLY SEAR

UNITED AUTO WORKERS V. JOHNSON CONTROLS

The Supreme Court's decision to hear *United Auto Workers v. Johnson Controls* put the issue of discrimination from exclusionary policies (so-called fetal protection policies) on the agenda again (Becker, 1986; Bertin, 1986; Williams, 1981) nearly 10 years after commentators called reproductive hazards "the occupational health issue of the 1980s" and after nearly a decade of stonewalling by the Equal Employment Opportunity Commission on the issue (Cooke and Kenney, 1988; U.S., Congress, House Education and Labor Committee, 1990). In 1977, a mere 13 years after Congress had outlawed sex discrimination in employment, Johnson Controls hired its first women for jobs with high lead exposure. It advised women who were planning to conceive not to take the jobs and required them to sign a waiver stating the company had informed them of the risks. After several women did become pregnant and registered blood leads higher than the Occupational Safety and Health Administration (OSHA) recommends, in 1982 Johnson Controls began to exclude all women who did not have proof of infertility from jobs in which *any* employee had recorded a high blood lead as well as from jobs that fed into high lead exposure jobs. Having learned from the public relations debacle of American Cyanamid, the company officially discouraged sterilization.

In 1984, the United Auto Workers (UAW) union filed a class action suit arguing that Johnson Controls' adoption of an exclusionary policy at its 14 battery manufacturing plants violated Title VII. Johnson Controls requested the district court grant it summary judgment—that the court dispense with a trial because there were no contested issues of fact or law. The UAW protested that two important facts were in dispute: whether fetuses were at risk from low levels of maternal exposure to lead and whether men's exposure endangered their reproductive capacity. The company and the union also disagreed about how the court should classify the exclusionary policy under the law. How the court chooses to classify the policy assigns the burden of proof between employers and workers and determines how hard it is for an employer to justify its policy. Title VII of the Civil Rights Act of 1964, as amended by the Pregnancy Discrimination Act of 1978, prohibits sex discrimination in employment. Sex discrimination includes discrimination because of pregnancy, childbirth, or related medical condition (Furnish, 1980). To justify excluding all women from a job, an employer must show that sex is a bona fide occupational qualification (BFOQ) for the job—that you cannot do the job if you are a woman. If, however, an employer adopts a "neutral" policy that excludes disproportionately more women than men, such as a height requirement, the employer must justify the policy as a business necessity.

Although the policies discriminate on their face, three circuit courts treated them as neutral, allowing the employer to justify them under the business necessity defense. In *Wright v. Olin* (697 F.2d. 1172 [4th Cir. 1982]), the Court of Appeals for the Fourth Circuit had analyzed a similar policy under the category of disparate impact and laid out guidelines for when such policies would be lawful under Title VII. First, a company would have to show that a significant risk to the fetus resulted from women's but not men's exposure. Second, the company would have to produce scientific evidence for its conclusions, although there need not be consensus. Third, the company would have to show there were no less discriminatory alternatives. In *Hayes v. Shelby Memorial Hospital* (726 F.2d. 1543 [11th Cir. 1984]), the Court of Appeals for the Eleventh Circuit applied the disparate impact analysis but concluded that Hayes had been the victim of discrimination because Shelby Memorial Hospital could not show that the radiation an X-ray technician received posed a significant risk to the fetus. The Court of Appeals for the Sixth Circuit in *Grant v. General Motors* (908 F.2d 1303 [6th Cir. 1990]), however, required General Motors to defend its policy under the rubric of disparate treatment.

The consequences of treating facially discriminatory exclusionary policies as if they were neutral (disparate impact) became more significant as the Supreme Court lessened the standard of justification for business necessity during the 1980s (*Wards Cove Packing Co. v. Atonio,* 1989). Because the Court's rulings had made it virtually impossible to challenge neutral employment policies that froze women in low-paid jobs, Congress fought to amend the law and eventually succeeded in passing the Civil Rights Act of 1991. As *UAW v. Johnson Controls* worked its way through the appeals process, however, the reduced standard of proof for disparate impact was in effect.

Both the district court and the court of appeals analyzed the exclusionary policy as if it were neutral, although it discriminated against women on its face, and applied the reduced standard of justification for business necessity. Both did so without a trial record since District Judge Robert Warren granted Johnson Controls' motion for summary judgment. The Court of Appeals for the Seventh Circuit affirmed, 7–4. The majority held, however, that Johnson Controls would have been entitled to summary judgment even if the company had had to defend its policy as a bona fide occupational qualification. Both courts accepted that lead posed a risk to a developing fetus and dismissed the evidence of the effects of lead on men's reproductive capacity.

In 1978, when OSHA developed standards of exposure for lead, it explicitly rejected permitting employers to exclude all women (29 C.F.R. § 1910.1044, 1978). Because of evidence that men's reproductive capacity was also at risk from high lead exposure, OSHA set a single standard for men and women. OSHA recommended that employers permit men and women planning to conceive to transfer out of high lead exposure jobs. Because of evidence that lead might harm a developing fetus, OSHA recommended that pregnant women not have blood lead levels that exceeded 30 µg/dl (micrograms per deciliter) Judge Warren, however, found convincing Johnson Controls' evidence that blood lead levels far below 30 µg/dl might injure children and extrapolated that fetuses were also at risk from very low levels of maternal levels of lead in the blood. (Several of the medical experts that Johnson Controls cited objected to how the company used their evidence.)

Four dissenting justices on the court of appeals, however, including Reagan-appointed conservatives of the "law and economics school," argued that summary judgment was inappropriate because important matters of fact and law were in dispute. Judge Easterbrook, in words perhaps intended to pique the attention of the Supreme Court, wrote: "[T]his is the most important sex-discrimination case this circuit has ever decided. It is likely the most important sex-discrimination case in any court since 1964 when Congress enacted Title VII" (886 F.2d 871, 920).

Both Judges Easterbrook and Posner wrote opinions contesting the majority's legal analysis. Policies that explicitly discriminate on the basis of sex, they argued, could only be defended under Title VII as a bona fide occupational qualification—not a business necessity. Judge Easterbrook paraphrased the district court's reasoning as "this *must* be a disparate impact case because an employer couldn't win it as a disparate treatment case" (910). Judge Easterbrook thought Johnson Controls' policy was excessively broad since few women would become pregnant.

Judge Cudahy complained of both the granting of summary judgment and the classification of the policy as disparate impact, calling the analysis "result-oriented gimmickry" (902). He mused over the gender of those who had the power to decide.

It is a matter of some interest that, of the twelve federal judges to have considered this case to date, none has been female. This may be quite significant because this case, like other controversies of great potential consequence, demands, in addition to command of the disembodied rules, some insight into social reality. What is the situation of the pregnant woman, unemployed or working for the minimum wage and unprotected by health insurance, in relation to her pregnant sister, exposed to an indeterminate lead risk but well-fed, housed and doctored? Whose fetus is at greater risk? Whose decision is this to make? We, who are unfortunately all male, must address these and other equally complex questions through the clumsy vehicle of litigation. At least let it be complete litigation focusing on the right standard. (902; while the appeal was pending before the Supreme Court, California state courts declared Johnson Controls' policy to be in conflict with California's fair employment laws [*Department of Fair Employment and Housing v. Globe Battery,* 1987; *Foster v. Johnson Controls,* 1990])

The Supreme Court echoed the dissenters, not the majority, on the court of appeals in its ruling. On March 20, 1991, the United States Supreme Court unanimously held that Johnson Controls' exclusionary policy discriminated against women. The only title VII defense for explicit sex discrimination is that sex is a bona fide occupational qualification for the job—that you cannot do the job if you are a woman. All nine justices agreed that Johnson Controls' exclusionary policy was facially discriminatory and the lower courts erred in granting the company summary judgment. Justice Blackmun argued that the three circuits had erred in treating exclusionary policies as neutral, allowing the employer to justify them under the business necessity defense.

Justice Blackmun went on, however, to say that employers could *never* justify an exclusionary policy as a BFOQ. Being potentially pregnant does not render women incapable of making batteries. Nor could the threat of tort liability of injured children justify the exclusion of fertile women. Noting OSHA's lead standard, Justice Blackmun concluded that if employers met established exposure standards and informed women of the risks, courts would not consider them negligent. Justice Blackmun, author of *Roe v. Wade,** wrote: "Decisions about the welfare of future children must be left to the parents who conceive, bear, support, and raise them rather than to the employers who hire those parents" (1207).

In a concurring opinion, Justice White, joined by Chief Justice Rehnquist and Justice Kennedy, thought employers might be able to defend a more narrowly tailored policy as a BFOQ. Justice White did, however, agree that summary judgment was inappropriate and that the policy constituted disparate treatment. The likelihood of a substantial tort liability could justify a BFOQ, but the burden would be on the employer to prove that threat existed. Justice White thought the BFOQ could include considerations of cost and safety, instead of merely whether women could perform the job. He did, however, believe that Johnson Controls had overstated the risk and that it should have considered less discriminatory alternatives to excluding all nonsterilized women.

Justice Scalia's concurring opinion dismissed the evidence on lead as irrelevant. Even if all employed women put their fetuses at risk, and men's exposure did not jeopardize the health of their offspring, Johnson Controls' policy was facially discriminatory because "Congress has unequivocally said so [in passing the Pregnancy Discrimination Act]" (1216). Those who find that result unsatisfactory should appeal to Congress to amend the law. Although he agreed with Justice Blackmun that any action required by Title VII could not give rise to tort liability, Justice Scalia thought that cost could be a defense for explicit discrimination. A prohibitive expense might justify excluding women from certain jobs, but the employer would bear the burden of proof.

By overturning the lower courts' rulings upholding exclusionary policies, the Supreme Court restores conventional sex discrimination doctrine. Judges can no longer create an exception to the narrow requirements of the BFOQ defense because they see employers' policies as benign—they cannot substitute their own standard of what is unreasonable for the law's definition of discrimination (Kenney, 1992). Beyond sending a clear message to employers that exclusionary policies violate Title VII, the ruling has four principal effects.

First, Justice Scalia's concurring opinion raises an important point for feminist legal thought. Justice Scalia argued that the Title VII prohibits employers from excluding fertile women from hazardous work, not because men face reproductive hazards from lead, too, but because the Pregnancy Discrimination Act (PDA) states unambiguously that employers may not exclude women from jobs because of their capacity to become pregnant. Justice Blackmun also refers to the plain language of the PDA, but Justice Scalia explicitly mentions that a comparison is not required. As feminist legal scholars have long maintained, pointing to decisions such as *General Electric Co. v. Gilbert* (1976) and its British equivalents (*Turley v. Allders Department Stores,* 1980; *Hayes v. Malleable Working Men's Club,* 1985; *Webb v. EMO Air Cargo,* 1994), the law incorporates a male standard (MacKinnon, 1987). Women can have the right to work only if they are just like men or can compare their circumstances to men. In *UAW v. Johnson Controls,* the Supreme Court declared unequivocally that whether women can compare themselves to men or not, the law forbids employers punishing women because they can bear children.

Second, *UAW v. Johnson Controls* is a victory for sex discrimination law, not because it solves the problem of reproductive hazards in the workplace but because it alters the terms of the debate. Rather than trying to make it appear safe by excluding women workers and ignoring the evidence about men, employers will have to make the workplace safe for men and women. Focusing only on whether employers could exclude women and whether women were different from men deflected attention, not only from the reproductive hazards from men's exposure but also from concerns about the effects of toxins on workers more generally. The United Auto Workers union and groups supporting them, such as the Women's Rights Project of the American Civil Liberties Union, did not seek the right of women to poison their offspring on the same terms as men but for all workers to have the right to a workplace free from hazards, reproductive or nonreproductive. The Supreme Court's decision in *UAW v. Johnson Controls* removed this impediment to focusing on the safety of the workplace, rather than the sex of the worker.

Third, the decision should help promote initiatives to break down job segregation by sex. Women run no danger of being excluded from low-paying hazardous jobs. The real solution, of course, is to clean up the workplace. The Supreme Court's decision is a powerful statement that women do not have to give up their right to bear children if they want to work. Ironically, most of the women employed by Johnson Controls had no intention of becoming pregnant: They were in their forties or fifties; they were celibate or on the pill; or their husbands had had vasectomies. (Only 2 percent of blue-collar workers older than 30 become pregnant each year [Stellman and Henifin, 1982, 138]). They resented not only having to be sterilized to keep their jobs but having this fact known by their coworkers who joked about neutering, veterinarians having a special, and lost femininity (Faludi, 1991, 443, 448).

Finally, the decision should have an impact on how the Equal Employment Opportunity Commission (EEOC) enforces Title VII. Under Chairman Clarence Thomas, the EEOC's policy was to do nothing about complaints on exclusionary policies. Now that the Supreme Court has ruled that exclusionary policies are unlawful sex discrimination, the EEOC can no longer justify its inaction by claiming to be mystified by tough legal and scientific issues ("EEOC Issues," 1991).

REFERENCES: Becker, Mary E. 1986. "From *Muller v. Oregon* to Fetal Vulnerability Policies." *University of Chicago Law Review* 53(fall):1219–73; Bertin, Joan E. 1986. Review of *Double Exposure: Women's Health Hazards on the Job and at Home,* ed. Wendy Chavkin. *Women's Rights Law Reporter* 9(winter):89–93; *Christman v. American Cyanamid,* Civ. Action No. 80–0024(P) (N.D. W.Va.) (complaint filed January 28, 1980); Cooke, Edmund D., Jr., and Sally J. Kenney. 1988. "Commentary: The View from Capitol Hill." In *Reproductive Laws for the 1990s,* ed. Sherrill Cohen and Nadine Taub. Clifton, NJ: Humana Press; *Department of Fair Employment and Housing v. Globe Battery,* FEP 83–84 K1–0262s L–33297 87–19 (September 1, 1987), 6; *Doerr v. B. F. Goodrich Co.,* 22 Fair Empl. Prac. Cas. (BNA) 345 (N.D. Ohio 1979); "EEOC Issues Guidance to Staffers on Biased Fetal-Protection Policies." *Daily Labor Report* 132 (July 10, 1991); Faludi, Susan. 1991. *Backlash: The Undeclared War Against American Women.* New York: Crown; "Fetal Protection Issues Remain After Ruling in *Johnson Controls.*" *Daily Labor Report* 17 (January 27, 1992): A1; *Foster v. Johnson Controls,* 267 Cal. Rpt. 158 (Cal. App. 4 Dist. 1990), *cert denied,* Supreme Court of California 1990 Cal. LEXIS 2107 (may 17, 1990); Furnish, Hannah Arterian. 1980. "Prenatal Exposure to Fetally Toxic Work Environments: The Dilemma of the 1978 Pregnancy Amendments to Title VII of the Civil Rights Act of 1964." *Iowa Law Review* 66:63–129; *General Electric Co. v. Gilbert,* 429 U.S. 125 (1976); *Grant v. General Motors,* 743 F. Supp. 1260 (N.D. Ohio 1989), *vacated and remanded,* 908 F.2d 1303 (6th Cir. 1990); *Hayes v. Malleable Working Men's Club and Institute,* [1985] ICR 703 (EAT); *Hayes v. Shelby Memorial Hospital,* 546 F. Supp. 259 (N.D. Ala. 1982), 726 F.2d 1543 (11th Cir. 1984), *rehearing denied,* 732 F.2d 944 (11th Cir. 1984); *International Union, United Automobile, Aerospace and Agricultural Implement Workers of America, UAW v. Johnson Controls, Inc.,* 680 F. Supp. 309 (E.D. Wis. 1988), *aff'd, en banc,* 886 F.2d 871 (7th Cir. 1989), 111 S. Ct. 1196 (1991); Kenney, Sally J. 1992. *For Whose Protection? Reproductive Hazards and Exclusionary Policies in the U.S. and Britain.* Ann Arbor: University of Michigan Press; MacKinnon, Catharine A. 1987. *Feminism Unmodified: Discourses on Life and Law.* Cambridge, MA: Harvard University Press; *Oil, Chemical and Atomic Workers, International Union v. American Cyanamid Co.,* 741 F.2d 444 (D.C. Cir. 1984); Randall, Donna M., and James F. Short, Jr. 1983. "Women in Toxic Work Environments: A Case Study of Social Problem Development.'' *Social Problems* 30(April): 410–24; *Secretary of Labor v. American Cyanamid Co.,* 9 O.S.H. Cas. (BNA) 1596 (1981); Stellman, Jeanne Mager, and Mary Sue Henifin. 1982. ''No Fertile Women Need Apply: Employment Discrimination and Reproductive Hazards in the Workplace.'' In *Biological Woman—The Convenient Myth: A Collection of Feminist Essays and a Comprehensive Bibliography,* ed. Ruth Hubbard, Mary Sue Henifin, and Barbara Fried. Cambridge, MA: Schenkman; *Turley v. Allders Department Stores Ltd.,* [1980] IRLR 4 (EAT); U.S., Congress. House. Committee on Education and Labor. 1990. *A Report by the Majority Staff on the EEOC, Title VII and Workplace Fetal Protection Policies in the 1980s.* 101st Cong., 2d sess. U.S., Congress. Office of Technology Assessment. 1985. *Reproductive Health Hazards in the Workplace.* Washington, D.C.: U.S. Government Printing Office; *Wards Cove Packing Co. v. Atonio,* 109 S. Ct. 2115 (1989); *Webb v. EMO Air Cargo (U.K.) Ltd.,* [1994] IRLR 482 (ECJ); Williams, Wendy W. 1981. ''Firing the Woman to Protect the Fetus: The Reconciliation of Fetal Protection with Employment Opportunity Goals Under Title VII.'' *Georgetown Law Journal* 69: 641–704; *Wright v. Olin,* 24 Fair Empl. Prac. Cas. (BNA) 1646 (W.D. N.C. 1980), 697 F.2d 1172 (4th Cir. 1982), *on remand,* 585 F. Supp. 1447 (W.D. N.C. 1984), *vacated without opinion,* 767 F.2d 915 (4th Cir. 1984); *Zuniga v. Kleberg County Hospital,* 78 E.E.O.C. Dec. (CCH) 4180 ¶ 6642 (November 14, 1974), C.A. No. 77-C-62 (S.D. Texas January 23, 1981), 692 F.2d 986 (5th Cir. 1982).

SALLY J. KENNEY

UNITED NETWORK FOR ORGAN SHARING

UNOS, a private, nonprofit organization located in Richmond, Virginia, administers the national Organ Procurement and Transplantation Network (OPTN) and maintains a scientific registry of all transplant recipients in the United States. In addition to coordinating the logistics of matching organs with patients, and collecting, analyzing, and publishing transplant data, UNOS also educates the public and health care professionals about the donation process and works to increase the number of organ donations.

Since September 1986, the U.S. Department of Health and Human Services has awarded UNOS a contract to design and operate these programs. UNOS grew out of the South-Eastern Organ Procurement Foundation, which in 1982 had established a centralized computer system for the registry of organ donors and recipients.

The National Organ Transplant Act of 1984 (P.L. 98–507) mandated a national system to oversee the equitable allocation of transplantable organs, and in 1986 the Task Force on Organ Transplantation recommended the establishment of the OPTN. The OPTN created by UNOS operates an around-the-clock patient waiting list and an organ matching system. All patients accepted into a transplant program are registered with UNOS, which maintains a centralized computer network linking all organ procurement* organizations and transplant centers.

When a donor organ becomes available, the health care facility contacts UNOS, which generates a ranked list of patients whom the organ might benefit.

UNOS ranks the patients according to a variety of criteria: tissue match, blood type, organ weight, length of time on the waiting list, medical urgency, and immune status. The distance between the organ and the potential recipient is also often a factor: Organs are generally offered first locally, then regionally (there are 11 UNOS regions), and then nationally. The exception to this involves patients waiting for a donor kidney: The national list is used, and kidneys are sent to perfectly matched patients anywhere in the country. There are two primary goals of this national organ-recipient matching system: to increase the probability of a successful transplant and to attempt to provide equitable access to a scarce resource.

The Scientific Registry, which began in October 1987, includes information on all recipients of solid organ transplants (kidney, heart, liver, heart-lung, pancreas, and small bowel) in the United States. Types of data include treatment, clinical variables (e.g., types of immunosuppressant, type of preservation), sociodemographic variables (e.g., patient age, race, and sex), patient survival rates, and graft survival rates. The registry tracks all transplant patients from the time of transplant through hospital discharge and then continues annually until the organ fails and/or the patient dies.

UNOS conducts regional and national meetings to discuss transplant policy, it publishes brochures, reference manuals, and a monthly report, *UNOS Update.* UNOS also maintains a toll-free hotline to distribute donor cards and answer questions (1-800-24-DONOR).

REFERENCES: Benenson, E. L. 1991. "UNOS: Evolution of the Organ Procurement and Transplantation Network." *Dialysis and Transplantation* 20: 495–496; Menzel, Paul T. 1994. "Rescuing Lives: Can't We Count?" *Hastings Center Report* 24: 22–23; Sanfilippo, F. P., et al. 1992. "Factors Affecting the Waiting Time of Cadaveric Kidney Transplant Candidates in the U.S." *Journal of the American Medical Association* 267: 247–252; Ubel, Peter A., et al. 1993. "Rationing Failure." *Journal of the American Medical Association* 270: 2469–2474.

DEBORAH R. MATHIEU

U.S. BIOTECHNOLOGY COMPANIES FORM ALLIANCES WITH ESTABLISHED PHARMACEUTICAL FIRMS

In 1990, the Swiss-based pharmaceutical giant Hoffman–La Roche spent $2.1 billion to purchase 60 percent of Genentech, a luminary among the frontline biotechnology companies, and thereby transformed Roche Holding Ltd., the parent company, from the fifteenth largest pharmaceutical firm into a leading force in the area of biopharmaceuticals. Genentech benefited by receiving an infusion of essential research and development (R&D) capital without having to compromise the company's research-priority culture. The Roche/Genentech deal epitomized a trend in the biopharmaceutical sector toward business collaborations—mergers and acquisitions, joint ventures, so-called strategic corporate alliances, including comarketing and codistribution affiliations, and controlling combinations—all geared to accommodate both vigorous research agendas and the substantial uncertainty associated with commercializing pharmaceutical products. Key considerations behind such arrangements are (1) securing capital, (2) obtaining technical skills from the partner, (3) reducing costs and time in bringing a product to market, (4) validating a technology, (5) acquiring business skills from the partner, and (6) accessing a needed technology. A corporate partner can provide a source of support that is independent of the vagaries of the equities market, permitting a biotech-intensive company to plan in relative freedom from the pressures of quarterly reports and the like. The same economic considerations also have prompted U.S. biotechnology companies to partner with foreign pharmaceutical companies as a means to establish a pathway for expanding into markets abroad and bypassing complex U.S. regulations. But the Genentech/Roche deal triggered concern at the White House Office of Science and Technology Policy over possible adverse consequences to the competitive position of U.S. biotechnology. This concern was heightened even further in 1993 by another alliance, this time involving Sandoz Pharmaceuticals Corporation, another Swiss firm, and the Scripps Research Institute. The agreement in question provided Scripps with $300 million in research funding from Sandoz and gave Sandoz the right to commercialize any or all of Scripps' research for a period of 20 years. A subsequent congressional hearing in March 1993, where fears were expressed over whether the Sandoz/Scripps deal was anticompetitive or violative of law governing the transfer to private industry of federally funded technology, led to the effective abandonment of the proposed agreement.

REFERENCES: Esposito, Robert S. 1993. "Global Perspective on Deals that Drive the BioPharmaceutical Industry." *Genetic Engineering News* 13(20): 14; Fitzpatrick, Linda. 1990. "Genentech's Merger with Roche Opens Up Some Opportunities for Others." *Genetic Technology News* 10: 2; Gebhart, Fred. 1990. "Industry Considers the Roche-Genentech Deal a Major Vote of Confidence for Biotechnology." *Genetic Engineering News* 10(3): 1; Macilwain, Colin. 1994. "Conflict-of-Interest Debate Stirs Mixed Reaction at NIH." *Nature* 367: 401; Miller, Debbie. 1993. "Scripps-Sandoz Deal Demonstrates Need for U.S. to Emphasize Commitment to Technology." *Genetic Engineering News* 13(9): 4; "Sandoz Backs Down on Scripps Deal." *Biotechnology Business News* (The Financial Times Limited), July 16, 1993; "Scripps Imposes Limits on Sandoz Deal." *Marketletter* (Ziff Communications Company), July 19, 1993; "Scripps-Sandoz Agreement Doesn't Serve Public Interest, NIH Director Asserts." *BNA Health Care Daily* (Bureau of National Affairs, Inc.), March 30, 1993.

STEPHEN A. BENT

V

VETERANS ADMINISTRATION

The Veterans Administration was organized in 1930 as an independent agency to administer and finance health care, pensions, and loan benefits for veterans of military service. In 1988, it became the Department of Veterans Affairs with cabinet-level status. This entry deals primarily with the health functions of the former Veterans Administration.

American politics has debated and overwhelmingly rejected government-administered and -operated hospitalization for 60 years with but one exception—the federal hospital system for veterans. With a minimum of controversy, the veterans' health program emerged from World War I as a federally funded and operated health service. Initially, veteran health benefits were provided by the War Risk Insurance Act of 1914 (P.L. 63–193), which required the government to supply "medical, surgical and hospital services" to injured veterans. A variety of incremental statutory changes between 1919 and 1924 specified additional governmental obligations. By 1930, Congress authorized the Veterans Administration and consolidated most medical activity within the VA (Thompson, 1981, 187).

Why did the formation of a U.S. government health care system meet with so little resistance? One observer argues (Stevens, 1991, 281–283) that the creation of the veteran health program was relatively uncontroversial because it was not viewed as a *health* policy. It was a *veteran's* policy and was framed initially like workman's compensation and disability programs. Veterans were a distinct, easily defined group. Many of them suffered injury in the service of their country. The need and the ethical imperative to provide health services to returning veterans were abundantly clear.

The initial benefits given to veterans were formulated by the Council of National Defense whose members ranged from progressive reformers such as Julia Lathrop and V. Everit Macy to academics from Columbia University (Adkins,

1967). Consistent with the progressive mind-set, the need of the veteran was cast in terms of the absence or the injury of fathers and the need for workman's compensation (soldiers working for the federal government) rather than health care. The perspective conformed to a general consensus in labor and industry at the time that workers' health insurance, life insurance, and workman's compensation were acceptable as part of an employer's cost of production, as contrasted to generalized, social insurance that both labor and industry then opposed. Health care for veterans was not seen as generalized health care but as compensation for work-related injuries.

One of the first difficulties in treating veterans following the armistice of November 1918 was finding hospitals for thousands of injured and ill veterans suddenly released from service. Compensation and medical care for the disabled and ill were provided for, but there were few hospital facilities. U.S. Public Health Service* hospitals, navy and army facilities, and civilian contracted hospitals were often overcrowded, unsuited for treatment of tuberculosis, and not designed to rehabilitate disabled soldiers or treat neuropsychiatric conditions or provide long-term care. Legally, neither the U.S. Public Health Service hospitals nor military hospitals were supposed to be treating civilians. To compound the problem, hospitals in the states were largely dependent on municipal and charitable support that either could not or would not meet veteran health needs.

The problem of veteran health care reflected overall problems inherent in creating a coherent national health policy. Hospitals were organized around local religious and municipal charities, and availability reflected local perceived needs. Hospitals in the South were segregated. Military hospitals were only for personnel currently in the military. The Public Health Service had just been formed by 1916 out of the old Marine Hospital Service but had few functions and fewer resources. Moreover, those returning to civilian life included claimants whose legitimacy as veterans having service-related medical needs was questionable. Some 70,000 men who had been drafted and who reported to duty but were released as unhealthy and unfit—mostly with tuberculosis—also claimed entitlement to medical treatment (Adkins, 1967, 92–102).

By 1919, two converging political forces promoted the development of the construction and federal administration of veteran hospitals. Local congressmen were eager to have veteran hospitals built in their own district and benefit from the federal investment. But they were less inclined to construct a coherent policy that would meet the medical needs of returning veterans. Conversely, the American Legion and Veterans of Foreign Wars were now well organized, growing rapidly in membership, and insisting on a national effort to treat returning soldiers. Veteran organizations publicized horror stories of shell-shocked veterans sent to institutions for the mentally retarded and of tuberculosis patients placed in institutions proximate to swampy areas. On the last day of the Woodrow Wilson administration, a bill authorizing over $18 million for veteran hospitals was signed (Stevens, 1991, 292).

The early 1920s was a period of considerable corruption, from Teapot Dome to the malfeasance in the Treasury Department regarding enforcement of prohibition. Some of this corruption reached the Veterans Bureau, which now housed the veterans hospital program. Charles R. Forbes, first director of the Veterans Bureau, was indicted for bribery and fraud and sent to prison. Consequently, the design and placement of the new hospitals were largely the work of distinguished outside consultants from the Red Cross, medical schools, and medical professional organizations. The consequence of professional planning from such consultants, relatively free from patronage and congressional demands for hospital placement in their districts, was an expansion of veteran hospitals based on need (Stevens, 1991, 293, 297). Placement was in areas where physical and mental rehabilitation and long-term care of veterans would most benefit. Wherever possible, VA hospitals were located proximate to medical schools to ensure quality of physicians and medical technology.

By the mid-1920s the justification for veteran health care had also changed. Originally, the rationale was that veteran's care was parallel to "workmen's compensation" rather than social insurance. But in 1924 an amendment to the original legislation permitted treating veterans for any condition, whether service related or not, as long as beds were available. In modern times, this resulted in estimates as high as 75 percent of all care not being service related (Thompson, 1981, 202). Objections to this being socialized medicine were forthcoming from professional medical associations, but unlike in other contexts, they were to no avail. This was a veterans program, not a health program.

The VA hospital complex benefited from the same rapid expansion of civilian hospital construction following World War II. Affiliation with medical schools was further strengthened, and the quality of VA hospitals improved. Similarly, as hospital costs became of concern to government in the late 1970s, so too did the cost of VA hospitals. By the 1980s solutions to control costs at the VA followed similar patterns for civilian hospitals: more outpatient treatment, prospective payment, and reduced capital expenditures. Government-administered and -financed veteran health care had always rested on the political bedrock of support for veterans, not for government health care. The national health care debate may result in greater acceptability of a general government responsibility for health care delivery. Coupled with the end of the cold war and a reduction of veterans with special service-related needs, veterans' medical programs may soon assume the character of services looking for a mission.

REFERENCES: Adkins, Robinson E. 1967. *Medical Care of Veterans.* Report prepared for the House Committee on Veterans Affairs. 90th Cong., 1st Sess. P.L. 63–193; Stevens, Rosemary. 1991. "Can the Government Govern? Lessons from the Formation of the Veterans Administration." *Journal of Health Politics, Policy and Law* 16:281–305; Thompson, Frank J. 1981. *Health Policy and the Bureaucracy: Politics and Implementation.* Cambridge, MA: MIT Press.

ROBERT P. RHODES

WEBSTER V. REPRODUCTIVE HEALTH SERVICES

In July 1986, five health care workers employed by the state of Missouri and two women's health clinics challenged a recently enacted statute, which included a preamble stating that human life begins at the moment of conception and that state law must be interpreted to provide "the unborn child . . . all the rights, privileges, and immunities available to other persons, citizens, and residents" of the state. The law prohibits the use of public funding, employees, or facilities in "encouraging or counseling" a woman to have an abortion not necessary to save her life, as well as the use of public employees or facilities in performing or assisting in these procedures; it also requires physicians to perform abortions at 16 weeks or greater gestation in a hospital and to determine "the gestational age, weight, and lung maturity" of any fetus suspected of being more than 20 weeks prior to performing an abortion. The U.S. District Court for the Western District of Missouri found all of the measures unconstitutional in March 1987 and permanently enjoined their enforcement.

The state of Missouri appealed to the U.S. Court of Appeals for the Eighth Circuit, which affirmed in part and reversed in part. Upholding only the prohibition on the use of public funds for performing or assisting abortions, the appellate court agreed with the district court's holdings that the preamble, hospitalization requirement, and viability testing mandate were invalid under the Supreme Court's holdings in *Roe v. Wade** and subsequent decisions. Although upholding the prohibition on the use of public funds for performing or assisting abortions, the appeals court struck down the prohibition on the use of public facilities or employees when no public moneys were expended for that purpose and found that the prohibition on the use of public funds, facilities, or employees to encourage or counsel a woman to have an abortion is unconstitutionally vague and violates the right to privacy. The state of Missouri appealed but did not seek review of the judgment against the hospitalization requirement or most of the abortion counseling prohibition.

On July 3, 1989, a 5–4 opinion of the U.S. Supreme Court (492 U.S. 490) reversed the decision by the U.S. Court of Appeals for the Eighth Circuit. The majority stated that it was unnecessary to reach the constitutionality of the preamble because it "does not by its terms regulate abortion or any other aspect of [the plaintiffs'] medical practice." Relying on *Poelker v. Roe, Maher v. Roe,* and *Harris v. McRae,** the Court upheld all of the provisions before it relating to public employees and facilities. Claiming to leave *Roe* "undisturbed," five justices also found the viability testing requirement valid because it "is reasonably designed to ensure that abortions are not performed where the fetus is viable—an end which all concede is legitimate—and that is sufficient to sustain its constitutionality." *Webster* marked the first time that only four justices—less than a majority—voted to uphold *Roe* in its entirety. Asserting that the case "affords us no occasion to revisit the holding of *Roe,*" the majority nonetheless indicated that it "would modify and narrow" that decision and its progeny if given the opportunity in future cases. *Webster* was also remarkable for the number of amicus or "friend-of-the-court" briefs that were filed, which are believed to have subsequently prompted the Supreme Court to revise the rules for such papers.

REFERENCES: Faludi, Susan. 1991. *Backlash, the Undeclared War Against American Women.* New York: Crown Books; Gerber Fried, Marlene, ed. 1990. *From Abortion to Reproductive Freedom: Transforming a Movement.* Boston: South End Press; Ginsburg, Faye. 1989. *Contested Lives: The Abortion Debate in an American Community.* Berkeley: University of California Press; Petchesky, Rosalind. 1990. *Abortion and Woman's Choice: The State, Sexuality, and Reproductive Freedom.* Evanston, IL: Northeastern Press; Tribe, Laurence. 1990. *Abortion and the Clash of Absolutes.* New York: W. W. Norton.

ANDREA MILLER

WOMEN'S HEALTH INITIATIVE

The largest research study ever funded by the National Institutes of Health (NIH),* the Women's Health Initiative (WHI) is a 15-year disease prevention study that hopes to enroll approximately 160,000 postmenopausal women between the ages of 50 and 79 to define preventive interventions and risk factors for the major causes of morbidity and mortality in this population: breast and colorectal cancer, coronary artery disease, and osteoporosis. The WHI is unique in that it is specifically designed to look at disease prevention in women, with special attention to the inclusion of minority women, groups that have traditionally been understudied by researchers.

The study design has three components: a set of controlled clinical trials of the interventions, a prospective observational study to identify predictors of disease, and a study to determine the best community approach to encourage more healthful behavior among women. Enrollment in the WHI began in 1993.

The clinical trials will focus on potential preventive interventions: hormone replacement therapy (to help reduce coronary artery disease and osteoporotic fractures), a low-fat diet (to decrease the risk of colorectal and breast cancer and coronary artery disease), and calcium with vitamin D supplementation (to lower the risk for osteoporotic hip fractures and colorectal cancer). Approximately 64,500 women will be randomized to a treatment or a control arm and be followed for an average of nine years. An observational study will complement the clinical trials. It will observe the health and habits of approximately 100,000 women to assess risk factors (e.g., weight and cholesterol level) for chronic disease and identify factors that optimize health.

The House Subcommittee on Appropriations expressed concern regarding the WHI's cost and complexity and asked the Institute of Medicine* (IOM) to review the study critically. The IOM's report, which focused mainly on the clinical trial, recommended that the WHI continue but with several modifications. The NIH adopted some of the IOM's recommendations—the informed consent measures were revised to give women a clearer understanding of the health risks and benefits of participation, for instance—and rejected others. The IOM suggested, for instance, that emphasis be shifted from studying the effects of diet on breast cancer to studying the effects of diet on coronary artery disease. The NIH declined to adopt this change on the grounds that data linking diet and coronary artery disease are already generally accepted, while the link between diet and breast cancer remains controversial and therefore is of greater public health interest. The NIH also took some of the IOM's recommendations under advisement. In response to the IOM's suggestion that the project be completed in 8 years instead of the proposed 15, the NIH established an independent Data and Safety Monitoring Board to conduct comprehensive assessments of the clinical trial at frequent intervals in order to ensure that the hypotheses are adequately tested and to prevent study continuation after confident answers have been found. In testimony in late April 1994, the director of NIH endorsed the WHI before the House Subcommittee on Appropriations and reported that all components of the WHI will move forward as planned.

REFERENCES: Bennett, J. Claude. 1993. "Inclusion of Women in Clinical Trials." *New England Journal of Medicine* 329: 288–292; Institute of Medicine. 1993. *An Assessment of the National Institutes of Health Women's Health Initiative.* Washington, D.C.: National Academy Press; Mastroianni, Anna C., et al., eds. 1994. *Women and Health Research.* Vol. 1–2. Washington, D.C.: National Academy Press.

ANA MARIA LOPEZ

Y

YORK V. JONES

In 1989, the Yorks, a married couple who had moved from Virginia to California, requested that the Jones Institute at Norfolk transport a single frozen embryo left over from three failed attempts at in vitro fertilization (IVF). The Norfolk Clinic refused to release the frozen embryo, claiming that the Yorks agreed to have it thawed for placement only in Norfolk. The Yorks sued in federal court for custody of their embryo and for damages for unlawful retention, breach of contract, and violation of civil rights.

In *York v. Jones* the Federal District Court for the Eastern District of Virginia found in favor of the Yorks, holding that neither the state's human subject research statute nor the terms of the original agreement between the parties undercut their property interest in the frozen embryo. The court held that the most reasonable reading of the consent form was that the Yorks retained dispositional custody including the right to remove the embryo from the Jones Institute. Had the consent form explicitly prohibited transfer, however, the program could have retained custody according to the ruling, which turned on the contractual—not ethical—issues. Shortly after the court ruling, the couple had the embryo transported to California for implantation.

REFERENCES: Walther, Deborah Kay. 1992. "Ownership of the Fertilized Ovum In Vitro." *Family Law Quarterly* 26(3): 235–36; *York v. Jones,* 717 F. Supp. 421 (E.D. Va. 1989).

See also **DAVIS V. DAVIS; IN VITRO FERTILIZATION (IVF).**

ROBERT H. BLANK

Appendix A: Chronology of Key Events, Court Cases, and Legislation

1863	Congress established the National Academy of Sciences
1876	Cruelty to Animals Act, the first law governing the use of animals in scientific research, passed in Britain
1904	National Confederation of State Medical Examining and Licensing Boards recommends uniform curriculum for all medical schools
1906	Congress passes Food and Drug Act
1916	National Research Council established by Congress
1927	Food, Drug and Insecticide Administration created; later to become the Food and Drug Administration
	Congress passes Caustic Poison Act, requiring warning labels
	Buck v. Bell, 274 U.S. 200
1930	National Institute of Health established
1932	Tuskegee Syphilis Study begins
1937	National Cancer Institute established
1938	Congress passes Food, Drug and Cosmetic Act
1942	*Skinner v. Oklahoma,* 316 U.S. 535
1944	Public Health Service Act established the Public Health Service
	National Institute of Health becomes the National Institutes of Health
1946	National Mental Health Act
	Hill-Burton Act provides grants for expansion and building of hospitals
	The Communicable Disease Center is created; it evolved into the Centers for Disease Control and Prevention
1947	National Institute of Mental Health established
1948	National Heart Act establishes the National Heart Institute (later to become the National Heart, Lung, and Blood Institute)

National Institute of Dental Research established

1949   Nuremberg Code created

1950   National Science Foundation created

National Institute of Arthritis and Metabolic Diseases established (later to become the National Institute of Arthritis and Musculoskeletal and Skin Diseases and the National Institute of Diabetes and Digestive and Kidney Diseases)

National Institute of Neurological Diseases and Blindness established (later to become the National Institute of Neurological Disorders and Stroke and the National Eye Institute)

1951   Congress begins investigation of safety of chemicals in foods and cosmetics

1952   Animal Welfare Institute founded

1953   James Watson and Francis Crick discover the structure of the DNA molecule

1954   First solid organ transplant (kidney)

1955   Joint Commission on Mental Health established to study the human and economic problems of mental health

National Institute of Allergy and Infectious Diseases established

1958   Food Additives Amendment to the Food, Drug and Cosmetic Act requires manufacturers to establish safety

1960   Color Additive Amendments to the Food, Drug and Cosmetic Act requires manufacturers to establish safety

1962   National Institute of Child Health and Human Development established

Kefauver-Harris Drug Amendments to the Food, Drug and Cosmetic Act require manufacturers to prove efficacy

Newborn screening for phenylketonuria (PKU) initiated

National Institute of General Medical Sciences established

1964   Declaration of Helsinki created

National Academy of Engineering established

Civil Rights Act, Title VII, protects against discrimination based on race, gender, religion, or national origin

1965   Social Security Act Amendments establish Medicare and Medicaid

Griswold v. State of Connecticut, 381 U.S. 479 (June 7)

1966   Animal Welfare Act

Public Health Service issues its first policy concerning the protection of human research subjects

1968   Uniform Anatomical Gift Act

Harvard Criteria for Determining Brain Death

First prenatal diagnosis of trisomy 21 performed via amniocentesis

Founding of Hastings Center Institute of Society, Ethics, and Life Sciences

National Eye Institute established

1969   First genetic counseling program established at Sarah Lawrence College in Bronxville, New York

1970   Occupational Safety and Health Act requires that health standards be set so as to protect the most susceptible worker

Institute of Medicine established

National Institute on Alcohol Abuse and Alcoholism established

Environmental Protection Agency established

1970–1972   State laws to foster sickle-cell screening are enacted

1971   Public Health Service regulations governing human research subjects are extended to all research supported by the Department of Health, Education, and Welfare

The first workshop on gene therapy is held

Paul Berg proposes transferring SV-40 genetic material into *E. coli*

1972   Enactment of National Sickle Cell Anemia Control Act

National Institute on Drug Abuse established

FDA begins review of over-the-counter drugs

Office of Technology Assessment established

Animal Welfare Act amended

Consumer Product Safety Act establishes the Consumer Product Safety Commission

Eisenstadt v. Baird, 405 U.S. 438 (March 22)

Congress established the End-Stage Renal Disease Program within Medicare

Tuskegee Syphilis Study is publicized and so ends

1973   Enactment of National Cooley's Anemia Control Act

Maryland creates a Commission of Hereditary Disorders

The first in vitro fertilization (IVF) procedure performed

Right to abortion determined by U.S. Supreme Court: *Roe v. Wade*, 410 U.S. 113, 93 S. Ct 705

Senate Committee on Labor and Public Welfare holds hearings on Depo-Provera (February 21)

Gordon Conference on nucleic acids (June 11–15)

Federal Rehabilitation Act protects against discrimination affecting those with handicaps

FDA announces intention to approve Depo-Provera for limited contraceptive use (October 9)

Alcohol, Drug Abuse, and Mental Health Administration established

1974   National Research Act passed, establishing the National Commission for the Protection of Human Subjects of Biomedical and Behavioral Research

National Health Planning and Resources Development Act (Public Law 93–641) initiates Certificate-of-Need programs

Office for Protection from Research Risks created by the Public Health Service

Congress passes United States Privacy Act

Recombinant DNA Advisory Committee (RAC) established by the National Institutes of Health (October 7)

FDA stays limited approval of Depo-Provera pending further review

1975   National Research Council report on *Genetic Screening*

National Institute on Aging established

Asilomar Conference on Recombinant DNA Molecule Research (February 24–27)

First meeting of the RAC (February 28)

National Commission for the Protection of Human Subjects of Biomedical and Behavioral Research published *Research on the Fetus*

First study conducted by the Centers for Disease Control to determine extent of organ shortage

Declaration of Helsinki revised

1976   *In re Quinlan,* 429 U.S. 922

Congress passes Medical Devices Amendments to the Food, Drug and Cosmetic Act

Congress passes National Genetic Disease Act

Federal regulations for funding of fetal research are promulgated (45 CFR 46.201–211)

National Commission for the Protection of Human Subjects of Biomedical and Behavioral Research publishes *Research Involving Prisoners*

Animal Welfare Act amended

Congress creates the Office of Science and Technology Policy to advise the executive branch

Guidelines for Research Involving Recombinant DNA Molecules (Guidelines) published at 41 *Fed. Reg.* 27902 (July 7)

1977   National Commission for the Protection of Human Subjects of Biomedical and Behavioral Research publishes *Research Involving Children*

1978   National Commission for the Protection of Human Subjects of Biomedical and Behavioral Research publishes *The Belmont Report*

Uniform Determination of Death Act

National Commission for the Protection of Human Subjects of Biomedical and Behavioral Research disbanded

Congress passes the Pregnancy Discrimination Act

Promulgation of the lead standard by the Occupational Safety and Health Administration

President's Commission for the Study of Ethical Problems in Medicine and Biomedical and Behavioral Research established by Congress

First revision of the RAC *Guidelines* published at 43 *Fed. Reg.* 60080 (1978) relaxes explicit bans of initial version (December 22)

FDA disapproves Depo-Provera for general marketing for contraception (June 30)

House Select Committee on Population holds hearing on FDA's disapproval of Depo-Provera (August 8–10)

1979   Establishment of the National Society of Genetic Counselors, Inc.

FDA orders a Public Board of Inquiry hearing on Depo-Provera (July 27)

Office of Recombinant DNA Activities established within the National Institutes of Health

DHEW Ethics Advisory Board issues report and conclusions on *HEW Support of Research Involving Human In Vitro Fertilization and Embryo Transfer*

DHEW issues *Healthy People: Surgeon General's Report on Health Promotion and Disease Prevention*

1980   People for the Ethical Treatment of Animals founded, the first American mass animals rights organization

Diamond v. Chakrabarty, 447 U.S. 303

Cohen and Boyer patent on first technique for the production of recombinant DNA

Women sterilized to keep their jobs at American Cyanamid Corporation file suit

Harris v. McRae, 448 U.S. 297 (June 30)

Joint letter from Protestant, Catholic, and Jewish religious leaders to President Jimmy Carter expressing concern over genetic engineering

1981   President's Commission for the Study of Ethical Problems in Medicine and Biomedical and Behavioral Research defines ''concept'' of death in its report *Defining Death*

Department of Health and Human Services revises regulations governing human research subjects

Payton v. Abbott Labs, 83 F.R.D. 382 (D. Mass.), class action suit by women exposed to DES

First reported in utero surgery on fetus

Genetic antidiscrimination law passed in Florida: Fla. Stat. Ann. 448.075 (West 1981)

Elizabeth Carr is first baby born in United States via in vitro fertilization

1982   President's Commission issues report *Splicing Life*

Development of enzyme-linked immunosorbent assay (ELISA) to detect antibodies to HIV

Successful wrongful life claim: *Maccash v. Burger,* 290 N.E.2d 825 (Va. 1982)

Oregon passes statute prohibiting psychosurgery in the state

Baby Doe born in Bloomington, Indiana (April 9)

DHHS publishes Notice to Health Care Providers: ''Discriminating Against Handicapped by Withholding Treatment or Nourishment'' *(Fed. Reg.* 47: 116)

Social Security Amendments and Tax Equity and Fiscal Responsibility Act establish diagnosis related groupings (DRGs)

1983   Creation of the federal Interagency Human Subjects Coordinating Committee

DHHS publishes its Interim Final Rule: ''Nondiscrimination on the Basis of Handicap'' *(Fed. Reg.* 48:45)

President's Commission publishes its report *Deciding to Forego Life-Sustaining Treatment*

American Academy of Pediatrics v. Heckler, 561 F. Supp. 395 (April 14) invalidates DHHS Interim Final Rule

Baby Jane Doe born in Port Jefferson, New York, suffering from spina bifida, hydrocephalus, microcephaly, and related complications

Congress passes Orphan Drug Act to encourage production of drugs for rare diseases

City of Akron v. Akron Center for Reproductive Health, 462 U.S. 416 (June 15)

President's Commission issues report *Screening and Counseling for Genetic Conditions*

Maternal and Child Health Bureau begins to fund multistate Councils of Regional Networks for Genetic Services

Office of Technology assessment report *Genetic Testing in the Workplace*

NIH approves Dr. Lindow's deliberate release experiment (June 1)

Resolution signed by 56 clerics and eight scientists sent to Congress urging no germ-line therapy

Kentucky v. Surrogate Parenting Associates, Inc. decided by the Kentucky Circuit Court, Franklin County

Successful wrongful life claim: *Turpin v. Sortini,* 31 Calif. 3d 220, 643 P.2d 954, 182 Calif. Rptr. 337

1984   Successful wrongful life claim: *Procanik v. Cillo,* 478 A.2d 755 (N.J. 1984)

The Child Abuse Amendments of 1984 (Public Law 8–457) become law on October 9

Deficit Reduction Act freezes physician payments per service for 15 months

National Organ Transport Act; establishment of the Organ Procurement and Transplantation Network (OPTN); sale of organs explicitly prohibited

Oil, Chemical and Atomic Workers, International Union v. American Cyanamid Co. decided by the Court of Appeals for the D.C. Circuit (August 24)

Foundation on Economic Trends v. Heckler, 587 F. Supp. 753 (D.D.C. 1984) decided (May 16)

First meeting of the RAC's Human Gene Therapy Working Group to respond to *Splicing Life* (October 12)

Office of Technology Assessment report *Human Gene Therapy—A Background Paper*

A Working Group on Human Gene Therapy is set up as part of the Recombinant DNA Advisory Committee

Public Law 98–551 establishes Council on Health Care Technology

NIH/FDA report finding no clear benefit from routine use of ultrasound for pregnant women

1985 Health Research Extension Act authorizes creation of the Biomedical Ethics Board

RAC publishes first version of *Points to Consider in the Design and Submission of Human Somatic-Cell Gene Therapy Protocols* (Points to Consider), 50 *Fed. Reg.* 2940 (January 22)

Foundation on Economic Trends v. Heckler, 756 F.2d 143 (D.C. Cir. 1985) decided (February 27)

Animal Welfare Act amended to require the establishment of Institutional Animal Care and Use Committees

First required request laws passed by Oregon and New York states

Consolidated Omnibus Budget Reconciliation Act creates Physician Payment Review Commission (PPRC)

Health Research Extension Act amends the Public Health Service Act

Orphan Drug Act amended to create National Commission on Orphan Diseases

National Institute of Arthritis and Musculoskeletal and Skin Diseases established

National Institute of Diabetes and Digestive and Kidney Diseases established

Office of Technology Assessment report *Reproductive Health Hazards in the Workplace*

Genetic antidiscrimination law passed in Louisiana: La. Rev. Stat. Ann. 23: 1001–1004 (West 1985)

DHHS issues Final Rule to implement the Child Abuse Amendments of 1984

American College of Obstetricians and Gynecologists issues liability alert to obstetricians concerning duty to inform patients about MSAFP testing

1986   California enacts a law requiring physicians to inform women about MSAFP screening for neural tube defects

U.S. Congress enacts legislation requiring hospitals to develop protocols to ensure that families are made aware of the donor option and reorganizes organ procurement organizations (OPOs) for greater efficiency

United Network for Organ Sharing is awarded the federal contract to operate the national organ procurement and transplantation network

Final Report of the Task Force on Organ Transplantation

Surrogate Parenting v. Com. Ex Rel. Armstrong decided by the Supreme Court of Kentucky

Thornburgh v. American College of Obstetricians and Gynecologists, 476 U.S. 747 (June 11)

Foundation on Economic Trends v. Thomas, 637 F. Supp. 25 (D.D.C. 1986) decided (March 6)

1986 version of the *Guidelines* (51 *Fed. Reg.* 16598) (1986) published (May 7)

Coordinated Framework for the Regulation of Biotechnology (51 *Fed. Reg.* 23302) is released (June 26)

Bowen v. American Hospital Association (106 S. Ct. 2101) invalidates 1984 DHHS Final Rule on Baby Doe (June 9)

1987   House Committee on Interior and Insular Affairs holds hearing on the use of Depo-Provera by the Indian Health Service (August 6)

Office of Technology Assessment report *Life-Sustaining Technologies and the Elderly*

Office of Technology Assessment report *Losing a Million Minds: Confronting the Tragedy of Alzheimer's Disease and Other Dementias*

Office of Technology Assessment report *New Developments in Biotechnology, 1*

National AIDS Demonstration Research Project begun to study and change the high-risk behaviors of injection drug users

Revision of Uniform Anatomical Gift Act

U.S. Patent and Trademark Office rules that multicellular organisms are patentable subject matter (April 7)

First deliberate release of a genetically engineered organism approved by the RAC (April 29)

Hybritech, Inc. v. Monoclonal Antibodies, Inc., 802 F2d 1367 (Fed. Cir. 1986)

Appointment of the Biomedical Ethics Advisory Committee (August)

FDA forces withdrawal of Gender Choice sex-preselection kit from the marketplace

1988   First gene transfer protocol approved

Policy guidelines on Reproductive and Fetal Hazards in the Workplace issued by Equal Employment Opportunity Commission

FDA approves cervical cap for general use

Office of Technology Assessment report *Infertility: Medical and Social Choices*

Office of Technology Assessment report *Mapping Our Genes: Genome Projects: How Big? How Fast?*

DHHS imposes moratorium on federal support for fetal tissue transplantation applications (March)

Human Fetal Tissue Transplantation Research Panel recommends restoration of federal funding for fetal tissue transplantation (September)

NIH Director's Advisory Committee unanimously approves lifting moratorium on fetal tissue transplantation (December)

Veterans Administration becomes Department of Veterans Affairs with cabinet-level status

Presidential Commission on the Human Immunodeficiency Virus Epidemic report to the president (June)

Initiation of Human Genome Project (National Institutes of Health and Department of Energy), with earmarked funding for ethical, legal, and social issues

Medicare Catastrophic Coverage Act (repealed in 1989)

In re Baby M., 537 A.2d 1227 (N.J. 1188)

Health Omnibus Programs Extension sets minimum standards for OPO performance

National Institute on Deafness and Other Communication Disorders created

AIDS Amendments to the Health Omnibus Programs Extension expand research, treatment, and prevention efforts

1989   Biomedical Ethics Advisory Committee expires

Congress passes Public Law 101–58 declaring the decade beginning January 1990 the ''Decade of the Brain''

Omnibus Reconciliation Act requires that the resource-based relative value scale (RBRVS) to determine physician payment by Medicare be in place by 1992

Webster v. Reproductive Health Services, 492 U.S. 490 (July 3)

Secretary of DHHS Louis Sullivan announces indefinite extension of the moratorium on fetal tissue transplantation

Genetic antidiscrimination law passed in North Carolina: N.C. Gen. Stat. 95–28.1

Institute of Medicine report *Medically Assisted Conception: An Agenda for Research*

The gene for cystic fibrosis is identified

First federally approved clinical gene transfer (May 22)

Agency for Health Care Policy and Research established

Declaration of Helsinki revised

1990   Forty-one states and the District of Columbia recognize whole brain death

DHHS proposes a "parallel track" for AIDS patients to receive unapproved drugs

Congress passes Nutrition Labeling and Education Act

Congress passes Safe Medical Devices Act

Regulations issued under the 1985 amendments to the Animal Welfare Act

House Committee on Education and Labor of the U.S. Congress issues its report *The EEOC, Title VII and Workplace Fetal Protection Policies in the 1980s*

Human Genome Project officially initiated

Successful wrongful life claim: *Pines v. Moreno,* 569 P.2d 203 (La. App. 1990)

Americans with Disabilities Act (ADA) of 1990 became federal law

Genetic antidiscrimination law passed in Oregon: Or. Rev. Stat 659.227 (Supp. 1990)

FDA approves the Norplant contraceptive system

First human gene therapy protocol approved by FDA

Office of Technology Assessment report *Genetic Monitoring and Screening in the Workplace*

Office of Technology Assessment report *Neural Grafting: Repairing the Brain and Spinal Cord*

Office of Technology Assessment report *Neurotoxicity: Identifying and Controlling Poisons of the Nervous System*

Ryan White Comprehensive AIDS Resources Emergency Act

1991   National Society of Genetic Counselors devised and adopted a code of ethics

Common Federal Rule for the Protection of Human Subjects

Auto Workers v. Johnson Controls, Inc., 111 S. Ct. 1196

President George Bush signs Public Law 101–126 reauthorizing the Child Abuse Amendments of 1984 (October 25)

The EEOC issues guidance on biased fetal protection policies (June)

Genetic antidiscrimination law passed in New Jersey: N.J. Stat. Ann. 10: 5–5(y) (West Supp. 1991)

Missouri passes statute that disallows referral for an abortion unless the mother's life is endangered by the continuation of the pregnancy: Mo. Ann. Stat. 191. 300–.380

Tennessee passes statute that disallows genetic prenatal diagnosis if there is no treatment (other than therapeutic abortion) available: Tenn. Code Ann. 68–5–504(a) (1991)

Supreme Court case limiting disclosure regarding abortion: *Rust v. Sullivan,* 500 U.S. 173

Louisiana law restricting abortion: 1991 La. Act 26

Darlene Johnson sentenced to three years' probation for felony child abuse on the condition she take Norplant; case appealed, *People v. Johnson,* FO15316 (Calif. Court of Appeals, 5th District, April 25, 1991), but dismissed when Ms. Johnson violated other conditions of her probation

DHHS issues *Healthy People 2000: National Objectives for Health Promotion and Disease Prevention*

1992   Alcohol, Drug Abuse and Mental Health Administration abolished

Substance Abuse and Mental Health Services Administration established

Formation of the American Board of Genetic Counseling, which is separate and distinct from the American Board of Medical Genetics

Genetic antidiscrimination law passed in New York: N.Y. Civ. Rights Law 48 (McKinney Supp. 1992)

Wisconsin law prohibiting genetic testing by employers: Act of Mar. 5, 1992, 1991 Wis. Laws 117

Discovery of a gene for Alzheimer's disease

NIH first applies for patents on cDNA Expressed Sequence Tags (ESTs)

Report in *JAMA* of the infant girl born to a woman after preimplantation genetic diagnostic testing for cystic fibrosis and IVF

NIH director grants compassionate plea for gene therapy application

Establishment of National Advisory Board on Ethics in Reproduction (NABER)

FDA approves Depo-Provera for general marketing

Planned Parenthood v. Casey, 112 S. Ct. 2791 (June 29)

1993   National Institute of Nursing Research established

National Institutes of Health begin enrolling women for the Women's Health Initiative, the largest research study ever funded by the NIH

President Bill Clinton issues executive order removing ban on the issue of fetal tissue for transplantation

Institute of Medicine report *Assessing Genetic Risks: Implications for Health and Social Policy*

Huntington's disease gene identified

Amyotrophic lateral sclerosis gene identified

Office of Technology assessment report *Biomedical Ethics in U.S. Public Policy*

President Clinton sends Health Security Plan to Congress (September)

NIH Revitalization Act removes requirement of Ethics Advisory Board approval for human embryo research

Bray v. Alexandria Women's Health Clinic, 113 S. Ct. 753 (January 13)

Creation of American Association of Bioethics

1994   Regulations issued under the 1985 amendments to the Animal Welfare Act upheld in court; court rules that animal rights groups have no legal standing to contest regulations

Current versions of *Guidelines* and *Points to Consider* for release of genetically engineered organisms published (*Fed. Reg.* 59: 34496) (July 5)

Creation of NIH Human Embryo Research Panel

Draft charter for National Bioethics Advisory Commission (NBAC) is published in *Federal Register* (August 12)

President Clinton establishes Special Advisory Committee on Human Radiation Experiments

1995   Office of Technology Assessment abolished by Congress

Institute of Medicine publishes *Society's Choices: Social and Ethical Decision Making in Biomedicine*

Appendix B: Directory of Major Sources of Information

This appendix is designed to provide the reader with an overview of sources of research materials, databases, and other information that might be helpful in studying biomedical policy. It must be noted that because biomedical policy is a yet-emerging focus for study and relevant materials come from a broad range of disciplines, the information provided here should be viewed as preliminary and noninclusive. The information provided here, however, reflects the diversity and richness of biomedical policy and provides a representative selection of the most critical sources of research material.

BIBLIOGRAPHIES

For over 20 years, the *Bibliography of Bioethics* has been published annually by the Kennedy Institute of Ethics at Georgetown University. Volume 20 was published in 1994 and edited by LeRoy Walters and Tamar Joy Kahn. This bibliography provides the most extensive source of bioethics literature and a reasonably comprehensive source of work relevant to biomedical policy across the spectrum of subjects in this encyclopedia. If supplemented by thorough searches of MEDLINE and LEXUS or other medical and legal databases, the researcher will cover most of the appropriate academic literature for studying biomedical policy in the United States. A search of U.S. government documents should complete coverage of appropriate materials. Several more specific bibliographies are also available for persons interested in particular policy areas.

In addition to the comprehensive *Index Medicus* published monthly by the National Library of Medicine, it also publishes two special bibliographic series of particular use for biomedical policy research. The *AIDS Bibliography* is a monthly listing of recent references to journal articles, books, and audiovisual materials. The *Current Bibliographies in Medicine* series contains between 15 and 20 bibliographies annually on distinct research topics in biomedicine ranging from "Cocaine, Pregnancy and the Newborn" to "Hospital Technology Assessment" to "Medical Waste Disposal." Individual titles can be obtained and ordered separately from the National Library of Medicine.

The National Reference Center for Bioethics Literature of the Kennedy Institute of Ethics publishes a series of "Scope Notes," which include summaries of committee statements and court cases as well as an annotated bibliography on specific research topics. These 15- to 20-page notes can be purchased from the library of the Center at 1-800-MED-ETHX. The Kennedy Institute of Ethics Library also published the *International Directory of Bioethics Organizations* in 1993, which provides information on almost 500 such organizations worldwide.

In 1993 the Department of Energy Office of Energy Research published a comprehensive bibliography on the ethical, legal, and social implications of the Human Genome Project. Compiled by Michael S. Yesley, this second edition contains over 5,600 entries. Researchers should note that an extensive collection of publications in the ELSI database is available for public use at the General Law Library of Los Alamos National Laboratory (FAX [505]665-4424). Topics in this database include behavior, counseling, discrimination, ethics, eugenics, law, patent, press, privacy, reproduction, screening, and therapy.

JOURNALS

Biomedical policy is a multidisciplinary area that crosses medicine, law, bioethics, and the social sciences. As a result, relevant articles can be found in a wide range of professional journals. List 1 below represents a selection of the most relevant journals for researchers of biomedical policy. List 2 contains journals that have published relevant articles on a more sporadic basis. In addition to these journals, most law journals increasingly are publishing articles and cases that will be useful in researching biomedical policy, particularly as it relates to the active legal dimensions.

1. These journals have significant policy-oriented content on a consistent basis:

> *AIDS and Public Policy Journal*
> *American Journal of Law and Medicine*
> *American Journal of Public Health*
> *Bioethics*
> *Environmental Health Perspectives*
> *Family Planning Perspectives*
> *Genetic Technology News*
> *Gene Watch*
> *Hastings Center Report*
> *Health Affairs*
> *Health Care Analysis*
> *Health Policy*
> *Health Services Research*
> *International Journal of Health Services*
> *International Journal of Technology Assessment in Health Care*
> *Issues in Law and Medicine*
> *Journal of Contemporary Health Law and Policy*
> *Journal of Epidemiology and Community Health*
> *Journal of Health Politics, Policy and Law*
> *Journal of Law, Medicine and Ethics*
> *Journal of Legal Medicine*
> *Journal of Medical Ethics*
> *Journal of Medicine and Philosophy*

Journal of the American Medical Association (JAMA)
Medical Care
Medical Law Review
Medicine and Health
Milbank Quarterly
Morbidity and Mortality Weekly Report
New England Journal of Medicine
Politics and the Life Sciences
Public Health Reports
Social Science and Medicine
Women's Health Issues

2. These journals have policy-oriented content on an occasional basis or through special issue symposia:

American Journal of Human Genetics
American Journal of Managed Health Care
American Journal of Medicine
British Medical Journal
Fertility and Sterility
Harvard Women's Law Journal
Health and Human Rights
Health Care Financing Review
Health Law and Ethics
Human Gene Therapy
Institute of Laboratory Animal Resources Review
Issues in Science and Technology
Journal of Behavioral Medicine
Journal of Clinical Ethics
Journal of Ethics, Law and Aging
Journal of Health and Human Resources Administration
Journal of Health and Social Behavior
Journal of Health Economics
Journal of Obstetrics and Gynecology
Journal of Religion and Health
Journal of Social Issues
The Lancet
New Scientist
New York State Journal of Medicine
Perspectives on Biology and Medicine
Policy Studies Journal
Policy Studies Review
Population Bulletin
Population Studies
Project Appraisal
Science, Technology and Human Values
Second Opinion
Signs
Sociology of Health and Illness

Theoretical Medicine
Trends in Health Care, Law and Ethics
Western Medical Journal
Women and Politics
Women's Rights Law Report
Women's Study International Forum

OTHER SOURCES OF RESEARCH MATERIALS

In addition to the sources listed in the references for each entry and found in bibli-ographies and journals discussed above, the reader should turn to the various reports and background papers of the U.S. Office of Technology Assessment and the Institute of Medicine. Over the past decade, these reports have addressed many of the substantive areas included here. The *Encyclopedia of Bioethics,* although focused on the ethical dimensions, provides authoritative coverage of the issues that underlie biomedical policy. The *Bioethics Yearbook* published by Kluwer Publishers also may be of interest in par-ticular topical areas. The three-volume series *Emerging Issues in Biomedical Policy,* edited by Robert Blank and Andrea Bonnicksen (Columbia, 1992–1994), provides more in-depth coverage of policy issues across a range of topical areas, as does the earlier volume *Biomedical Technology and Public Policy,* edited by Robert Blank and Miriam Mills (Greenwood, 1989).

The following is a selected list of contacts for organizations that have published reports or provide databases for issues in U.S. health and biomedical policy.

Agency for Health Care Policy and Research
Public Health Service
2101 East Jefferson Street
Rockville, MD 20852

American Society of Law, Medicine and Ethics
765 Commonwealth Avenue, 16th Floor
Boston, MA 02215

Association of Academic Health Centers
1400 Sixteenth Street, N.W.
Washington, D.C. 20036

Center for Health Economics Research
300 Fifth Avenue
Waltham, MA 62154

Center for Health Policy Research
Suite 800
2021 K Street, N.W.
Washington, D.C. 20006

Center for the Health Professions
1388 Sutter Street
San Francisco, CA 94109

The Commonwealth Fund
Harkness House

One East 75th Street
New York, NY 10021

Group Health Association of America
129 20th Street, N.W.
Washington, D.C. 20036

Harvard School of Public Health
677 Huntington Avenue
Boston, MA 02115

Hastings Center
255 Elm Road
Briarcliff Manor, NY 10510

Health Care Technology Institute
225 Reinekers Lane, Suite 220
Alexandria, VA 22314

Health Insurance Association of America
1025 Connecticut Avenue, N.W.
Washington, D.C. 20036

Henry J. Kaiser Foundation
2400 Sand Hill Road
Menlo Park, CA 94025

Howard Hughes Medical Institute
4000 Jones Bridge Road
Chevy Chase, MD 20815

Institute of Medicine
National Academy of Sciences
2101 Constitution Avenue
Washington, D.C. 20418

Milbank Memorial Fund
One East 75th Street
New York, NY 10021

National Academy for State Health Policy
50 Monument Square
Suite 502
Portland, ME 04101

National Clearinghouse on Health Indices
National Center for Health Statistics
Room 1070, 6525 Belcrest Road
Hyattsville, MD 20782
(301) 436-7035

National Library of Medicine
8600 Rockville Pike
Bethesda, MD 20894
(800) 272-4787

Office on Women's Health
Public Health Service
200 Independence Avenue, S.W., Room 730-B
Washington, D.C. 20201

Public Policy Institute
American Association of Retired Persons
601 E. Street, N.W.
Washington, D.C. 20049

RAND/UCLA Center for Health Study Policy
1700 Main Street
Santa Monica, CA 90407

Robert Wood Johnson Foundation
P.O. Box 2316
Princeton, NJ 08543-2316

U.S. Office of Technology Assessment
600 Pennsylvania Avenue, S.E.
Washington, D.C. 20510

Index

Page numbers in **bold type** refer to main entries in the encyclopedia.

About the Editors and Contributors

EDITORS

ROBERT H. BLANK (Editor-in-Chief) holds the chair of Political Science at the University of Canterbury in Christchurch, New Zealand. His research interests center on the legal and public policy aspects of biomedical technologies. Among his numerous books and articles on biomedical policy are *Rationing Medicine* (1988), *Regulating Reproduction* (1990), *Fertility Control* (1991), *Mother and Fetus* (1992), *Fetal Protection in the Workplace* (1993), *Medicine Unbound* (1994), and *Biomedical Policy* (1995).

JANNA C. MERRICK (Editor-in-Chief) is Associate Dean for Academic Affairs and Professor of Government and International Affairs at the University of South Florida at Sarasota. Her research deals primarily with public policy issues relating to pregnant women and young children. Her recent publications include *Human Reproduction, Emerging Technologies, and Conflicting Rights* (1995), coauthored with Robert H. Blank; *The Politics of Pregnancy* (1993), coedited with Blank; and *Compelled Compassion: Government Intervention in the Treatment of Critically Ill Newborns* (1992), coedited with Blank and Arthur L. Caplan. She has contributed articles to *Politics and the Life Sciences, The Journal of Legal Medicine,* and *Policy Studies Review.*

JAMES BOPP, JR. (Section Editor) is president of the National Legal Center for the Medically Dependent and Disabled, Inc.; general counsel for the National Right to Life Committee, Inc.; and editor-in-chief of *Issues in Law & Medicine.* He practices law in Terre Haute, Indiana, and has published numerous articles. His research interests include bioethics, constitutional rights, and disability rights, especially as they affect the issues of abortion, assisted suicide, euthanasia, infanticide, and withdrawal of essential medical care, including withdrawal of nutrition and hydration.

BARRY A. BOSTROM (Section Editor) is vice president of the National Legal Center for the Medically Dependent and Disabled, Inc.; executive editor of *Issues in Law & Medicine*; and an attorney in Terre Haute, Indiana. His interests include medical ethics, assisted suicide, and euthanasia, topics he has addressed in articles appearing in *Issues in Law & Medicine*.

DEBORAH R. MATHIEU (Section Editor) is Associate Professor of Political Science at the University of Arizona. Her research focuses on medical ethics and health policy. She is the author of *Preventing Prenatal Harm: Should the State Intervene?* (1991) and the editor of *Organ Substitution Technology: Ethical, Legal, and Policy Issues* (1988). She has written a number of journal articles, including contributions to the *Journal of Social Philosophy*, *Constitutional Political Economy*, the *Arizona State Law Review*, the *Harvard Journal of Law and Public Policy*, and *Politics and the Life Sciences*.

PAULINE VAILLANCOURT ROSENAU (Section Editor) is Associate Professor at the School of Public Health, Houston Medical Science Center. She was a professor at the University of Quebec in Montreal for 20 years before joining the School of Public Health in 1993. Her last two books, *Health Care Reform in the Nineties* (1994) and *Post-Modernism in the Social Sciences* (1992) received *Choice* Outstanding Academic Book Awards. Her current research includes the social and policy consequences of the new gene technology and comparative international health systems in industrialized countries.

CONTRIBUTORS

ROBERT M. ARNOLD, Center for Medical Ethics, University of Pittsburgh

BENEDICT M. ASHLEY, Professor Emeritus of Moral Theology, Aquinas Institute of Theology, St. Louis Bertrand Priory

MICHAEL J. ASTRUE, Biogen, Inc., Cambridge, Massachusetts

DANIEL AVILA, National Legal Center for the Medically Dependent and Disabled, Inc., Terre Haute, Indiana

STEPHEN A. BENT, Foley & Lardner, Washington, D.C.

ROBERT A. BOHRER, California Western School of Law, San Diego, California

ANDREA L. BONNICKSEN, Department of Political Science, Northern Illinois University

DANIEL CALLAHAN, The Hastings Center, Briarcliff Manor, New York

RICHARD M. CHAPMAN, Legal Department, Landmark Graphics, Houston, Texas

JACQUELINE L. COLBY, Department of Philosophy, University of Alaska

RICHARD E. COLESON, Attorney, Bopp, Coleson and Bostrom, Terre Haute, Indiana

CHRISTOPHER M. DeGIORGIO, Los Angeles County/USC Medical Center; and Clinical Neurophysiology Laboratory and Epilepsy Program, Los Angeles, California

WILLIAM F. DENNY, Chair, Institutional Review Board, Health Sciences Center, University of Arizona

JOSEPH C. d'ORONZIO, Columbia University College of Physicians and Surgeons, New York

TIM DUVALL, Department of Political Science, University of Arizona

RICHARD FENIGSEN, Willem-Alexander Hospital, 's-Hertogenbosch, the Netherlands (1972–1990)

JULIANNA S. GONEN, Group Health Association of America, Washington, D.C.

GERALD GOODMAN, Texas Children's Hospital, Houston, Texas

WILLIAM C. GREEN, Department of Geography, Government and History, Morehead State University

CURTIS E. HARRIS, American Academy of Medical Ethics, Oklahoma City, Oklahoma

JACQUELINE T. HECHT, Department of Pediatrics, University of Texas, Houston Health Science Center, Houston, Texas

MICHAEL D. HINDS, Attorney, Gaithersburg, Maryland

DALE JAMIESON, Department of Philosophy, University of Colorado

KAREN ORLOFF KAPLAN, Choice in Dying, New York

MARSHALL B. KAPP, Office of Geriatric Medicine and Gerontology, Wright State University, Dayton, Ohio

SALLY J. KENNEY, Humphrey Institute for Public Affairs, University of Minnesota

KRIS A. LARSON, The Hemlock Society U.S.A., Eugene, Oregon

AMANDA LEWIS, Department of Molecular and Cellular Biology, University of Arizona

ANA MARIA LOPEZ, Arizona Cancer Center, University of Arizona

CHARLES R. McCARTHY, Kennedy Institute of Ethics, Georgetown University

BARRY McKEE, Attorney, Stillwater, Minnesota; represented Oliver Wanglie in the 1991 Hennepin County, Minnesota case in *In re Wanglie*

PATRICIA GAIL McVEY, School of Public Health, University of Texas Health Science Center, Houston, Texas

THOMAS J. MARZEN, National Legal Center for the Medically Dependent and Disabled, Inc., Indianapolis, Indiana

ERIC M. MESLIN, Center for Bioethics, University of Toronto

ANDREA MILLER, Center for Reproductive Law and Policy, New York, New York

PHILIP D. MORAN, Attorney, Salem, Massachusetts

ROBERT M. NELSON, Children's Hospital of Wisconsin, Milwaukee, Wisconsin

GILBERT S. OMENN, School of Public Health and Community Medicine, University of Washington

PHILIP R. REILLY, Shriver Center, Waltham, Massachusetts

ROBERT P. RHODES, Department of Political Science, Edinboro University

CHERYLON ROBINSON, Division of Social and Policy Sciences, University of Texas at San Antonio

LAINIE FRIEDMAN ROSS, Department of Pediatrics and the MacLean Center for Clinical Medical Ethics, University of Chicago

MARY R. SCHLACHTENHAUFEN, Rice University, Houston, Texas

MOLLY SEAR, Center for Medical Ethics, University of Pittsburgh

LAURA A. SIMINOFF, Center for Medical Ethics, University of Pittsburgh

LYNN D. WARDLE, J. Reuben Clark Law School, Brigham Young University, Provo, Utah

WALTER M. WEBER, Litigation Counsel, The American Center for Law and Justice, Washington, D.C.

CATHERINE WICKLUND, Cooper Hospital, Department of Pediatrics, Divisions of Genetics, UMDNJ, Camden, New Jersey

LAURA R. WOLIVER, Department of Political Science, University of South Carolina

ISBN 0-313-28641-8

90000>

EAN

9 780313 286414

HARDCOVER BAR CODE